Current Trends in Orthodontics

Edited by Farid Bourzgui

Published in London, United Kingdom

Current Trends in Orthodontics
http://dx.doi.org/10.5772/intechopen.94803
Edited by Farid Bourzgui

Contributors
Lahcen Ousehal, Asmaa El Mabrak, Mohamed El Fatmi Kadri Hassani, Soukaina Sahim, Hajar Bouzid, Hakima Aghoutan, Siddharth Sonwane, Sagar S. Bhat, Ameet V. Revankar, Shrinivas M. Basavaraddi, Guilherme Nakagawa dos Santos, Charles Lenzi de Araujo, Romeu Cassiano Pucci da Silva Ramos, David Andrade, Ana Norton, Viviana Macho, Rui Andrade, Miguel Palha, Sandra Bussadori, Lurdes Morais, Maria-João Palha, Manuela Santos, Cristiane Barros André, Bruno Pasqua, José Rino Neto, Fábio Dupart Nascimento, Suvetha Siva, Sukanya Dhanapal, Janani Ravi, Chandhini Suresh, Shreya Kishore, Agharsh Chandrasekaran, Harshavardhan Kidiyoor, H.P. Naga Deepti, Nandakishore Rajgopal, Betsy Sara Thomas, Mohan Alexander, Farid El Quars, Carla A. Evans, Kristin Moore, David Musich, Donald Taylor, Budi Kusnoto, Tara Emerick, Maria Grace Costa Viana, Tejashri Pradhan, Aarti Sethia, Mehmet Akin, Leyla Cime Akbaydogan, Dalal Elmoutawakkil, Nabil Hacib, Farid Bourzgui, Rania Fastani, Salwa Khairat, Mohamed El Had, Samir Diouny, Zineb Serhier, Mohamed Bennani Othmani, Amanda Nadia Ferreira

First published in London, United Kingdom, 2022 by IntechOpen
IntechOpen is the global imprint of INTECHOPEN LIMITED, registered in England and Wales, registration number: 11086078, 5 Princes Gate Court, London, SW7 2QJ, United Kingdom
Printed in Croatia

British Library Cataloguing-in-Publication Data
A catalogue record for this book is available from the British Library

Additional hard and PDF copies can be obtained from orders@intechopen.com

Current Trends in Orthodontics
Edited by Farid Bourzgui
p. cm.

This title is part of the Dentistry Book Series, Volume 9
Topic: Prosthodontics and Implant Dentistry
Series Editor: Sergio Alexandre Gehrke
Topic Editor: Wen Lin Chai
Associate Topic Editor: Ghee Seong Lim

Print ISBN 978-1-83969-963-4
Online ISBN 978-1-83969-964-1
eBook (PDF) ISBN 978-1-83969-965-8
ISSN 2631-6218

For EU product safety concerns:
IN TECH d.o.o., Prolaz Marije Krucifikse Kozulić 3, 51000 Rijeka, Croatia,
info@intechopen.com or visit our website at intechopen.com.

IntechOpen Book Series

Dentistry

Volume 9

Aims and Scope of the Series

This book series will offer a comprehensive overview of recent research trends as well as clinical applications within different specialties of dentistry. Topics will include overviews of the health of the oral cavity, from prevention and care to different treatments for the rehabilitation of problems that may affect the organs and/or tissues present. The different areas of dentistry will be explored, with the aim of disseminating knowledge and providing readers with new tools for the comprehensive treatment of their patients with greater safety and with current techniques. Ongoing issues, recent advances, and future diagnostic approaches and therapeutic strategies will also be discussed. This series of books will focus on various aspects of the properties and results obtained by the various treatments available, whether preventive or curative.

Meet the Series Editor

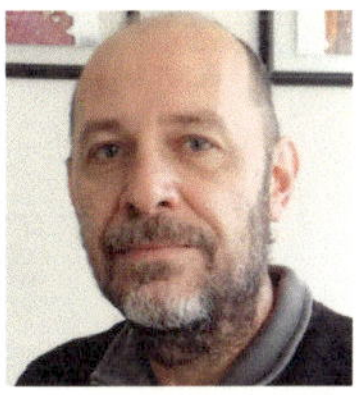

Dr. Sergio Alexandre Gehrke is a doctorate holder in two fields. The first is a Ph.D. in Cellular and Molecular Biology from the Pontificia Catholic University, Porto Alegre, Brazil, in 2010 and the other is an International Ph.D. in Bioengineering from the Universidad Miguel Hernandez, Elche/Alicante, Spain, obtained in 2020. In 2018, he completed a postdoctoral fellowship in Materials Engineering in the NUCLEMAT of the Pontificia Catholic University, Porto Alegre, Brazil. He is currently the Director of the Postgraduate Program in Implantology of the Bioface/UCAM/PgO (Montevideo, Uruguay), Director of the Cathedra of Biotechnology of the Catholic University of Murcia (Murcia, Spain), an Extraordinary Full Professor of the Catholic University of Murcia (Murcia, Spain) as well as the Director of the private center of research Biotecnos – Technology and Science (Montevideo, Uruguay). Applied biomaterials, cellular and molecular biology, and dental implants are among his research interests. He has published several original papers in renowned journals. In addition, he is also a Collaborating Professor in several Postgraduate programs at different universities all over the world.

Meet the Volume Editor

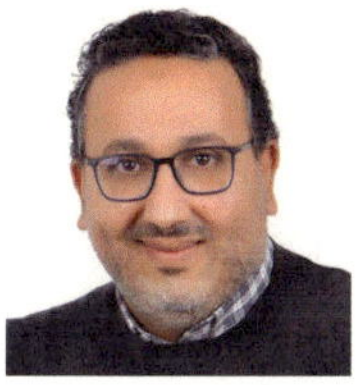

Prof. Farid Bourzgui obtained his DMD and his DNSO option in Orthodontics at the School of Dental Medicine, Casablanca Hassan II University, Morocco, in 1995 and 2000, respectively. Currently, he is a professor of Orthodontics. He holds a Certificate of Advanced Study type A in Technology of Biomaterials used in Dentistry (1995); Certificate of Advanced Study type B in Dento-Facial Orthopaedics (1997) from the Faculty of Dental Surgery, University Denis Diderot-Paris VII, France; Diploma of Advanced Study (DESA) in Biocompatibility of Biomaterials from the Faculty of Medicine and Pharmacy of Casablanca (2002); Certificate of Clinical Occlusodontics from the Faculty of Dentistry of Casablanca (2004); University Diploma of Biostatistics and Perceptual Health Measurement from the Faculty of Medicine and Pharmacy of Casablanca (2011); and a University Diploma of Pedagogy of Odontological Sciences from the Faculty of Dentistry of Casablanca (2013). He is the author of several scientific articles, book chapters, and books.

Contents

Preface

In recent years, the practice of orthodontics has undergone major technological developments, including artificial intelligence. It is now more important to develop the necessary skills to understand the functioning and impact of these technologies on orthodontics. This should help identify gaps in our understanding of emerging technologies and new trends.

Artificial intelligence and digitalization are powerful tools that offer solutions to unresolved and poorly managed challenges. New trends in orthodontics make use of the advances that are being made in digital and clinical research. The finesse and sophistication of the techniques used in this discipline should allow the practice of orthodontics to defy the laws of nature.

This book explores current trends in orthodontics.

Section 1 consists of four chapters that focus on current evidence on tooth movement. Chapter 1 discusses biomarkers in saliva and gingival crevicular fluid during orthodontic treatment. Chapter 2 highlights the symbiosis between orthodontics and periodontics. Chapter 3 provides an update on some current methods of accelerating orthodontic dental movements. Chapter 4 explores the risk of root resorption during orthodontic treatment.

Section 2, which deals with digitization and workflow, includes four chapters that address issues related to modelization, workflow in an orthodontic practice, and the use of digital set-up for both orthodontic and orthognathic surgery planning.

Section 3 is dedicated to orthodontic techniques. It contains seven chapters covering recent trends in clinical techniques such as the use of bone screws, the predictability of orthodontic movement by aligner, the role of the orthodontist in the management of sleep apnea, and the assessment of orthodontic pain perception.

The final section deals with early treatment and includes three chapters highlighting the importance of the place of clinical treatments in our therapeutic arsenals.

I am grateful to the contributing authors for the science, creativity, time, and effort they put into their chapters.

Farid Bourzgui, D.M.D. MSc
Professor,
Department of Orthodontics,
Dental School,
Hassan II University of Casablanca,
Casablanca, Morocco

Section 1

Current Evidence on Tooth Movement

Chapter 1

Orthodontic Therapeutic Biomarkers in Saliva and Gingival Crevicular Fluid

Sagar S. Bhat, Ameet V. Revankar and Shrinivas M. Basavaraddi

Abstract

Several biologically active substances representing the bone deposition and resorption processes are released following damage to periodontal tissue during orthodontic movement. Biomarkers are by definition objective, quantifiable characteristics of biological processes. The analysis of saliva/salivary fluid and Gingival crevicular fluid (GCF) may be an accepted way to examine the ongoing biochemical processes associated with bone turnover during orthodontic tooth movement and fixed orthodontic treatment pain. Assessing the presence of these salivary physiological biomarkers would benefit the clinician in appropriate pain diagnosis and management objectively of various problems encountered during the orthodontic procedures and for better outcome of biomechanical therapy. Due to lack of standardized collection procedure, even though well accepted by patients, saliva is often neglected as a body fluid of diagnostic and prognostic value. A literature search was carried out in major databases such as PubMed, Medline, Cochrane library, Web of Science, Google Scholar, Scopus and EMBASE for relevant studies. Publication in English between 2000 to 2021 which estimated Saliva markers as indicators of orthodontic tooth movement was included. The list of biomarkers available to date was compiled and is presented in table format. Each biomarker is discussed separately based on the available and collected evidences. Several sensitive salivary and GCF biomarkers are available to detect the biomechanical changes occurring during orthodontic tooth movement and pain occurring during fixed orthodontic therapy. Further focussed research might help to analyze the sensitivity and reliability of these biomarkers or cytokines, which in turn can lead to the development of chairside tests to assess the pain experienced by patients during orthodontic therapy and finally the outcome of the fixed orthodontic therapy.

Keywords: fixed orthodontic therapy, molecular biomarkers, saliva, GCF, objectivity

1. Introduction

Biomarkers are—quantifiable criteria of biological processes that provide indications objectively. During the orthodontic procedure, the analysis of saliva/salivary fluid and Gingival crevicular fluid (GCF) may be examined to monitor biological process/progress.

In the orthodontic treatment, emphasis is on the point of patient care for the best results, by growth modification of the craniofacial region along with alveolar bone remodeling during fixed orthodontic procedure [1]. Induction of biologically active compounds occur inside the periodontium due to the orthodontic treatment which eventually induces cellular response in different microenvironment for biological response [1]. Orthodontic treatment is considered successful by three major factors namely periodontal health, oral hygiene and optimal orthodontic forces [1, 2]. Availability of newer techniques have reduced lateral effects like, pain, periodontal diseases, abbreviate the treatment period and limit iatrogenic damages like root resorption and development of nonvital teeth. The sequential events that occur following the orthodontic tooth movement (OTM) can be illustrated by the released molecules, regarded as biomarkers [1, 2]. Biomarkers are attributes that can be quantified, these can the indicators of biological processes which may be normal or pathogenic and/or other metabolic processes [3, 4]. Other important features of the biomarkers are specificity and sensitivity, which will have the ability to notify the biological conditions/changes occurring during any process/procedures [4]. Adequate knowledge about the cellular and biological processes makes it easier to understand the biological mechanics that can shorten the treatment time avoiding the detrimental effects linked to the orthodontic treatment due to its objective characteristics [3, 4].

In the orthodontic treatment, emphasis is on the point of patient care for the best results, by growth modification of the craniofacial region along with alveolar bone remodeling during fixed orthodontic procedure [1]. Induction of biologically active compounds occur inside the periodontium due to the orthodontic treatment. This induces cellular response in different microenvironment for biological response [1]. Orthodontic treatment is considered successful by three major factors namely periodontal health, oral hygiene and optimal orthodontic forces [1, 2]. Availability of newer techniques have reduced lateral effects like, pain, periodontal diseases, abbreviate the treatment period and limit iatrogenic damages like root resorption and development of nonvital teeth. The sequential events that occur following the orthodontic tooth movement (OTM) can be illustrated by the released molecules, regarded as biomarkers [1, 2]. Biomarkers are attributes that can be quantified, these can be the indicators of biological processes which may be normal or pathogenic and/or other metabolic processes [3, 4]. Other important features of the biomarkers are specificity and sensitivity, which will have the ability to notify the biological conditions/changes occurring during any process/procedures [4]. Adequate knowledge about the cellular and biological processes makes it easier to understand the biological mechanics that can shorten the treatment time avoiding the detrimental effects linked to the orthodontic treatment due to its objective characteristics [3, 4].

Forces induced by orthodontic therapy stimulates periodontium cells to release many chemical intermediaries like cytokines. The cytokines contribute immensely in the periodontal and alveolar bone remodeling, bone resorption and new bone deposition [5]. During the process of bone metabolism, the biomarkers are released into the circulation which indicates bone remodeling activity comprising of both osteoblastic deposition and osteoclastic resorption. Systemic circulation in the orthodontic patients indicates the skeletal maturity, this can be detected using biomarkers. And their detection locally, in saliva and gingival crevicular fluid (GCF), indicates the advancement of orthodontically induced alveolar bone remodeling [4]. Many research studies have been executed, suggestive of presence of array of molecules indicating the skeletal growth turnover. The assessment of molecular biomarkers of bone remodeling in the body fluids such as saliva, GCF etc., would guide the clinicians to arrive at a better treatment plan for orthodontic therapy at the ideal time and estimate the advent of the treatment [4, 5].

Saliva is considered a medium for the microbes and transport, which is affected by status of oral health and the quantity and types of bacteria present in the oral cavity. It is also comprising of innate immune factors and various salivary defense proteins. The fixed orthodontic therapy induces site-specific bone resorption and formation and cytokines which are released from periodontal ligament (PDL) cells.

The complex combination of serum, host inflammatory cells, structural cells of oral bacteria and the periodontium leads to the formation of the GCF which arises from the plexus of gingival blood vessels in the gingival corium, lying underneath to the epithelial lining of the dentogingival space. It can be isolated from healthy sulcus as well [3, 5].

The origination of GCF components is from blood, subgingival plaque and host tissues. Presence of the transudate of the gingival interstitial fluid due to the osmotic gradient in the healthy periodontium is observed. There will be a steady increase in the volume with inflammation and greater capillary permeability [6]. Previously GCF was known as continuous transudate but currently it is considered as inflammatory transudate [7]. GCF comprises of host-derived substances which includes cytokines, antibodies, tissue degradation products and enzymes [8]. The inflammatory exudate increases by more than 5-fold during the inflammatory conditions, such as periodontal disease and gingivitis [9].

Orthodontic forces result in a condition which can be described as a consequence of the orthodontic force, a condition persists that involves a series of inflammation and repair intended at converting it into normal tissues and [10] according to some reports GCF reflects the immune reactions arising from both orthodontic force application and periodontitis [11, 12].

Nowadays many biomarkers are detected using saliva. It was recently discovered that several new isoforms for Nerve Growth Factor (NGF), Brain derived Neurotropic Factor (BDNF) and Calcitonin gene-related peptide (CGRP) were found in the saliva [3]. Identification of these isoforms can be utilized to develop subtle ways that can be considered to be methods to detect and analyze markers related to pain. The nuclear factor kappa B ligand and of the nuclear factor kappa B/osteoprotegerin (RANK/RANKL/OPG) signaling pathway being one of the several key factors that initiated the commencement of osteoclasts. The recruitment, differentiation and survival of osteoclasts are facilitated by the osteoblasts [12] which secretes a molecular biomarker RANKL. Induction of differentiation of immature osteoclasts into functional cells are due to the binding of RANKL with RANK (expressed at the surface of the osteoclast). Osteoblasts produce OPG which acts as a soluble receptor for RANKL. This inhibits the terminal stages of osteoclast differentiation [12].

Pain and discomfort are inevitable during orthodontic treatment [13]. Conventionally, the degree of pain is assessed subjectively using many pain scales [14]. Assessing pain objectively using salivary physiological biomarkers would benefit the clinician for appropriate pain diagnosis and management [13, 15]. The role of saliva in the diagnostic and prognostics is side-lined due to unavailability of a standardized collection procedure, even though well accepted by patients [3].

The neuropeptide, NGF protects the neurons and regenerates them. It plays an important role in hyperalgesia and its concentration increases during inflammation which is up regulated in response to noxious stimuli [16]. The occurrence and development of pain and hyperalgesia are credited to be due to the role of CGRP and BDNF. CGRP and BDNF has been implicated in migraine and headache based on increased saliva and plasma concentrations during active pain periods [16, 17].

Only a few studies have investigated the levels of these above-mentioned neuropeptides in saliva [16–18]. Several patients describe much longer periods of pain and discomfort which are common during the first 1 or 2 days of the orthodontic treatment. Scheurer et al. reported that even after 7 days of insertion of a fixed appliance, 25% of all investigated patients still reported pain [19]. According to measurements at 4 h and 24 h, the intensity of pain generally increases with time, but falls to normal levels after 7 days of the orthodontic treatment [19]. Biomarkers can be used to characterize the sequential events following OTM. The rate, amount, and the activity of the released substances/biomarkers indicates the activity of individual cells and the metabolic activity involved in the tissues and organs [1]. These potential biological markers can be collected from different tissue samples. The sampling is done as per the required biomarker and the biological processes to be studied [1, 20]. Several possible biomarkers representing many of these biological changes during specific phenomenon like pain experienced during orthodontic treatment pain, bone remodeling, inflammation and root resorption have also been proposed [20]. The clinical application can be developed from the knowledge of biomarkers that can accelerate the orthodontic treatment as well.

2. Phases of orthodontic tooth movement (OTM)

There are two types of tooth movement namely: OTM and Physiological tooth movement. The physiological tooth movement occurs slowly in the cancellous bone in buccal direction or the cortical bone [21]. In contrast, OTM can occur both rapidly or slowly, it depends on the rate, physical characteristics and amount of the force application and the biological response of the Periodontal Ligament (PDL) [22]. The orthodontic force application can change the dental and paradental tissues, including the PDL, alveolar bone, dental pulp and gingiva resulting in pressure and tension sites at the tooth region [23].

Perinetti et al. [24] through their research study state that, one bone remodeling cycle involves four main phases namely: activation, bone resorption, reversal, and bone formation. Recent studies have exhibited that several enzymes are expressed during these phases which have been designated as biomarkers during bone remodeling namely Tartrate-resistant Acid Phosphatase (TRAP), Alkaline Phosphatase (ALP), Lactate Dehydrogenase (LDH), Aspartate Aminotransferase (AST), and many more.

Orthodontic therapy involves the supervision, guidance and correction of growing and maturing dentofacial structures which is based on the principle that if the teeth is subjected to prolonged pressure, consequently it will lead to remodeling of the bone. This OTM is exemplified by the remodeling of dental and paradental tissues [21].

In 1962, Burstone [25] stated the three phases of tooth movement, when rates of tooth movement are plotted against time:

1. Initial phase

2. Lag phase

3. Post-lag phase.

Phase I (initial)	24 h–2 days Initial tooth movement within the socket	Acute inflammatory response Vasodilation-migration of leucocytes-release of cytokines-cell signaling molecules (metabolic products of paradental remodeling)
Phase II (arrest)	20–30 days Movement stops	Chronic inflammation Continuation of migration of leucocytes Paradental remodeling
Phase III (acceleration)	40 days of accelerated tooth movement after initial force application	Another period of acute inflammation superimposing the on-going chronic inflammation
Phase IV (linear)	Overall tooth movement	Recruitment of macrophages, fibroblasts, osteoblasts, and osteoclasts Alkaline phosphatase activity

Table 1.
Phases of orthodontic tooth movement [27].

1. Initial phase: is described by immediate and quick movement which occurs in time period between 24 h to 48 h after the preliminary orthodontic force application to the tooth. This rate is largely recognized to the tooth movement in the PDL space.

2. Lag phase: The duration of this phase lasts up to 20–30 days which relatively shows little to no tooth movement. In this phase the region in which compression is applied, such region demonstrates the PDL hyalinisation. No subsequent tooth displacement occurs until the cells remove the necrotic tissues completely.

3. Post-lag phase: follows the lag phase, where the rate of tooth movement increases [26].

Pilon et al. [27, 28] divided the curve of tooth movement into four phases (**Table 1**). The GCF of tooth movement contain the biomarkers that indicate these phases and signaling pathways. Considerable increased levels of concentrations of cytokines responsible for inflammation and prostaglandins are observed.

The tissue changes that are involved during OTM includes compression region (which involves osteoblasts), tension region (which involves osteoclasts), pulp tissues and dental root [29]. Several possible biological factors or biomarkers representing these biological changes during particular phenomenon that is, bone remodeling. Inflammation and root resorption, have been identified. Similarly, lactic acid dehydrogenase (LDH) and dentin sialophosphoprotien (DSPP) are also potentially observed. A research study suggests that using sampling from four different sampling procedures, that is, saliva, GCF, tissue (biopsy), and serum, the biomarkers indicative of the ongoing biological processes can be identified [29]. The suggested amount and concentration of biomarkers during OTM are the best and practical sampling or testing procedure indicative of the biological phenomenon. The amount of precise force application and duration that should be used for each tooth during OTM can be decided based on the knowledge of these biomarkers. Ultimately, it produces an optimal treatment with mild side effects or accelerate the treatment [29].

3. Saliva and biomarkers

Most of the laboratory diagnostic procedures involves the analysis of the cellular and biochemical constituents of the blood. Saliva can be used in the diagnosis of several diseases. This can be feasible and valuable for children and older adults due to the ease of collection of the fluid [30]. Saliva can be classified into two types: gland-specific saliva and whole saliva. It is feasible to collect saliva specific to different glands from individual salivary glands namely: parotid, submandibular, sublingual and minor salivary glands. Since the secretions from both the submandibular and sublingual salivary glands enter the oral cavity only through single duct known as Wharton's duct [31], hence collection of the saliva from submandibular and sublingual glands separately is challenging.

Orthodontists generally aims to gain ideal orthognathic conditions with fewer treatment times i.e.; shorter treatment time with longer treatment intervals with fewer appointments [32]. Conversely, when heavier force is applied to accelerate tooth movement, the oxygen tension in the periodontium will be conceded due to reduced vascular supply [33]. This will risk or expose the healthy supporting alveolar bone and periodontal structure leading to the slow progress of the treatment. In order to supervise the orthodontic tooth movement in a non-invasive approach in human beings, the alterations that appear during the examination of the profile and levels of various cytokines, enzymes, growth factors, and proteoglycans in saliva and GCF. Evidences support the elevated levels of several biomarkers or cytokines, that is, interleukin (IL)-1β, IL-6, epidermal growth factor (EGF), prostaglandin (PG) and proteoglycans, in the saliva and GCF [34–36]. Components of GCF namely ALP, TRAP, LDH and AST have been recognized to be potential biomarkers during OTM [37–40]. Study conducted by Shahrul et al. [41] showed that ALP, TRAP, and LDH also existed in saliva. Orthodontic treatment using a surface-enhanced laser desorption/ionization time of flight mass spectrometry (SELDI-TOF MS) approach the effects of the orthodontic treatment on salivary proteins has been performed as per the study by Zhang et al. [42]. The outcome of this approach determined the relatively low molecular weight proteins but not the identity of these proteins. Only the expression profile was cross-examined.

Saliva has protective and anti-microbial properties and contains a variety of growth factors [43, 44]. Saliva helps in the easy digestion of the food since it has lubricating functions [45]. The role of saliva and different salivary constituents responsible for its functions are summarized below in **Table 2** [30].

Salivary protein concentration ranges from 2 to 5 mg/mL which constitutes about 3% of the protein concentration of blood. Numerous proline-rich glycoproteins, immunoglobulin A and amylase are the major secretory proteins of the parotid glands, other antibacterial salivary proteins include lysozymes, peroxidases and lactoferrin. Submandibular and sublingual glands contribute mucous glycoproteins to oral fluid. Pathological analysis can be carried out using the saliva produced by specific glands. Since saliva contains constituents of other serum, whole saliva is used for the diagnosis of systemic diseases. The gingival fluid flows into the oral cavity. The constituents of gingival fluid can be derived from the local vasculature of the salivary glands. Analysis of saliva perhaps be useful for the diagnosis of different hereditary disorders, endocrine disorders, malignant, autoimmune and infectious diseases, as well as in the assessment of therapeutic levels of drugs and in the monitoring of illicit use of drugs.

Evaluation of the fluids from the individual salivary glands can help in detecting the infection and obstruction. Mixture of oral fluids can be present in the whole saliva or mixed. This may include the secretions from both the major and minor salivary glands including several constituents of non-salivary origin. The fluids of non-salivary origin may include expectorated bronchial and nasal secretions, GCF, serum and blood derivatives from oral wounds [46–49].

Functions salivary components involved:

1. Protective functions
   - Lubrication—Mucins, proline-rich glycoproteins, water.
   - Antimicrobial—Amylase, complement, defensins, lysozyme, lactoferrin, lactoperoxidase, mucins, cystatins, histatins, proline-rich glycoproteins, secretory IgA, secretory leukocyte protease inhibitor, statherin, thrombospondin.
   - Growth factors—Epidermal growth factor (EGF), Transforming growth factors (TGF-α), TGF-β, fibroblast growth factor (FGF), insulin-like growth factor (IGF-I & IGF-II), Nerve growth factor (NGF).
   - Mucosal integrity—Mucins, electrolytes, water.
   - Lavage/cleansing—Water.
   - Buffering—Bicarbonate, phosphate ions, proteins.
   - Remineralization—Calcium, phosphate, statherin, anionic proline-rich proteins.
2. Food- and speech-related functions:
   - Food preparation—Water, mucins.
   - Digestion—Amylases, lipase, ribonuclease, proteases, water, mucins.
   - Taste—Water, gustin.
   - Speech—Water, mucins.

Table 2.
The major functions of saliva [30].

Evaluation of the systemic disorders is done by the salivary analysis of the whole saliva collected with or without stimulation. There are two procedures to collect the saliva using stimulation, they are gustatory stimulation (i.e., application of citric acid on the subject's tongue [50]; or by masticatory action (i.e., from a subject chewing on paraffin). Constituents, pH and concentration of the fluid depends on the quantity of saliva collected by the stimulation method. Unstimulated saliva is collected without gustatory, masticatory, exogenous or mechanical stimulation. The factors that affect the salivary flow rate depends on the degree of hydration, olfactory stimulation, exposure to light, body positioning, seasonal and diurnal factors. There are two appropriate methods to collect the saliva, they are by the draining or drooling method, in which saliva can drip off the lower lip. In the second methods which is the spitting method the subject expectorates saliva into a test tube [51].

Specialized epithelial cells make up the salivary glands, based on their structure, these cells can be divided into two specific regions: the ductal and acinar regions. During the primary salivary secretion, the ductal cells actively absorb most of the Na^+ and Cl^- ions and secrete small amounts of K^+ and HCO_3^- and some proteins. This modifies the primary salivary secretion into a hypotonic final salivary secretion when it enters the oral cavity [52].

In the acinar region most of the protein synthesis and secretion takes place, this is where the oral fluid is generated as well. The amino acids enter the acinar cells through active transport. After the intracellular protein synthesis, secretory stimulation releases most proteins, these are stored in storage granules [53, 54]. Description of three models for acinar fluid secretion area are available, which include the active passage of anions into the lumen and passage of osmotic gradient water from the interstitial fluid to the salivary lumen [55, 56]. Fluid obtained at the initial stage is isotonic in nature. This is derived from the local vasculature whereas the acinar cells are water-permeable, and the ductal cells are impermeable. The autonomic nervous system(sympathetic and parasympathetic system) controls the salivary secretion and its signaling mechanism involves the binding of neurotransmitter (primarily acetylcholine and norepinephrine) to plasma membrane receptors and signal transduction *via* guanine nucleotide-binding regulatory proteins (G-proteins) and activation of intracellular calcium signaling mechanisms [52, 57–59]. A few diagnostic uses of saliva like viral infections, including hepatitis and HIV, and in the detection of certain endocrine disorders have been demonstrated.

Certain markers in the serum cannot be relied upon but with the salivary samples, the levels of certain markers are consistent than its manifestation. The components of the biomarker molecules and normal saliva have similar physicochemical characteristics. Hence the diffusion of lipophilic molecules into the saliva is easier than the lipophobic molecules. The molecules involved in the biological processes reach the saliva through different mechanisms. Hence extraction of molecules using the methods such as ultrafiltration and active transport have also been proposed for many substances recently. Whereas previously passive diffusion was the most common mechanism for drugs and hormones.

For accurate diagnosis, an appropriate relationship must be established between the biomarker concentration in serum and its concentration in saliva. Normalcy in the salivary gland function is necessary for the collection of salivary molecules or cytokines with diagnostic value. The flow rate of the saliva and its concentration is expected to vary between individuals and in the same individual under various conditions. Erratic collection of the serum markers is possible in the whole saliva due to the oral wounds and through GCF flow. Effectiveness of such samples may be questionable as these parameters may interfere in the correct diagnosis based on the salivary constituents [60]. Apart from some of the systemic disorders, other factors like the medications and radiation will affect salivary gland function, the quantity and consequently the composition of saliva [61, 62]. The whole saliva may contain some proteolytic enzymes that come from the host and there may be presence of enzymes derived from the oral microorganisms [63]. These enzymes can affect the stability, consistency and reliability of certain diagnostic biomarkers. Degradation of some molecules happened during intracellular diffusion into saliva. The diagnostic functional value of the marker may be affected by any condition or medication.

Despite the limitations of saliva to be used for diagnostic purposes, it is becoming popular as per the evidences suggested by many recent researches. Commercially available salivary diagnostic tests are currently being used by patients, researchers, and clinicians. Objective and qualitative detection that is the detection of the presence or absence of a biomarker using saliva is possible but it is not a feasible option for the quantitative diagnosis. Saliva also plays a major role in eliciting and monitoring the hormone levels, especially steroids which facilitates repeated sampling in short time intervals, which may be particularly important for hormone monitoring and avoiding patient and clinician compliance problems.

Nevertheless, before a salivary diagnostic test can replace more conventional methods, the diagnostic values of a new salivary test must be compared with the gold-standard. The effectiveness of a new test must be determined in terms of specificity, sensitivity, reproducibility and the correlation with an established disease diagnostic criterion.

The known functions of proteins identified by proteomic analysis are summarized in **Table 3**. Using the proteomics approaches, these proteins have been identified previously [32, 64, 65]. There has been no reports of the changes in the protein

Protein	Known function
Protein S100-A9 (S100 calcium-binding protein A9) (Calgranulin-B)	i. Calcium-binding protein. ii. At the sites of wounding, it promotes phagocyte migration and infiltration of granulocytes. iii. Takes part as a proinflammatory mediator in acute and chronic inflammation.
Serum albumin precursor	i. It binds with water, $Ca2^+$, Na^+, K^+, fatty acids, hormones, bilirubin, and drugs. ii. The main function is to regulate the colloidal osmotic pressure of blood. iii. Major zinc transporter in plasma.
Immunoglobulin J chain	i. Links two monomer units of either IgM or IgA. ii. Helps in binding IgM or IgA to a secretory component.
Ig alpha-1 chain C region	i. A major immunoglobulin class in the body secretions. ii. Serves as a defence against local infection and prevents access of foreign antigens.
Cysteine-rich secretory protein 3 precursor (CRISP-3)	i. Innate immune response ii. Potential biological marker for prostate cancer
Hemoglobin subunit beta (Hemoglobin beta chain) (Beta-globin)	Role in the transportation of oxygen from the lung to the various peripheral tissues.
14-3-3 protein σ (Stratifin) (Epithelial cell marker protein 1)	i. An adapter protein. ii. Results in the modulation of the activity of the large number of binding partners.

Table 3.
Summary of identified proteins and their known functions [30].

expression in relation to the orthodontic treatment, tooth movement and its forces. The **Table 3** lists the functions of proteins and their predictive role in the OTM.

3.1 Protein S100-A9

During acute and chronic inflammation Protein S100-A9 (S100-A9) is a calcium-binding protein that functions as a proinflammatory mediator. It is found in high concentration in an inflamed tissue. Previous research described that S100-A9 was concerned in chondrocytic and osteoblastic maturation, matriceal calcification and was noticeable in osteoclasts [66]. Therefore, the presence of osteoclast indicates an active process of bone resorption. It is also been stated that it regulates cartilage destruction and joint inflammation during antigen-induced arthritis [67]. A recent study showed an obvious downregulation of S100-A9 protein, this indicates that there may not be an involvement of the protein during bone resorption in fixed orthodontic tooth movement. Its involvement may be in the inflammatory conditions as suggested by the data from the previous study. As per the study, on day 14 of the treatment, the inflammatory process was not active. The orthodontic treatment for 14 days resulted in the downregulation of this above protein indicated by the suppression of inflammation.

3.2 Immunoglobulin J chain (IgJ)

Immunoglobulin J chain (IgJ) is a constituent of IgA or IgM, whereas Ig Alpha-1 chain C region (IgAC) is a major immunoglobulin class in the body secretions.

Both are common elements of the immune response in humans. Acute inflammatory responses were noticed in the periodontal tissues surrounding the mechanically stressed teeth, in the early phase of the OTM [24]. Recent study also exhibited an obvious downregulation of both IgAC and IgI after 14 days of the fixed orthodontic therapy. Previous study also did not show any increase of LDH after 14 days of orthodontic activation [41]. After these studies researchers suggested that no further inflammation had occurred at that period.

3.3 Cysteine-rich secretory protein 3 precursor (CRISP-3)

CRISP-3 shows the presence of the exocrine secretion and secretory granules of neutrophil in them. It has notable functions in innate immunity [68] and it is a potential biological marker for prostate cancer [69]. According to the results from the recent study after 14 days of orthodontic treatment, the presence of this protein was noticed. There is not much clarity regarding its relationship with orthodontic tooth movement.

3.4 Serum albumin precursor (ALB)

ALB and hemoglobin subunit beta (HBB) are serum proteins. These serum proteins are responsible for the increase in subjects with periodontal disease [70]. ALB is considered as a major zinc transporter in the plasma which regulates the colloidal osmotic pressure of blood [71]. The HBB is a subunit of hemoglobin containing two beta units and four subunits with two alpha. Transport of oxygen from the lung to different peripheral tissues involves the alpha and beta subunit carrying an ion-containing molecule (heme) in each of them [72]. HBB is commonly found in the red blood cells (RBCs) but its function(s) in saliva is still unknown. Recent study showed that ALB was present only at day 0 of treatment. And its role(s) in orthodontic tooth movement is also still unclear.

3.5 Protein: 14-3-3 σ

On Day 0, an adaptor protein—14-3-3 σ also known as epithelial cell marker protein 1 or stratafin (SFN) was found to be present. This binds to many partners and results in the modulation of the activity of the binding partner(s). In several types of human cancers, loss of protein 14-3-3 σ expression has been observed suggesting its role as a tumor suppressor protein [73]. However, there is lack of evidence on the role of SFN protein in inflammation or bone resorption and formation, and the role(s) it may play during fixed orthodontic tooth movement.

Orthodontic and dentofacial orthopedic therapeutic appliances used in the treatment and correction of various maxillofacial and dento-maxillary anomalies with skeletal and dental problems most frequently believe that the orthodontic force application of high intensity can induce a localized inflammatory process around the tooth and tooth supporting structures. Due to the presence of this inflammatory process there is an increased synthesis of free radicals secondarily produced which is followed by the oxidative stress [74]. In the literature till date, there are very limited number of human studies and evidences on the oxidative stress and oxidative damage that may occur due to an aseptic inflammation in tissues caused because of orthodontic tooth movements [74].

A recent study performed in 2009 by Olteanu et al. [60] compared and determined the amount of oxidative stress markers in the saliva of patients, they were treated using orthodontic appliances for a predefined stipulated time period. The time periods that were predefined for determination were: before and after 1 h of treatment, 24 h and 7 days after the initiation of the treatment. At 24 h, maximum variation was observed in the concentrations of the saliva markers of the oxidative stress for ceruloplasmin and malondialdehyde (MDA). And for the hydrogen donors at one hour respectively, and at the 7 days from the placing of an appliance, the concentrations of markers were similar to the values observed in the initial phase of the tests. Concentration of saliva markers for oxidative stress showed changes but this cannot prove pathological processes prevalent in the patients with orthodontic appliances at the level of the oral cavity.

Recently, the research study performed using saliva by Ozcan et al. [75] had the objective to evaluate the changes in some oxidative stress markers for the determining of oxidative stress damage that occurs in the process of bone and tissue remodeling, including dysfunction of periodontal tissue caused by orthodontic tooth movement. At certain time intervals, the unstimulated saliva samples of patients with fixed orthodontic appliances were collected. The time intervals followed were: just before treatment, at the 1st month of treatment and at the 6th month of treatment. Investigations were conducted using spectrophotometric method to detect nitric oxide (NO) and MDA. The TNF-α, IL-1β, and 8-OHdG levels were detected using ELISA method. In the results, at any of the predefined time period, the study did not show any significant change in the saliva in all biochemical parameters. In another study involving the unstimulated saliva samples of individuals with fixed orthodontic appliances, there were no significant differences observed when compared to the control group in kynurenine concentration [76]. And the data presented in the study at least at the first 6 months of the treatment indicate that orthodontic materials and orthodontic tooth movement used in orthodontic treatment do not cause oxidative damage in the oral cavity.

4. Pain and tooth movement

Nowadays many biomarkers are detected using saliva. It was recently discovered that several new isoforms for Nerve Growth Factor (NGF), Brain derived Neurotropic Factor (BDNF) and Calcitonin gene-related peptide (CGRP) were found in the saliva [3]. Identification of these isoforms can be utilized to develop subtle ways that can be considered to be methods to detect and analyze markers related to pain.

Pain and discomfort are inevitable during orthodontic treatment [6]. Conventionally, the degree of pain is assessed subjectively using many pain scales [7]. Assessing pain objectively using salivary physiological biomarkers would benefit the clinician for appropriate pain diagnosis and management [6, 8].

These potential biological markers can be collected from different tissue samples. The sampling is done as per the required biomarker and the biological processes to be studied [1, 9]. Several possible biomarkers representing many of these biological changes during specific phenomenon like pain experienced during orthodontic treatment pain, bone remodeling, inflammation and root resorption have also been proposed [20]. The clinical application can be developed from the knowledge of biomarkers that can accelerate the orthodontic treatment as well.

Development of objective markers of nociception and pain helps in diagnosis of pain and its management. Standardization of pain assessment objectively is important to avoid bias in research studies. Tools that are sensitive and specific to pain fulfilling certain criteria's like being observer-independent, not reliant on the patient's ability to communicate and not influenced by disease characteristics are needed in developing an objective method of pain assessment [13]. A review by Cowen et al. [13] states that the objective biomarkers of nociception or pain which have been validated for clinical use, although there are currently promising strategies like monitoring changes in the autonomic nervous system, biopotentials, neuroimaging and composite algorithms. There is a serious need for theoretically promising and clinically useful objective marker for assessment of pain. Restricted use of physiological markers as 'objective' measures of pain and nociception is due to the lack of evidence in support of its use as biomarker. Biomarker research in saliva for pain and nociception as part of clinical phenotyping should be watched closely.

Fleming et al. [14] suggests that unlike the bracket type, the subjective pain experience at 4 h, 24 h, 3 days, and 7 days following fixed orthodontic appliance placement [14]. The subjective pain was recorded using Visual Analog Scale (VAS) [14].

In cross sectional study conducted by Jasim et al. [3], the levels of nerve NGF, CGRP and BDNF were determined using novel western blotting-based technology using Capillary Isoelectric Focussing (CIEF) Immunoassay. Glutamate and substance P (SP) was determined using ELISA. Numerous new isoforms were found for NGF, CGRP and BDNF in saliva. In expression and chemiluminescence levels, the isoform pattern showed significant difference between different collection methods. In this study, new sensitive methods to study pain related markers in saliva were developed. And this study was the first to:

1. detect NGF, CGRP, BDNF, Glutamate and S P (SP) in five different salivary types,

2. to develop a new protocol/method for analysis of different isoforms of NGF, CGRP and BDNF,

3. show quantifiable levels of several isoforms of NGF, CGRP and BDNF in human saliva, and finally.

4. establish a correlation between the glutamate level in stimulated whole saliva and plasma.

Activation of the orthodontic appliance induces painful sensations due to the inflammatory process, this occurs as part of the tooth movement related to tissue remodeling. It is established that the immunoreactive neuron C-fos is involved in the transmission of nociceptive information expressed bilaterally in the lateral parabranchial nucleus. And ipsilaterally in the trigeminal subnucleus caudalis past the initial 24 h of orthodontic force application. Similarly, fos-like immunoreactive neurons were distributed in other brain regions such as the neocortex, thalamic nucleus and dorsal raphe [77]. Nociceptive information by tooth movement is modulated and transmitted in several regions of the brain. Endogenous pain control systems are activated by these stimuli, including descending monoaminergic pathways [78].

Initial studies suggested that through dopaminergic and serotonergic systems, the nociception is nociception is regulated [77]. Subsequently, another experiment performed showed an increase in serotonin turnover in the medulla, indicating the bulbospinal serotonergic pathway activation by nociceptive neurological response [78]. Therefore, an indirect nociceptive mechanism operating during tooth movement occurs that suggests a continuous and delayed nociceptive response, which is expected to regulate the masticatory function during active tooth movement.

A recent case report published data on administration of MK-801 in rats (a non-competitive antagonist of N-methyl-Daspartate receptors), intraperitonially before tooth movement. The results suggested the N-methyl-D-aspartate receptors blockade along with neuronal suppression of sensory nuclear complex of the trigeminal nerve branch. Subsequently, these effects were found to increase the neuronal activity in the descending antinociceptive system, including dorsal raphe nucleus, nuclear raphe magnus, ventrolateral PAG, and Edinger-Westphal nucleus. Following, during orthodontic tooth movement, these results indicated a pharmacological way to decrease pain perception [79].

Salivary biomarkers as a measure has the potential to be an objective approach and a diagnostic tool for the studies related to pain. However, there is a need of estimating the different collection methods and develop more profound techniques for analysis. These biomarkers have a crucial part in objectively assessing the pain.

5. Gingival crevicular fluid (GCF) and biomarkers

GCF is an exudate that can be collected from the gingival sulcus in periodontium, which provides a prospective source of factors or biomarkers associated with the changes and destruction in the underlying periodontium that generally occurs during the orthodontic force application during fixed orthodontic treatment [80].

Due to its non-invasive nature and ease of repetitive sampling from the same site with the help of filter paper strips, gingival washings, platinum loops and micropipettes, GCF is commonly collected for the examination and check the levels and concentration of these biomarkers during the orthodontic force application. This fluid is easily available as that of saliva in the oral cavity and is usually used to analyze various biochemical markers [80].

The importance of GCF biomarkers in periodontal effects is tabulated in **Table 4**.

GCF which can be described as a transudate or an exudate arises at the gingival margin where its flow rate is of 0.05–0.20/min which indicates gingival inflammation [81]. Various biochemical markers such as prostaglandin production and the action of various extracellular and intracellular factors, such as IL-6, IL-1, TNF, epidermal growth factors, cathepsin, aspartate aminotransferease, microglobulin, alkaline phosphatase, and lactate dehydrogenase are analysed by this GCF.

Various cell mediators or enzymes are produced due to the remodeling changes in the PDL and the alveolar bone that can be used as the biomarkers of orthodontic treatment [66, 82]. The initial works conducted by Embery, Waddington [83] and Last et al. [84], proved the presence of many proteoglycan, tissue proteins and GAGs in GCF and also reported presence of chondroitin-4-sulphate in GCF from the pressure side of tooth movement. Biological alteration is caused in deep-seated tissues due to that the increase in chondroitin-4-sulphate since the orthodontic model is a nonplaque and non-disease-related process.

Uematsu et al. [85, 86] found elevated levels of IL-1, IL-6, TNF, epidermal growth factors, TGF 2 and microglobulin during the orthodontic treatment in the GCF. Lee et al. [87] and Grieve et al. [88] also reported stated the similar finding for IL-1, and

Inflammatory mediators
• Protein E2 (P E2) -bone resorption
• Substance P (S P) (neuropeptide)-bone resorption
• Epidermal growth factor (EGF)-bone resorption
• Transforming growth factor (TGF)-bone remodeling
• RANKL - stimulation of osteoclastic differentiation
• Osteoprotegerin-inhibition of osteoclastic differentiation
• Granulocyte macrophage colony stimulating factor-bone turn over
• α2 microglobulin-enhancer of IGF-1
• IL 1β, 2, 6, 8-bone remodeling
• Myeloperoxidase–enzyme in PMN-inflammation
Metabolic products of paradental remodeling
• Hyaluronic acid (GAG)-indicator of breakdown of gingival tissue
• Chondroitin sulfate (GAG)-indicator of breakdown of alveolar bone and
• PDL
• Pentaxrin-3 (TNF stimulated gene14)-marker of inflammation
• Osteocalcin-bone turnover
• Insulin growth factor-regulators of cell differentiation and apoptosis
• Pyridinoline, deoxypyridinoline-indicators of bone metabolism
• N-telopeptide-bone resorption
• Dentin matrix protein-root resorption
Enzymes
• Acid phosphatase- bone resorption
• Alkaline phosphatase-bone formation
• Aspartate amino transferase-cell necrosis
• CathepsinB-extracellular matrix degradation
• Matrix metalloproteins (1, 2 and 8)-breakdown denatured collagen
• β glucuronidase-marker of granule release by PMN
• Lactate dehydrogenase-indicator of cell death

GCF, Gingival crevicular fluid; IGF-1, Insulin-like growth factor-1; GAG, Glycosaminoglycans; PMN, Polymorphonuclear neutrophil; TNF, Tumor necrosis factor; PDL, Periodontal ligament.

Table 4.
List of GCF biomarkers and their role in orthodontic tooth movement.

PGE2. Lowney et al. [89] for TNF. Griffiths et al. [90] demonstrated the presence of osteocalcin in GCF from teeth which is subjected to the orthodontic treatment force application. A recent study by Insoft et al. [91] also found an increased level of alkaline phosphatase during the first 3 weeks of orthodontic treatment, whereas acid phosphatase increased in successive weeks. Perinetti et al. [92] also determined the aspartate aminotransferase along with the alkaline phosphatase activity in GCF. Orthodontic force application induced an increase in the lactate dehydrogense activity in GCF as per a recent study by Serra et al. [93]. After the study it is proposed to be a sensitive factor or biomarker for periodontal metabolism. Sugiyama et al. [82] suggested that cathepsin B involved in ECM degradation and reported its increase in the amount in GCF.

After an orthodontic force presentation for 4–8 h Apajalahti et al. [94] found a significantly higher amount of MMP-8 in GCF. They suggested that MMP-8 reflects the enhanced periodontal remodeling, this is the effect of increased expression and activation of GCF. From the studies, it was concluded that presence of such markers in GCF during the orthodontic studies are useful in identifying the bone-remodeling activities. Therefore, GCF can be considered a promising topic for future research, as these investigations have already begun to provide an insight into the progressive aspects of remodeling.

According to the QUOROM statement suggestions, a systematic review was conducted by Allgayer et al. [95] in 2014 by strictly adhering to the guidelines suggested by PROSPERO [95]. Several key databases namely PubMed, Embase, Cochrane library, MEDLINE, and Web of Science were searched in May 2014 using the MESH terms 'Orthodontics, Corrective', 'IL-17', or 'helper 17 cell', or 'helper T Cells', or 'TH 17', 'IL 17', 'IL-23', 'crevicular fluid', 'IL 23', and using the free text terms 'GCF, gingival crevicular fluid, regulatory proteins, tooth displacement, cytokines, inflammatory factors, root resorption and canine distalization', and, by reference tracking an additional search was performed. The search results from each database were compiled, combined and the duplicate results were eliminated (**Table 5**).

The results of this systemic review provide an insight by identifying the 115 potentially relevant studies. **Table 5** below represents an overview of the outcomes. Among these studies, further analysis of the titles, abstracts, and full texts revealed that for this systematic review the major 25 studies were relevant [95]. Many studies were performed on mixed samples of young adults and adolescents, and two related studies reported the levels of GCF cytokines in different age groups (**Table 5**). More than 20 subjects were found to be recruited for only 3 studies. Out of 25 studies, seventeen of them used the maxillary canine as their study tooth, and the orthodontic force system was distalization of the canine with either continuous arch wires or sectional wires. The other eight studies addressed insertion of separation elastics (two), Hyrax appliance (two), aligning movement (three), and cervical headgear (one).

MMPs are considered to be the main endogenous chemical mediators of the pathologic destruction of tissues in periodontitis [96]. Extensive research studies have been performed to assess the levels of MMPs in GCF [97] and saliva and also, they have been found to be elevated in patients suffering with periodontitis compared to subjects with healthy periodontium. Additionally, after the periodontal therapy there was drastic decrease in the levels of MMPs in GCF. The levels of MMP-8, 9 MMP-3,10 and MMP-13,11,12 have been linked with the periodontal disease progression in GCF. MMPs also play a dominant role in the remodeling process of PDL during orthodontic tooth movement.

A study in dogs by Redlich et al. [96, 98] suggests an increase in the activity of MMP-1 and mRNA levels in the compression side of the gingiva during orthodontic tooth movement. Similarly, a study performed on rats also demonstrates an increased expression of MMP-13, mRNA, and MMP-8 in the PDL during active tooth movement [13]. Using MMP inhibitors orthodontic tooth movement can be prevented or delayed in mice and rats [96, 98]. A few studies performed on humans [96] have enumerated the presence of MMPs in GCF during orthodontic tooth movement and have stated the alterations in their levels during the orthodontic force application. Additionally, in orthodontic patients treated with fixed appliances, the total collagenase activity in the GCF has been revealed to be 10-fold that of control GCF [99].

Surprisingly, it is found that the effects of orthodontic force application on teeth affected by periodontal disease has not been significantly studied. However, a few

Reference/article	Sample (n) Age (yr)	Sampling (points)	Method	Cytokine	Peak	Results
Alikhani et al 2014	20 19.5-33.1	0, 24 h, 28 d	Canine distalization	IL-1β, IL-1α, IL-6, IL- 8, TNF, MCP-1		Tend to increase
Enhos et al 2014	20 18+-3	0, 24, 48, 168 h, 30 d	Canine distalization	RANKL OPG		OPG and RANKL levels vary as a result of force application
Gastel et al 2011	24 14+-1	0, 365 d	Headgear	IL-2 IL-4 IL-6 IL-8 IL-10 GM-CSF INF TNF MCP-1 IP-10		No significant alteration No significant alteration Tend to increase Tend to increase No significant alteration No significant alteration No significant alteration No significant alteration No significant alteration No significant alteration
Tzannetou 2008	9 10-18	0, 24 h, 7 d, 14 d, 21 d	Hyrax RME	IL-1β		Increased during active RME; remained high in retention phase
Karacay et al 2007	10 15+-1	0, 1, 24, 168 h	Canine distalization	TNF-α	1 d	Hybrid: no change with time Distraction: higher than hybrid
Iwasaki 2006	10 15+-4	0, 1, 3, 7, 14, 28, 42, 56, 70, 84 d	Canine distalization	IL-1β IL-1ra		Tooth movement rate relate to IL-1 gene polymorphisms
Dudic 2006	18 9-14	-7 d, 0, 1 min, 1 h, 1 d, 7 d	Separation elastics	IL-1β PGE2 SP	1 d 1 d 1 d	Higher levels at tension sites Higher levels at tension sites
Basaran 2006	18 16-19	0, 7 d, 21 d, 6 mns, +7 d, +21 d	Canine distalization	IL-1β TNF-α		Tend to increase Tend to increase

Reference/article	Sample (n) Age (yr)	Sampling (points)	Method	Cytokine	Peak	Results
Kawasaki 2006	15 15+-3 15 31+-4	0, 1, 24, 168 h	Canine distalization	RANKL OPG	1 d 1 d	Lower ratio in adults Lower ratio in adults
Nishijima 2006	10 15+-2	0, 1, 24, 168 h	Canine distalization	RANKL OPG	1 d 1 d	No change at 1 h or 168 h No change at 1 h or 168 h
Basaran 2006	17 17+-2	0, 7 d, 21 d, 6 mns, +7 d, +21 d	Canine distalization	IL-2 IL-6 IL-8		Tend to increase at 7 d, back at 21 d Tend to increase at 7 d, back at 21 d Decrease at 7 d, back to baseline at 21 d
Giannopoulou 2006	18 9-14	0, 1, 24, 168 h	Separation elastics	IL-1β PGE2	1 d	Associated with pain at 24 h Weak association with pain at 1 h
Yamaguchi 2006	9 22-2	0, 1, 4, 8, 24, 72, 120, 168 h	Canine distalization	IL-1β	1 d	Correlated with P-substance
Toia 2005	6 10-13	0, 4 h, 10 d	Aligning	IGF	4 h	Decreased 10 d after time-dependent decrease
Hoshino-Itoh 2005	10 23+-3	0, 1, 24, 168 h	Canine distalization	PAI	1 d	Increased only at 24 h Increased only at 24 h
Iwasaki 2005	10 10-30	-28, -14, 0, 1, 3, 14, 28, 42, 56, 70, 84 d	Canine distalization	IL-1β IL-1ra		The ratio of both correlate with the rate of tooth movement
Tuncer 2005	10 15-17	0, 1, 24 h, 6 d, 10 d, 30 d	Canine distalization	IL-8		Tend to increase in early phase
Lee 2004	10 18-22	0, 1, 24, 168 h	Canine distalization	IL-1β PGE2	1 d 1 d	Continuous: 168 h back to baseline Interrupted: higher level at reactivation Continuous: 168 h back to baseline Interrupted: remained high for 1 wk

Reference/article	Sample (n) Age (yr)	Sampling (points)	Method	Cytokine	Peak	Results
Ren 2002	43 10-14 41 21-27	0, 24 h	Aligning	IL-6 PGE2		Upregulated in both age groups Increased only in youngsters Increased only in adults
Iwasaki 2001	7 12-16	-28, -14, 0, 1, 3, 14, 28, 42, 56, 70, 84 d	Canine distalization	IL-1β IL-1ra		28 d periodic changes, no site difference No periodicity, no site difference
Tzannetou 1999	9 10-18	0, 24 h, 7 d, 14 d, 21 d	Hyrax RME	IL-1β		Increased during active RME; remained high in retention phase
Uematsu 1996	12 14	0, 1, 24, 168 h	Canine distalization	IL-1β IL-6 TNF-α	1 d 1 d 1 d	No change at 1 h or 168 h No change at 1 h or 168 h No change at 1 h or 168 h No change at 1 h or 168 h
Uematsu 1996	12 14	0, 1, 24, 168 h	Canine distalization	TGF-β1	1 d	No change at 1 h or 168 h
Lowney 1995	20 12-36	0, 5 min	Canine distalization	TNF-α		More than twofold increase
Grieve 1994	10 24-27	0, 1, 24, 48, 168 h	Aligning	TNF-α PGE	1 d 1 d	Increased at 1 h, back to baseline at 168 h Stay high at 48 h, back to baseline at 168 h

Table 5.
A brief insight on those studies assessing biomarkers or the cytokines in gingival crevicular fluid (GCF) in orthodontics.

retrospective and longitudinal studies [97, 99] indicated that the orthodontic force application can be tolerated by periodontally compromised teeth without any additional damage to the periodontium.

6. Conclusion

Present dissertation deals with brief insight into the biomarkers, connected to orthodontic treatment and progression. Suitable biomarkers may be used to distinguish the sequence of events following OTM. Biophysical mechanisms are involved in the displacement of tooth in the periodontal space and shift of stimulus from continuous force application. The assessment of these biological mechanisms can be done by the evaluation of rate and amount of synthesis of biomarkers in periodontium. This knowledge of the ongoing process occurring in periodontal tissues during orthodontic and dentofacial orthopedic therapies in turn may help us to make proper choice of mechanical orthodontic loading, the amount of orthodontic force application during the treatment and period of treatment may be shortened. It also helps to avoid adverse consequences such as bone loss or root resorption associated with orthodontic treatment. The essential goal is to develop a screen test based on these factors or biological markers that could be used non-invasively and easily by the orthodontist at chairside to monitor the ongoing process and detect early root resorption. Several sensitive, salivary biomarkers are available to detect the biomechanical changes occurring during orthodontic tooth movement and pain occurring during fixed orthodontic therapy. Further focussed research might help to analyze the sensitivity and reliability of these biomarkers (cytokines), which in turn can lead to the development of chairside tests to assess the pain experienced by patients during orthodontic therapy and finally the outcome of the fixed orthodontic therapy. There is an enormous scope for research in this field which may be a boon for future orthodontic treatment and modalities.

Conflict of interest

None.

Author details

Sagar S. Bhat*, Ameet V. Revankar and Shrinivas M. Basavaraddi
Department of Orthodontics and Dentofacial Orthopaedics, SDM College of Dental Sciences and Hospital, SDM University, Dharwad, Karnataka, India

*Address all correspondence to: sagarbhat1994@yahoo.co.in

References

[1] Nagarajan D, Usha K, Rao GU, Vijjayakanth M, Jayanthy M, Sabarigirinathan C, Sriramaprabu G, Vinayagavel K, Amit K. Biomarkers in Orthodontics. Int J Oral Health Med Res 2015;2(3):88-90.

[2] Karacay S, Saygun I, Bengi AO, Serdar M. Tumor Necrosis Factor–α Levels during Two Different Canine Distalization Techniques. Angle Orthod. 2007 Jan;77(1):142-147.

[3] Jasim H, Carlsson A, Hedenberg-Magnusson B, Ghafouri B, Ernberg M. Saliva as a medium to detect and measure biomarkers related to pain. Scientific reports. 2018 Feb 19;8(1):3220.

[4] Taba M, Kinney J, Kim AS, Giannobile WV. Diagnostic biomarkers for oral and periodontal diseases. Dental Clinics. 2005 Jul 1;49(3):551-571.

[5] Alhadlaq AM, Patil S. Biomarkers of orthodontic tooth movement in gingival crevicular fluid: a systematic review. J Contemp Dent Pract. 2015 Jul 1;16(7):578-587.

[6] Yamaguchi M. RANK/RANKL/OPG during orthodontic tooth movement. Orthodontics & craniofacial research. 2009 May;12(2):113-119.

[7] Delima AJ, Van Dyke TE. Origin and function of the cellular components in gingival crevice fluid. Periodontology 2000. 2003 Feb;31(1):55-76.

[8] Cimasoni G. Method of collection. Crevicular fluid updated. 1983 Basel.

[9] Kowashi Y, Jaccard F, Cimasoni G. Sulcular polymorphonuclear leucocytes and gingival exudate during experimental gingivitis in man. Journal of periodontal research. 1980 Apr;15(2):151-158.

[10] Meikle MC. The tissue, cellular, and molecular regulation of orthodontic tooth movement: 100 years after Carl Sandstedt. Eur J Orthod. 2006 Jun 1;28(3):221-240.

[11] Ren Y, Hazemeijer H, de Haan B, Qu N, de Vos P. Cytokine profiles in crevicular fluid during orthodontic tooth movement of short and long durations. J Perio. 2007 Mar 1;78(3):453-458.

[12] Ren Y, Maltha JC, Van' t Hof MA, Von den Hoff JW, Kuijpers-Jagtman AM, Zhang D. Cytokine levels in crevicular fluid are less responsive to orthodontic force in adults than in juveniles. Journal of clinical periodontology. 2002 Aug;29(8):757-762.

[13] Cowen R, Stasiowska MK, Laycock H, Bantel C. Assessing pain objectively: the use of physiological markers. Anaesthesia. 2015 Jul;70(7): 828-847.

[14] Fleming PS, Dibiase AT, Sarri G, Lee RT. Pain experience during initial alignment with a self-ligating and a conventional fixed orthodontic appliance system: a randomized controlled clinical trial. Angle Orthod. 2009 Jan;79(1): 46-50.

[15] Hawker GA, Mian S, Kendzerska T, French M. Measures of adult pain: Visual Analog Scale for Pain (VAS Pain), Numeric Rating Scale for Pain (NRS Pain), McGill Pain Questionnaire (MPQ), Short-Form McGill Pain Questionnaire (SF-MPQ), Chronic Pain Grade Scale (CPGS), Short Form-36 Bodily Pain Scale (SF-36 BPS), and Measure of Intermittent and Constant

Osteoarthritis Pain (ICOAP). Arthritis Care & Research. 2011;63(S11): S240-S252.

[16] Jang, M.-U., Park, J.-W., Kho, H.-S., Chung, S.-C., & Chung, J.-W. (2010). Plasma and saliva levels of nerve growth factor and neuropeptides in chronic migraine patients. Oral Diseases, 17(2), 187-193.

[17] Zidverc-Trajkovic J, Stanimirovic D, Obrenovic R, Tajti J, Vécsei L, Gardi J, Németh J, Mijajlovic M, Sternic N, Jankovic L. Calcitonin gene-related peptide levels in saliva of patients with burning mouth syndrome. J Oral Path Med. 2009 Jan;38(1):29-33.

[18] Mandel AL, Ozdener H, Utermohlen V. Identification of pro-and mature brain-derived neurotrophic factor in human saliva. Arch Oral Bio. 2009 Jul 1;54(7):689-695.

[19] Scheurer PA, Firestone AR, Bürgin WB. Perception of pain as a result of orthodontic treatment with fixed appliances. Eur J Orthod. 1996 Jan 1;18(1):349-357.

[20] Krishnan V, Davidovitch Z. On a path to unfolding the biological mechanisms of orthodontic tooth movement. J Dent Res. 2009 Jul;88(7):597-608.

[21] Wahab RA, Kasim NA, Senafi S, Jemain AA, Abidin IZ, Shahidan MA, Ariffin SH. Enzyme activity profiles and ELISA analysis of biomarkers from human saliva and gingival crevicular fluid during orthodontic tooth movement using self-ligating brackets. Oral health Dent. Manage.2014;13: 194-199.

[22] Maltha JC, Van Leeuwen EJ, Dijkman GE, Kuijpers-Jagtman AM. Incidence and severity of root resorption in orthodontically moved premolars in dogs. Orthodontics & craniofacial research. 2004 May;7(2):115-121.

[23] Krishnan V, Davidovitch ZE. Cellular, molecular, and tissue-level reactions to orthodontic force. Am J Orthod Dentofacial Orthop. 2006 Apr 1;129(4):469-4e1.

[24] Perinetti G, Paolantonio M, D'Attilio M, D'Archivio D, Tripodi D, Femminella B, Festa F, Spoto G. Alkaline phosphatase activity in gingival crevicular fluid during human orthodontic tooth movement. Am J Orthod Dentofacial Orthop. 2002 Nov 1;122(5):548-556.

[25] Burstone CJ. The biomechanics of tooth movement. Vistas in orthodontics. 1962:197-213.

[26] Dolce C, Malone JS, Wheeler TT. Current concepts in the biology of orthodontic tooth movement. Semin Orthod2002 Mar 1 (Vol. 8, No. 1, pp. 6-12). WB Saunders.

[27] Pilon JJ, Kuijpers-Jagtman AM, Maltha JC. Magnitude of orthodontic forces and rate of bodily tooth movement. An experimental study. Am J Orthod Dentofacial Orthop. 1996 Jul 1;110(1):16-23.

[28] Van Leeuwen EJ, Maltha JC, Kuijpers-Jagtman AM. Tooth movement with light continuous and discontinuous forces in beagle dogs. Eur J Oral Sci. 1999 Dec;107(6):468-474.

[29] Zainal Ariffin SH, Yamamoto Z, Abidin Z, Megat Abdul Wahab R, Zainal Ariffin Z. Cellular and molecular changes in orthodontic tooth movement. Sci World J. 2011;11:1788-1803.

[30] Kaufman E, Lamster IB. The diagnostic applications of saliva—a review. Critical Reviews in oral biology & medicine. 2002 Mar;13(2):197-212.

[31] Navazesh M. Methods for collecting saliva. Annals of the New York Academy of Sciences. 1993 Sep;694(1):72-77.

[32] Streckfus CF, Storthz KA, Bigler L, Dubinsky WP. A comparison of the proteomic expression in pooled saliva specimens from individuals diagnosed with ductal carcinoma of the breast with and without lymph node involvement. Journal of oncology. 2009;

[33] Ellias MF, Zainal Ariffin SH, Karsani SA, Abdul Rahman M, Senafi S, Megat Abdul Wahab R. Proteomic analysis of saliva identifies potential biomarkers for orthodontic tooth movement. Sci World J. 2012;2012.

[34] Grieve III WG, Johnson GK, Moore RN, Reinhardt RA, DuBois LM. Prostaglandin E (PGE) and interleukin-1β (IL-1β) levels in gingival crevicular fluid during human orthodontic tooth movement. Am J Orthod Dentofacial Orthop. 1994 Apr 1;105(4):369-374.

[35] Uematsu S, Mogi M, Deguchi T. Interleukin (IL)-1β, IL-6, tumor necrosis factor-α, epidermal growth factor, and β2-microglobulin levels are elevated in gingival crevicular fluid during human orthodontic tooth movement. J Dent Res. 1996 Jan;75(1):562-567.

[36] Waddington RJ, Embery G. Proteoglycans and orthodontic tooth movement. J Orthod. 2001 Dec;28(4):281-290.

[37] Perinetti G, Varvara G, Salini L, Tetè S. Alkaline phosphatase activity in dental pulp of orthodontically treated teeth. Am J Orthod Dentofacial Orthop. 2005 Oct 1;128(4):492-496.

[38] Shibutani T, Murahashi Y, Tsukada E, Iwayama Y, Heersche JN. Experimentally induced periodontitis in beagle dogs causes rapid increases in osteoclastic resorption of alveolar bone. J Perio. 1997 Apr 1;68(4):385-391.

[39] Serra E, Perinetti G, D'Attilio M, Cordella C, Paolantonio M, Festa F, Spoto G. Lactate dehydrogenase activity in gingival crevicular fluid during orthodontic treatment. Am J Orthod Dentofacial Orthop. 2003 Aug 1; 124(2):206-211.

[40] Rohaya MA, Hisham ZS, Khazlina K. Preliminary study of aspartate aminotransferase activity in gingival crevicular fluids during orthodontic tooth movement. J Applied Sci. 2009;9(7):1393-1396.

[41] Ariffin SH, faiz ellias M, Wahab RM, Bakar Y, Senafi S. Profil aktiviti laktat dehidrogenase, asid fosfatase rintang tartarat dan alkalin fosfatase pada air liur semasa rawatan ortodontik. Sains Malaysiana. 2010 Jun;39(3):405-412.

[42] Zhang J, Zhou S, Zheng H, Zhou Y, Chen F, Lin J. Magnetic bead-based salivary peptidome profiling analysis during orthodontic treatment durations. Biochemical and biophysical research communications. 2012 May 18;421(4):844-849.

[43] Zelles T, Purushotham KR, Macauley SP, Oxford GE, Humphreys-Beher MG. Concise review: saliva and growth factors: the fountain of youth resides in us all. J Dent Res. 1995 Dec;74(12):1826-1832.

[44] Shugars DC, Wahl SM. The role of the oral environment in HIV-1 transmission. J Am Dent Asso. 1998 Jul 1;129(7):851-858.

[45] Mandel ID. The functions of saliva. J Dent Res. 1987 Feb;66(1_suppl):623-7.

[46] FDI Working Group 10, Core (1992). Saliva: its role in health and disease. Int Dent J 42:287-304.

[47] Fox PC. Saliva composition and its importance in dental health. Compendium (Newtown, Pa.). Supplement. 1989(13):S457.

[48] Mandel ID, Wotman S. The salivary secretions in health and disease. Oral sciences reviews. 1976(8):25-47.

[49] Sreebny LM (1989). Salivary flow in health and disease. Compend Suppl 13:461-469.

[50] Mandel ID. Salivary diagnosis: more than a lick and a promise. Journal of the American Dental Association (1939). 1993 Jan;124(1):85-7.

[51] Navazesh M. Methods for collecting saliva. Annals of the New York Academy of Sciences. 1993 Sep;694(1):72-77.

[52] Baum BJ. Principles of saliva secretion. Annals of the New York Academy of Sciences. 1993 Sep;694(1): 17-23.

[53] Young JA, Van Lennep EW. 1978. The process of secretion of organic products.

[54] Castle D. Cell biology of salivary protein secretion. In: Dobrosielski-Vergona K, editor. Biology of the salivary glands. Boca Raton, FL: CRC Press Inc.; 1993. pp. 81-104

[55] Turner RJ. Mechanisms of fluid secretion by salivary glands. Annals of the New York Academy of Sciences. 1993 Sep;694(1):24-35.

[56] Turner RJ, Paulais M, Manganel M, Lee III S, Moran A, Melvin JE. Ion and water transport mechanisms in salivary glands. Critical Reviews in Oral Biology & Medicine. 1993 Apr;4(3):385-391.

[57] Baum BJ. Principles of saliva secretion. Annals of the New York Academy of Sciences. 1993 Sep;694(1):17-23.

[58] Ambudkar IS. Regulation of calcium in salivary gland secretion. Critical Reviews in Oral Biology & Medicine. 2000 Jan;11(1):4-25.

[59] Bailey B, Klein J, Koren G. Noninvasive methods for drug measurement in pediatrics. Pediatric Clinics of North America. 1997 Feb 1;44(1):15-26.

[60] Olteanu C, Muresan A, Daicoviciu D, Tarmure V, Olteanu I, Keularts IM. Variations of some saliva markers of the oxidative stress in patients with orthodontic appliances. Fiziologia-Physiology. 2009 Sep 1;19(3).

[61] Sreebny LM, Schwartz SS. A reference guide to drugs and dry mouth–2nd edition. Gerodontology. 1997 Jul;14(1):33-47.

[62] Fox PC. Acquired salivary dysfunction: drugs and radiation. Annals of the New York Academy of Sciences. 1998 Apr;842(1):132-137.

[63] Chauncey HH (1961). Salivary enzymes. J Am Dent Assoc 63:361-369.

[64] Fleissig Y, Deutsch O, Reichenberg E, Redlich M, Zaks B, Palmon A, Aframian DJ. Different proteomic protein patterns in saliva of Sjögren's syndrome patients. Oral diseases. 2009 Jan;15(1):61-68.

[65] Vitorino R, Lobo MJ, Ferrer-Correira AJ, Dubin JR, Tomer KB, Domingues PM, Amado FM. Identification of human whole saliva protein components using proteomics. Proteomics. 2004 Apr;4(4):1109-1115.

[66] Zreiqat H, Howlett CR, Gronthos S, Hume D, Geczy CL. S100A8/S100A9 and their association with cartilage and bone. J Mol Histo. 2007 Oct 1;38(5):381-391.

[67] Van Lent PL, Grevers L, Blom AB, Sloetjes A, Mort JS, Vogl T, Nacken W, Van Den Berg WB, Roth J. Myeloid-related proteins S100A8/S100A9 regulate joint inflammation and cartilage destruction during antigen-induced arthritis. Annals of the rheumatic diseases. 2008 Dec 1;67(12):1750-1758.

[68] Udby L, Sørensen OE, Pass J, Johnsen AH, Behrendt N, Borregaard N, Kjeldsen L. Cysteine-rich secretory protein 3 is a ligand of α1B-glycoprotein in human plasma. Biochemistry. 2004 Oct 12;43(40):12877-12886.

[69] Kosari F, Asmann YW, Cheville JC, Vasmatzis G. Cysteine-rich secretory protein-3: a potential biomarker for prostate cancer. Cancer Epidemiology and Prevention Biomarkers. 2002 Nov 1;11(11):1419-1426.

[70] Gonçalves LD, Soares MR, Nogueira FC, Garcia C, Camisasca DR, Domont G, Feitosa AC, de Abreu Pereira D, Zingali RB, Alves G. Comparative proteomic analysis of whole saliva from chronic periodontitis patients. Journal of proteomics. 2010 May 7;73(7):1334-1341.

[71] Ianzer D, Konno K, Xavier CH, Stöcklin R, Santos RA, de Camargo AC, Pimenta DC. Hemorphin and hemorphin-like peptides isolated from dog pancreas and sheep brain are able to potentiate bradykinin activity in vivo. Peptides. 2006 Nov 1;27(11):2957-2966.

[72] Lu J, Stewart AJ, Sadler PJ, Pinheiro TJ, Blindauer CA. Albumin as a zinc carrier: properties of its high-affinity zinc-binding site. 2008: 1317-1321.

[73] Suárez-Bonnet A, de las Mulas JM, Herráez P, Rodríguez F, de los Monteros AE. Immunohistochemical localisation of 14-3-3 σ protein in normal canine tissues. The Veterinary Journal. 2010 Aug 1;185(2):218-221.

[74] Buczko P, Zalewska A, Szarmach I. Saliva and oxidative stress in oral cavity and in some systemic disorders. J Physiol Pharmacol. 2015 Feb;66:1-7.

[75] Atuğ Özcan SS, Ceylan I, Özcan E, Kurt N, Dağsuyu İM, Canakci CF. Evaluation of oxidative stress biomarkers in patients with fixed orthodontic appliances. Disease markers. 2014;2014.

[76] Szarmach IJ, Buczko P, Tankiewicz-Kwedlo A, Kasacka I, Tankiewicz J, Pawlak D. The concentration of kynurenine and anthranilic acid in saliva of patients with fixed orthodontic appliances. Pol J Environ Stud. 2007;16:125-127.

[77] Roberts WE, Huja S, Roberts JA. Bone modeling: biomechanics, molecular mechanisms, and clinical perspectives. Semin Orthod2004 Jun 1 (Vol. 10, No. 2, pp. 123-161). WB Saunders.

[78] Yamashiro T, Fukunaga T, Kabuto H, Ogawa N, Takano-Yamamoto T. Activation of the bulbospinal serotonergic system during experimental tooth movement in the rat. J Dent Res. 2001 Sep;80(9):1854-1857.

[79] Hattori Y, Watanabe M, Iwabe T, Tanaka E, Nishi M, Aoyama J, Satoda T, Uchida T, Tanne K. Administration of MK-801 decreases c-Fos expression in the trigeminal sensory nuclear complex but increases it in the midbrain during experimental movement of rat molars. Brain research. 2004 Sep 24;1021(2): 183-191.

[80] Gaur A, Maheshwari S, Verma SK. Detection of molecular biomarkers as a

diagnostic tool in the planning and progression of orthodontic treatment. J Orofacial Sci. 2017 Jul 1;9(2):80.

[81] Ferguson DB. Oral bioscience. Churchill livingstone: China; 1999

[82] Sugiyama Y, Yamaguchi M, Kanekawa M, Yoshii M, Nozoe T, Nogimura A, Kasai K. The level of cathepsin B in gingival crevicular fluid during human orthodontic tooth movement. Eur J Orthod. 2003 Feb 1;25(1):71-76.

[83] Waddington RJ, Embery G. Proteoglycans and orthodontic tooth movement. J Orthod. 2001 Dec;28(4): 281-290.

[84] Last KS, Stanbury JB, Embery G. Glycosaminoglycans in human gingival crevicular fluid as indicators of active periodontal disease. Arch Oral Bio. 1985 Jan 1;30(3):275-281.

[85] Uematsu S, Mogi M, Deguchi T. Interleukin (IL)-1β, IL-6, tumor necrosis factor-α, epidermal growth factor, and β2-microglobulin levels are elevated in gingival crevicular fluid during human orthodontic tooth movement. J Dent Res. 1996 Jan;75(1):562-567.

[86] Uematsu S, Mogi M, Deguchi T. Increase of transforming growth factor-β1 in gingival crevicular fluid during human orthodontic tooth movement. Arch Oral Bio. 1996 Nov 1;41(11):1091-1095.

[87] Lee KJ, Park YC, Yu HS, Choi SH, Yoo YJ. Effects of continuous and interrupted orthodontic force on interleukin-1β and prostaglandin E2 production in gingival crevicular fluid. Am J Orthod Dentofacial Orthop. 2004 Feb 1;125(2):168-177.

[88] Grieve WG III, Johnson GK, Moore RN, Reinhardt RA, Dubois LM. Prostaglandin E (PGE) and interleukin-1 beta (IL-1beta) levels in gingival crevicular fluid during human orthodontic tooth movement. Am J Orthod Dentofacial Orthop 1994;105: 369-374.

[89] Lowney JJ, Norton LA, Shafer DM, Rossomando EF. Orthodontic forces increase tumor necrosis factor α in the human gingival sulcus. Am J Orthod Dentofacial Orthop. 1995 Nov 1;108(5):519-524.

[90] Griffiths GS, Moulson AM, Petrie A, James IT. Evaluation of osteocalcin and pyridinium crosslinks of bone collagen as markers of bone turnover in gingival crevicular fluid during different stages of orthodontic treatment. J clinical perio. 1998 Jun;25(6):492-498.

[91] Insoft M, King GJ, Keeling SD. The measurement of acid and alkaline phosphatase in gingival crevicular fluid during orthodontic tooth movement. Am J Orthod Dentofacial Orthop. 1996 Mar 1;109(3):287-296.

[92] Perinetti G, Paolantonio M, D'Attilio M, D'Archivio D, Dolci M, Femminella B, Festa F, Spoto G. Aspartate aminotransferase activity in gingival crevicular fluid during orthodontic treatment. A controlled short-term longitudinal study. J Perio. 2003 Feb 1;74(2):145-152.

[93] Serra E, Perinetti G, D'Attilio M, Cordella C, Paolantonio M, Festa F, Spoto G. Lactate dehydrogenase activity in gingival crevicular fluid during orthodontic treatment. Am J Orthod Dentofacial Orthop. 2003 Aug 1;124(2):206-211.

[94] Apajalahti S, Sorsa T, Railavo S, Ingman T. The in vivo levels of matrix metalloproteinase-1 and-8 in gingival crevicular fluid during initial

orthodontic tooth movement. J Dent Res. 2003 Dec;82(12):1018-1022.

[95] Allgayer S, Macedo de Menezes L, Rinaldi L, Roennau M. Cytokines in crevicular fluid and orthodontic force: a systematic review. Revista Odonto Ciência. 2017 Jun 1;32(2).

[96] Redlich M, Rahamim E, Gaft A, Shoshan S. The response of supraalveolar gingival collagen to orthodontic rotation movement in dogs. Am J Orthod Dentofacial Orthop. 1996 Sep 1; 110(3):247-255.

[97] Alhashimi N, Frithiof L, Brudvik P, Bakhiet M. Orthodontic tooth movement and de novo synthesis of proinflammatory cytokines. Am J Orthod Dentofacial Orthop. 2001 Mar 1;119(3):307-312.

[98] Redlich M, Reichenberg E, Harari D, Zaks B, Shoshan S, Palmon A. The effect of mechanical force on mRNA levels of collagenase, collagen type I, and tissue inhibitors of metalloproteinases in gingivae of dogs. J Dent Res. 2001 Dec;80(12):2080-2084.

[99] Capelli Junior J, Kantarci A, Haffajee A, Teles RP, Fidel Jr R, Figueredo CM. Matrix metalloproteinases and chemokines in the gingival crevicular fluid during orthodontic tooth movement. Eur J Orthod. 2011 Mar 9;33(6):705-711.

Chapter 2

Orthodontics and the Periodontium: A Symbiotic Relationship

Betsy Sara Thomas and Mohan Alexander

Abstract

The force applied by the orthodontist to facilitate the orderly movement of teeth to their new position may have deleterious effects on the most important structure involved in the procedure—the periodontium. This chapter endeavors to provide an overview of the biological processes that play a role in achieving the patient's as well as the orthodontist's objective.

Keywords: accelerated tooth movement, inflammation, periodontal ligament, alveolar bone, cytokines

1. Introduction

The art and science of orthodontics have certainly come a long way from the era of treatment using removable appliances, which mainly produced tipping movements of the teeth, to the fixed appliances that bring about bodily movements of the teeth to their desired destination. But this has not been a journey without hiccups. The quest for the perfect smile or the ideal occlusion has been marred by quite a few stories of botched-up cases, which, sometimes, could be the result of unscientific methods being utilized to achieve the promised results. But it also seems to be a story of due respect not being accorded to the most important structure in the treatment process—the periodontium. This chapter discusses the relationship that the periodontium (*and the periodontist*) shares with the specialty of orthodontics, one which, at times, tends to be taken for granted.

2. Theories of tooth movement

The force applied to the teeth during orthodontic treatment results in remodeling of the alveolar bone. The exact mechanism of how this force is converted to biological activity has not been elicited till now. Various theories try to explain this phenomenon:

1. Bone-bending/biological electrical

2. Pressure-tension

3. Neurogenic inflammation

4. Fluid-flow sheer stress

Whatever be the mechanism, it seems obvious that it is the periodontium that plays a big role in achieving the treatment goals.

3. The periodontium

The periodontium has two main functions: protection and attachment. The former function is carried out by the gingiva and the latter by its three remaining parts, namely the cementum, periodontal ligaments, and the alveolar bone. It is only the gingiva that is visible in the oral cavity, the rest being covered and protected by it.

3.1 Gingiva

The primary function of the gingiva is protection, as stated earlier. Orthodontic treatment tends to be associated with gingivitis in many patients. As the presence of plaque is one of the main factors in the development of gingivitis, it could be the interference of the orthodontic brackets and elastics with effective removal of dental plaque, which might be resulting in gingivitis. However, it has been shown that because of orthodontic treatment a shift in the composition and type of bacteria can occur [1]. According to J. van Gastel, et al. [2], fixed orthodontic treatment may result in localized gingivitis, which rarely progresses to periodontitis. E. Bimstein and A. Becker [3] state that, following placement of a fixed appliance, a small amount of gingival inflammation will be visible, which could be transient in nature and does not lead to attachment loss, in the majority of the patients.

Gingival recession is considered to be one of the more common complications of orthodontic tooth movement (OTM). But in a study conducted among 205 orthodontic patients, Morris JW, et al. [4] found that "orthodontic treatment is not a major risk factor for the development of gingival recession." They further state that "although greater amounts of maxillary expansion during treatment increase the risks of post-treatment recession, the effects are minimal."

3.2 Cementum

Any treatment procedure that a human being undergoes, whether surgical or medical, can have side effects or risks involved, and orthodontic treatment is no exception. Similar to other medical procedures, the aim in orthodontics is also to minimize the risks involved in the maximum number of patients possible.

Microscopic resorption of the cementum of erupted as well as unerupted teeth is a common phenomenon. This occurs without involving the underlying dentin in the majority of cases. The resorption may be caused by local or systemic factors or can be idiopathic. Trauma from occlusion, malaligned erupting teeth, periapical as well as periodontal infections, replanted or transplanted teeth, orthodontic movement, etc. are the local factors that may result in cementum resorption. According to some authors [5–7], root resorption is the most common side effect of orthodontic treatment and occurs within 6 months of commencement of the treatment. Anja Pejicic, et al. [8] have described three degrees of severity of orthodontically induced root resorption (OIRR): the first degree wherein there is only surface resorption of the cementum which will regenerate or remodel fully. The second degree shows deep resorption with cementum and outer dentin layers involved and this is usually repaired with cementum. In this, the original shape of the root may or may not be achieved following the repair. In their third degree, there is full resorption of the apical hard tissues evidenced by shortening of the root.

Biologic as well as mechanical factors have been highlighted as probable causes of OIRR, with tooth root morphology, abnormal root shape, previous history of trauma or root resorption, genetic and systemic factors, endodontic treatment, habits and oral health, etc. likely to be the biologic factors. Mechanical factors could be the amount of apical displacement, the magnitude of force applied, duration of treatment, whether it is continuous or intermittent force, type, extent and direction of tooth movement, etc., according to Anja Pejicic, et al. There are studies [9–12] that suggest that it is the trauma due to over-compression of the periodontal ligament that causes OIRR. It seems to be an accepted fact that orthodontic movements are not entirely translatory due to mechanical laws. This results in the concentration of orthodontic forces at the apical region. During OTM, hyalinization does occur because it is virtually impossible to prevent the occlusion of blood vessels totally. Because of this, root resorption might begin at the hyalinized region of the necrotic periodontal ligament. As hyalinized necrotic tissue develops in almost 100% of patients during orthodontic treatment, some authors believe that root resorption occurs in almost every orthodontic patient [13, 14]. It is believed that the aggressiveness of the resorbing cells, the vulnerability and sensitivity of the tissues involved and individual variation and susceptibility will decide the extent of resorption [8].

The use of light orthodontic force has been shown to minimize the extent of root resorption, especially with horizontal and vertical displacement. This could be because the apical third of the root is covered with cellular cementum, whereas the coronal third is covered with acellular cementum. Because of the increased proliferation activity, cells of the cellular cementum might be easily damaged, whereas the slowly dividing cells of the acellular cementum might be more resistant to those forces [15–17].

Nitric oxide (NO), the intra- and the intercellular signal molecule, is synthesized by the activity of neuronal, endothelial, and inducible isoforms of NO synthases (NOSs). The primary sensor of NO is soluble guanylate cyclase (sGC). It plays a very important part in many physiological as well as pathological processes and conditions and also in NO signaling. The enzymatic activity of sGC is boosted when NO binds to it. In inflammation, sGC is oxidized and becomes insensitive to NO. Inflammation of the periodontium induces the resorption of cementum by cementoclasts and the resorption of the alveolar bone by osteoclasts. Korkmaz Y, et al. think that if medication can be used to activate sGC in periodontal tissues of patients suffering from periodontitis in nitric oxide and heme-independent manner, it could result in a novel treatment to stop cementum resorption for such patients. They reached this conclusion after studying the α1- and β1-subunits of sGC in cementoclasts of healthy and inflamed human periodontium using double immunostaining for CD68 and cathepsin K. They compared this with those of osteoclasts from the same sections and noticed that under inflammatory conditions, cementoclasts showed a decreased staining intensity for both the subunits [18].

Yufei Xie, Ning Zhao, and Gang Shen [19] investigated the anti-resorptive mechanisms of cementocytes during orthodontic tooth movement. They concluded that under fluid-flow sheer stress, cementocytes stimulate the differentiation of osteoblasts and inhibit the activation of osteoclasts, showing greater potential for bone protection than alveolar bone osteocytes. And according to them, "cementocytes might play an important role in preventing one of the most common complications of orthodontic treatment – root resorption."

According to Alberto Consolaro [20], teeth with OIRR do not need:

1. restraints, as they do not become mobile or painful. If either of these symptoms is present, he suggests that other etiological factors like recently removed orthodontic braces, trauma from occlusion, bruxism, cervical bone loss, bone loss due to periodontitis, etc. should be looked for.

2. endodontic treatment as the dental pulp does not undergo ischemia, infarction, or necrosis during the orthodontic movements.

3. replacement with dental implants, as the cervical third of the root is responsible for 60% of periodontal support.

3.3 The alveolar bone

The alveolar bone is a mineralized connective tissue and is made up of around 67% inorganic material by weight. The inorganic content is primarily calcium and phosphate, with the mineral content being typically in the form of hydroxyapatite crystals. Around 20% of the alveolar bone consists of organic material, containing both collagen and non-collagenous materials. Water constitutes the rest of the weight of the alveolar bone- ~ 15% [21]. The inner wall of the tooth socket, known as the alveolar bone proper, contains many openings through which the periodontal ligament connects with the neurovascular bundles of the cancellous bone. The interdental bone or septum is made up of cancellous supporting bone within cortical walls.

Adjacent to the PDL space is a plate of compact bone called the lamina dura, whereas the majority of alveolar bone is trabecular in nature. The alveolar bone contains many different types of cells such as adipocytes, endothelial cells, macrophages, osteoclasts, osteoblasts and osteocytes. But the crucial detail of maintaining the function as well as homeostasis of the alveolar bone is carried out by the last three types of cells. There are some differences between the osteoblasts which form bone, and the osteoclasts, which resorb bone. The former (and the osteocytes) descend from mesenchymal cells, whereas the latter originates from the monocyte or hematopoietic cells. At the same time, the osteoclasts are formed by the fusion of multiple monocytes and thus are multinucleated while the osteoblasts are mononucleated. Type I collagen, which is the most abundant protein in vertebrates, can be made by both fibroblasts and osteoblasts and it is this collagen that forms the structural and mechanical matrix of the alveolar bone. The osteoblasts contain the master switch Runx2, which helps in the differentiation of osteoblasts from the progenitor mesenchymal cells [21]. As age advances, there is a disproportion between bone deposition and resorption and this is because the number of osteoblasts decreases as we age [22]. While apposition of bone is taking place, osteoblasts get enclosed in the mineralized bone and these cells are known as the osteocytes. A lacuna can form around such an osteocyte by deposition of minerals such as calcium carbonate, hydroxyapatite and calcium phosphate, during bone formation. The lacunae connect with each other through canaliculi, which are narrow channels through which the dendrites of osteocytes correspond using gap junctions. The bone-resorbing osteoclasts express various substances such as osteoprotegerin (OPG), chloride channel 7 (ClCN7), cathepsin K, and tartrate-resistant acid phosphatase (TRAP). Bone matrix proteins such as elastin, collagen, and gelatin are catabolized by the protease cathepsin K, whereas ClCN7 maintains osteoclast neutrality by shuffling chloride ions through the cell membrane. OPG, though a member of the TNF receptor family, is secreted and acts as a cytokine.

Among all the periodontal tissues, alveolar bone is the least stable because it is in a constant state of flux. Local factors that cause internal remodeling include age-related changes as well as functional requirements on the tooth. Mechanical strains caused by orthodontic movements are thought to be resulting in physiologic bone adaptation together with minor injuries to the periodontium, which are reversible [23]. The pressure-tension theory of tooth movement proposes that a tooth moves in the periodontal space by creating a pressure and tension side. According to this theory, the tooth shifts its position within the periodontal ligament (PDL) space, resulting in PDL compression in some areas and PDL tension in others within a few seconds of force loading and this is brought about by chemical, rather than electric, signals as the stimulus for cellular differentiation and ultimately tooth movement. Bone resorption occurs at the compression side and bone formation at the tension side, with blood flow being decreased on the compression side and is maintained or increased on the tension side. Within minutes of force being applied, the alteration in blood flow changes the oxygen tension and the chemical environment by releasing biologically active agents such as prostaglandins and cytokines [24]. This happens especially if there is sustained force. This alteration results in less oxygen levels on the pressure side due to compression of the periodontal ligament and vice versa. It has been observed that low oxygen tension causes decreased adenosine triphosphate (ATP) activity [25]. These changes act on cellular differentiation and activity, bringing about bone resorption at the compression side and bone formation at the tension side. Schwarz (1932) correlated the tissue response to the magnitude of force, with capillary blood pressure. If the force exceeds the pressure of ~20–25 g/cm^2 of the root surface, tissue necrosis can occur due to the strangulated periodontium [26]. It has been shown that with the application of heavy force, blood flow tends to be cut off resulting in cell death under compression. According to Al Ansari et al., these cell deaths also include some osteocytes and osteoblasts in the adjacent alveolar bone. This causes acute inflammatory response with the release of chemokines that could attract other inflammatory and precursor cells into the extravascular space from the blood vessels. According to Taddei et al., during orthodontic movement, the chemokines known as monocyte chemo-attractant protein-1 (MCP-1) is released attracting the monocytes. These monocytes become either macrophages or osteoclasts once they exit the bloodstream and enter into the tissue. The release of other inflammatory mediators is also seen within the first few hours of tooth movement.

If the cessation of blood flow occurs because of heavy orthodontic force being applied, a delayed differentiation or recruitment of osteoclasts from adjacent bone marrow space also may occur resulting in "undermining resorption" that removes the lamina dura next to the compressed PDL. This is because no osteoclast differentiation occurs within the compressed PDL space. Under such a condition, tooth movement will take place only after this "undermining resorption" is completed, meaning only after a week or two. This also explains why tooth movement occurs within 2 to 3 days when light force is applied, because the light force will only reduce the blood flow permitting the quick recruitment of osteoclasts either from within the periodontal ligament space or from blood. This will result in the removal of the lamina dura by the process of "frontal resorption." At the same time, it is a fact that tooth movement is a result of a combination of "undermining" as well as "frontal" resorption. This is because some degree of hyalinization almost always occurs as it is virtually impossible to clinically prevent the occlusion of blood vessels completely [24].

3.4 The periodontal ligament

Yes, the force applied by the orthodontic appliance provides the impetus for the tooth to move. But without the PDL it would be impossible for the teeth to move through the bone and reach their intended destination, in an orderly manner. The PDL, like all ligaments in the body, connects the hard tissue structures, either the cementum of adjacent teeth to each other or the cementum of the tooth to the alveolar bone.

The PDL also connects with the neurovascular bundles of the cancellous bone through the alveolar bone proper *via* the numerous openings. The PDL is a dense fibrous connective tissue structure that consists of collagenous fiber bundles, cells, vascular and neural elements, and interstitial fluid. Its primary function is to support the teeth in their sockets and at the same time allow them to withstand considerable masticatory forces. The average width of the PDL space is around 0.2 mm, with the space decreasing as age advances. The space is occupied mostly by Type 1 collagen bundles and is the thinnest near the middle third of the root. These collagen fibers are mainly divided into principal, accessory, and elastic fibers. Sharpey's fibers are the term used for the terminal portion of these fibers that insert in the alveolar bone and cementum. The principal fibers can be subdivided into the transseptal fiber (or interdental ligament) and alveolodental ligament. Some authors consider the transeptal fibers as gingival fibers because they do not have an osseous attachment. These fibers connect the cementum of adjacent teeth, with their duty being maintaining the alignment of teeth, and the alveolodental ligament group of fibers helping teeth withstand compression forces during mastication. The accessory fibers prevent rotation of the tooth and run from the alveolar bone to cementum in different planes, in a tangential manner. Many cells occupy the PDL space, namely 1) synthetic cells like fibroblasts that make up to around 60% of the total PDL cell population, osteoblasts, and cementoblasts; 2) resorptive cells such as osteoclasts, cementoclasts; 3) progenitor cells including undifferentiated mesenchymal cells; 4) defense cells such as macrophages, mast cells, and lymphocytes; and 5) remnants of the epithelial root sheath of Hertwig, which are epithelial cells. The PDL space also contains interstitial fluid, which is contributed by the circulatory system [24]. This helps the PDL space to transmit the masticatory forces (which can range from 70 to 150 newtons) etc., onto teeth, thus acting as a shock absorber.

Some of the more frequent complications of orthodontic treatment are dehiscence or fenestration of the alveolar bone. These can result in root exposure, gingival recession, and relapse of the condition.

4. Inflammation and orthodontic tooth movement

As discussed earlier, tooth loading, physiologic or otherwise, causes areas of compression and tension on the soft tissues surrounding the teeth also—the PDL, nerves, blood vessels, etc. In the PDL, there is an intimate relationship of the nerve endings with the blood vessels. Neurotransmitters such as calcitonin gene-related peptide (CGRP) and substance P are released when the nerve endings get distorted and these cause vasodilation and increased permeability of the blood vessels resulting in plasma leakage [23, 26]. OTM is achieved by the remodeling of the PDL and alveolar bone. These remodeling activities and the movement of the teeth result in an aseptic inflammatory process with the consequent increase in mediators such as prostaglandins (PGs), interleukins (ILs. IL-6, IL-7 & IL-17), the tumor necrosis factor (TNF)-α superfamily, and the receptor activator of nuclear factor (RANK)/RANK ligand (RANKL)/osteoprotegerin (OPG).

Current scientific literature suggests that arachidonic acid (AA) pathway plays a very important role in many human diseases such as cardiovascular problems, carcinogenesis as well as inflammatory conditions such as asthma, arthritis. Periodontists have been exploring the role of AA in periodontitis for some time, it being an inflammatory condition. AA can be metabolized by three specific enzyme systems, that is, cyclooxygenases, lipoxygenases, and cytochrome P450 (CYP) enzymes. One of the derivatives of the AA cascade—the prostaglandins (PGs) are produced within seconds of cell injury. PGE2 is the most abundantly seen PG in various tissues and is known for its all-around physiologic and pathological actions. It increases vascular permeability and chemotactic actions by acting as a vasodilator and at the same time, it increases bone resorption and osteoclast formation. An increase in PGs levels in the PDL and alveolar bone has been reported by Ngan, et al. [27], during orthodontic treatment. PGE2 levels in the gingival crevicular fluid (GCF) increased during OTM, according to Shetty et al. [28]. Leiker et al. [29] demonstrated that exogenous prostaglandins enhanced the rate of OTM in rats. The administration of PGE or prostaglandin receptor EP4 also enhanced the rate of tooth movement [30, 31]. It has also been demonstrated that indomethacin, a specific inhibitor of prostaglandin synthesis, reduces the rate of OTM in rats [31, 32]. As mentioned earlier, the cytokines also increase during OTM. IL-β in particular is involved with inflammation and stimulates bone resorption. It has been reported that IL-1β is produced by both macrophages and neutrophils, and is increased in inflamed gingival tissues. IL-6 is a multifunctional cytokine produced by immune cells and induces osteoclastic bone resorption. IL-17 is an inflammatory cytokine that is produced by activated T cells and it has been reported that IL-17 induces osteoclastogenesis from monocytes.

RANK ligand (RANKL) and its receptor RANK are present on osteoblasts and precursor osteoclasts, respectively. They are considered to be the key factors that stimulate osteoclast formation and osteoclastogenesis. RANKL is required for osteoclast formation with macrophage-colony-stimulating factor (MCSF) from precursor monocyte/macrophages. Osteoprotegerin (OPG) inhibits RANK–RANKL interactions [24]. It binds to RANKL and prevents RANK–RANKL ligation. Therefore, OPG prevents osteoclast differentiation and activation. Kanzaki et al. demonstrated that compression forces upregulate RANKL expression through induction of COX-2 in human PDL cells *in vitro*. They also [33] demonstrated that the amount of rat experimental tooth movement is accelerated by the transfer of the RANKL gene to the periodontal tissue, while it is inhibited by OPG gene transfer. Additionally, compression force increases RANKL and decreases OPG secretion in human PDL cells *in vitro*. The GCF levels of RANKL are increased, and the levels of OPG are decreased in experimental canine movement. Therefore, it is suggested that the RANK–RANKL system is directly involved in the regulation of orthodontic tooth movement.

All these studies suggest that these and other inflammatory cytokines may be intricately entwined with one another during OTM, and may play important roles in bone remodeling. But studies on OIRR seem to suggest that these mediators might also be the cause for the most common complication in orthodontics-root resorption.

5. Accelerated orthodontic tooth movement

A systematic review of prospective studies on the duration of orthodontic treatment suggests that the duration of orthodontic treatment varies widely but takes less than 2 years to complete, on average [34]. Most patients would like their treatment to be done in a much shorter period and in addition, longer treatment periods might increase the chances of root resorption, decalcification, etc. This has resulted in orthodontists as well as manufacturers trying to shorten the duration by using various methods to accelerate OTM (AOTM). Some of the techniques advocated in this quest to accelerate OTM are as follows:

A. Those aimed at altering orthodontic mechanics

1. Limited orthodontic treatment.
2. Self-ligating and varying bracket designs
3. Customized appliances

B. Altering biological response to force

1. Medications such as corticosteroids, vitamin D3, parathyroid hormone, thyroxin, prostaglandins, platelet-rich plasma.
2. Micro-vibration
3. Low-intensity Laser
4. Photobiomodulation aka low-level light therapy
5. Electromagnetic fields
6. Direct electrical current

C. Surgical methods

1. Micro-osteoperforations
2. Piezocision
3. Corticotomies
4. Osteotomies/PDL distraction
5. Surgery first

Miles P [35] reviewed the studies involving the aforesaid techniques and was of the opinion that the technique of photobiomodulation may be of benefit but suggested that since there is limited evidence to support it, more studies will be needed before it can be applied routinely. With regard to the use of corticotomy, also he says that only low-level evidence is available and he concludes his review by suggesting that rigorous, well-designed randomized controlled trials with longer follow-up periods are necessary for all the techniques before they can be recommended.

The effects of most of the above AOTM procedures on the periodontium do not seem to have been studied in detail. The more commonly performed and studied one seems to be the corticotomies, *viz.*, the periodontally accelerated osteogenic orthodontics (PAOO).

5.1 Periodontally accelerated osteogenic orthodontics

In 2001, Wilcko, et al. [36] introduced the "periodontally accelerated osteogenic orthodontics" (PAOO) technique that they claimed shortened the duration of orthodontic treatment. This involved flap design, selective decortication, alveolar augmentation, membrane coverage, and closure using sutures. They radiographically assessed the presence of transient demineralization followed by remineralization at the corticotomy level. According to them, reversible osteopenia occurs both within the alveolar bone proper and on the surface and with this, the collagenous bony matrix also moves with the root in the same direction as the OTM. Once the OTM is completed and the teeth are retained in their predetermined position, remineralization of the matrix takes place. They claim that this demineralization-remineralization is complete in adolescents but not so much in adults and termed it the "regional acceleratory phenomenon" (RAP) of bone remodeling. They thought that this "bone matrix transportation" had made it possible to design a surgical approach, which permits extraction space closure in 3 to 4 weeks. The duration of RAP is claimed to last for 3–4 months by these authors and the amount of tooth movement during this period was double around 1 mm/month, in animal studies conducted by Iino S, et al. [37].

5.2 History of osteotomies/corticotomies to speed up tooth movement

The use of techniques to speed up orthodontic tooth movement by utilizing alveolar surgery has a history dating back to more than a century. But it is Heinrich Kole [38] who has been credited with refining the process. He proposed the idea of accelerating orthodontic movements by displacing bone blocks, more than 6 decades ago. He hypothesized that it was the cortical bone that slowed the orthodontic movement of teeth and so why not weaken it by osteotomizing it? He advocated buccal and lingual interdental corticotomies together with supra-apical horizontal osteotomies connecting the two vertical cuts. Though accelerated orthodontic movements were achieved, he encountered quite a few complications like the non-vitality of teeth. It should be noted that Kole achieved the tooth movements using removable appliances fitted with adjustable screws. Others tried to build on this technique with Duker in 1975 [39] sparing the crestal bone in his corticotomies and Suya [40] replacing the supra-apical osteotomy with a corticotomy in 1991.

According to T. Gellee, et al. [41], PAOO also allows larger tooth displacements, a reduction in the risk of root resorption, and a gain in stability after the removal of orthodontic devices.

6. Periodontal therapy and orthodontics

According to the American Association of Orthodontists, one in four orthodontic patients is an adult. Some studies suggest that almost 40% of the patients are adults. As more and more adult patients seek orthodontic treatment for various reasons, it can be challenging for the orthodontist to tailor his/her techniques to the specific patient. Many of these patients might have underlying periodontal problems that can affect the treatment process as well as its outcome. The periodontist can play an active role in ensuring the success of the orthodontic treatment—in adult patients or adolescents. This role can be before, during, or after the orthodontic treatment.

6.1 Pretreatment

A thorough periodontal examination/charting is of utmost importance for every orthodontic patient, especially if skeletal growth has been completed. This is to identify and manage active conditions such as gingivitis and periodontitis as well as conditions that result in deficiency of soft or hard tissues or both. In ideal conditions, and with good oral hygiene, gingival health can be maintained with as little as 1–2 mm of keratinized gingiva. But soft tissue grafting might be indicated under the following circumstances:

1. when the buccal displacement of the roots is planned during the treatment or when treatment might result in thinning of the gingiva.

2. chronically inflamed areas of keratinized gingiva or no area of keratinized gingiva where the alveolar mucosa prevents optimal plaque control.

3. minimal areas of attached gingiva compromised by a shallow vestibule or frenum pull.

4. advancing gingival recession.

The techniques that are available to correct these conditions include the following:

1. Laterally or coronally advanced pedicle grafts.

2. Coronally advanced flaps alone or in conjunction with barrier membranes or enamel matrix proteins.

3. Free gingival grafts.

4. Subepithelial connective tissue autografts.

5. Allografts.

Every patient should undergo professional plaque removal and root debridement before the start of the treatment. Oral hygiene instructions should be reinforced because it has been shown that orthodontic bands, elastics, etc., tend to retain plaque, resulting in gingivitis, which may then proceed to periodontitis. Orthodontically induced remodeling process may have a positive effect on bone, so extensive osseous surgery is usually not indicated at this time. But sometimes osseous surgery might be indicated in the following conditions:

1. **osseous craters**—these two-wall defects are mainly on the mesial and distal surfaces of the roots. If they are shallow craters (4–5 mm pocket depth), they might be left alone but more extensive ones might have to be treated.

2. **3-wall intra-bony defects**—these may be treated using bone grafts with or without membranes. Even though autografts are considered the gold standard for bone grafts, allografts also have been proven to give good results.

3. **Furcation defects**—this might be treated by open flap debridement followed by placement of the graft, etc., depending on the severity of the defect.

4. **Crown lengthening**—when the clinical crown is small, there might be a need to lengthen the crown utilizing gingivectomy procedures alone or in combination with osseous resection and apical repositioning of the gingiva.

The American Academy of Periodontology's systematic review on whether periodontal phenotype modification therapy (PhMT) involving hard tissue augmentation (PhMT-b) or soft tissue augmentation (PhMT-s) has clinical benefits for patients undergoing orthodontic treatment concluded that PhMT *via* corticotomy with particulate bone grafting (PhMT-b along with CAOT) may provide clinical benefits of augmenting periodontal phenotype, accelerating tooth movement, expanding the scope of incisor movement, and enhancing post-orthodontic stability of the mandibular anterior teeth. This study also says that the benefits of PhMT-s alone during orthodontic treatment remain undetermined because of the limited studies available [42].

6.2 During orthodontic treatment

The maintenance of oral hygiene during treatment is of paramount importance. During each visit reinforcement of oral hygiene instructions have to be carried out along with motivating the patient to do so. Periodontal evaluation every 6 months and radiographic examination once in a year would be ideal. Procedures like frenectomy might have to be carried out during the treatment period if the orthodontist feels that diastema closure, etc. are being hampered by an aberrant frenum.

6.3 Post-orthodontic phase

Regular periodontal charting should be carried out in patients who have completed their treatment. Depending on the case, circumferential supracrestal fiberotomy (CSF) may have to be carried out during the end part of the treatment or after the treatment is over. This is expected to release the tension on the supra-alveolar fibers following tooth de-rotation, thereby reducing the relapse risk. Reham Al-Jasser, et al. [43] in their study found that "post-treatment rotational relapse of anterior teeth subjected to CSF was minimal and statistically insignificant after 1 year of follow-up."

7. The periodontally compromised patient and orthodontics

Most orthodontists may be worried about carrying out orthodontic treatment in periodontally compromised patients and with good reason. At the same time, studies show that a large percentage (~65%) of patients with moderate to severe periodontitis are interested in such treatment for esthetic and functional changes caused by pathologic tooth migration [44].

Many questions need to be answered in these periodontally compromised patients who opt for orthodontic treatment. Some of the findings of a comprehensive search on PubMed focusing on "ortho-perio treatments" are as follows [45]:

1. Best time to start orthodontic treatment following periodontal therapy.

   According to the authors, in periodontally compromised cases that have undergone periodontal therapy, it is better to start orthodontic treatment as follows:

   1. 3 to 6 months after non-surgical/surgical periodontal treatment and

   2. 9 to 12 months after regenerative surgical procedures.

2. Acceptable periodontal status for orthodontic treatment

   It is important to achieve low rates of full-mouth plaque and bleeding on probing after active periodontal treatment with scores <25% of previous ones. They recommend that these low scores (i.e., optimal plaque control without clinical gingival inflammation) be reached and maintained during the entire phase of orthodontic therapy and they think that without these conditions, orthodontic tooth movement should be discontinued.

3. Biologic efficacy of orthodontic treatment

   A combined periodontist-orthodontist diagnostic and treatment endeavor in periodontally compromised patients can result in improved masticatory efficiency by a more balanced occlusion brought about by a realignment of the migrated teeth. The realignment may also result in the periodontal structures being better able to carry out their assigned functions.

According to Lindhe J and Ericsson I [46], a healthy periodontium with reduced height has a capacity similar to that of a normal periodontium to adapt to traumatizing occlusal forces. Wennström JL, et al. [47] state that sites with the horizontal bone loss after periodontal therapy will not be negatively influenced by the type of tooth movement once the individualized orthodontic mechanics are established (i.e., an appropriate ratio force/% remaining periodontal support). According to Polson A, et al., if teeth are moved through or into vertical bone defects, it can increase the rate of destruction of these periodontal structures. At the same time, if the OTM into infrabony pockets is done after successful elimination of subgingival infection, it will not result in adverse effects. They concluded that this movement/treatment will not bring about changes in the periodontal ligament attachment level; instead, the formation of a long junctional epithelium is what will be achieved [48].

According to Melsen B, et al. [49], "orthodontic intrusion at healthy sites can lead to new cementum formation and new collagen attachment, whereas for sites lacking proper oral hygiene, results vary from a moderate new attachment development to a worsening of the alveolar bone loss." And in a subsequent study, Melsen B [50] recommends that "the intrusion movement should be carefully planned as it can increase the risk of other adverse effects not desired in patients with a reduced periodontium, such as alveolar process reduction and root resorption."

Cassio Volponi Carvalho, et al. [51] studied the effects of orthodontic movement in the periodontal tissues of 10 adult patients with aggressive periodontitis and compared them with 10 patients with healthy periodontium. They evaluated the probing pocket depth, clinical attachment level, bleeding on probing, and dental plaque index before, during and 4 months after orthodontic treatment. They found improvement in all the above parameters, 4 months after orthodontic treatment.

Despite advances in therapeutics as well as our increased knowledge of the biological effects of orthodontic treatment, it might be better to avoid OTM in conditions such as uncontrolled infection/inflammation, inadequate anchorage, conditions where periodontal health might not improve despite periodontal therapy.

8. Conclusion

This chapter has attempted to portray the roles the periodontium, inflammation, and periodontal therapy play during the planning and execution of orthodontic treatment as well as once it is completed. It also discusses orthodontics in the periodontally compromised patient. There is a huge void in our knowledge about various aspects of the orthodontic movement of teeth and their effects on the periodontium. It is also evident that for the long-term success of orthodontic treatment, especially in the periodontally compromised patient, joining forces of the orthodontist and the periodontist would benefit patients as well as both the specialties.

Conflict of interest

The authors declare no conflict of interest.

Author details

Betsy Sara Thomas[1] and Mohan Alexander[2]*

1 Faculty of Dentistry, Department of Periodontology, MAHSA University, Bandar Saujana Putra, Selangor, Malaysia

2 Faculty of Dentistry, Department of Oral and Maxillofacial Surgery, MAHSA University, Bandar Saujana Putra, Selangor, Malaysia

*Address all correspondence to: mohan@mahsa.edu.my

References

[1] Petti S, Barbato E, Simonetti D'Arca A. Effect of orthodontic therapy with fixed and removable appliances on oral microbiota: A six-month longitudinal study. New Microbiologica. 1997;**20**(1): 55-62

[2] van Gastel J, Quirynen M, Teughels W, Carels C. The relationships between malocclusion, fixed orthodontic appliances and periodontal disease. A review of the literature. Australian Orthodontic Journal. 2007;**23**(2):121-129

[3] Bimstein E, Becker A. Malocclusion, orthodontic intervention, and gingival and periodontal health. In: Periodontal and Gingival Health and Diseases: Children, Adolescents, and Young Adults. London, UK: Martin Dunitz Ltd; 2001

[4] Morris JW, Campbell PM, Tadlock LP, Boley J, Buschang PH. Prevalence of gingival recession after orthodontic tooth movements. American Journal of Orthodontics and Dentofacial Orthopedics. 2017 May;**151**(5):851-859

[5] Smale I, Artun J, Behbehani F, Doppel D, et al. Apical root resorption six and 12 months after initiation of fixed orthodontic appliance therapy. The Angle Orthodontist. 2005;**75**:919-926

[6] Harris EF. Root resorption during orthodonic therapy. Seminars in Orthodontics. 2000;**6**:183-94. 3

[7] Harris EF, Boggan BW, Wheeler DA. Apical root resorption in patients treated with comprehensive orthodontics. The Journal of the Tennessee Dental Association. 2001;**81**:30-33

[8] Pejicic A, Bertl M, Čelar A. Extent and prognosis of apical root resorption due to orthodontic treatment A systematic literature review. Journal of Stomatology & Occlusion Medicine. 2012;**5**:147-154. DOI: 10.1007/s12548-012-0056-5

[9] Brezniak N, Wasserstein A. Root resorption after orthodontic treatment: Part 1. Literature review. American Journal of Orthodontics and Dentofacial Orthopedics. 1993a;**103**:62-6.

[10] Brezniak N, Wasserstein A. Root resorption after orthodontic treatment: Part 2 Literature review. American Journal of Orthodontics and Dentofacial Orthopedics. 1993b;**103**:138-46.

[11] Brezniak N, Wasserstein A. Orthodontically induced inflammatory root resorption. Part I: The basic science aspects. The Angle Orthodontist. 2002a;**72**:175-9.

[12] Brezniak N, Wasserstein A. Orthodontically induced inflammatory root resorption. Part II: The clinical aspects. The Angle Orthodontist. 2002b;**72**:180-184

[13] Brudvik P, Rygh P. Root resorption beneath the main hyalinised zone. European Orthodontic. 1994;**16**:249-63.

[14] Reitan K. Initial tissue behavior during apical root resorption. The Angle Orthodontist. 1974;**44**:68-82

[15] Owman-Moll P, Kurol J, Lundgren D. Repair of orthodontically induced root resorption in adolescents. The Angle Orthodontist. 1995;**65**:403-408

[16] Winter BU, Stenvik A, Vandevska-Radunovic V. Dynamics of orthodontic root resorption and repair in human premolars: a light microscopy study. European Journal of Orthodontics. 2009;**31**(4):346-351

[17] Beck BW, Harris EF. Apical root resorption in orthodontically treated subjects: analyses of edgewise and light wire mechanics. American Journal of Orthodontics and Dentofacial Orthopedics. 1994;**105**:350-361

[18] Korkmaz Y, Puladi B, Galler K, Kämmerer PW, Schröder A, Gölz L, et al. Inflammation in the Human Periodontium Induces Downregulation of the α1- and β1-Subunits of the sGC in Cementoclasts. International Journal of Molecular Sciences. 2021;**22**:539. DOI: 10.3390/ijms22020539

[19] Xie Y, Zhao N, Shen G. Anti-resorptive effects of cementocytes during orthodontic tooth movement. Tropical Journal of Pharmaceutical Research November. 2018;**17**(11):2291-2298

[20] Alberto Consolaro. Orthodontic Insight. https://doi.org/10.1590/2177-6709.25.2.018-023.oin

[21] Schroeder HE. The Periodontium. Springer-Verlag, Berlin Heidelberg: Springerz; 1986. p. 152

[22] Ducy P, Schinke T, Karsenty G. The osteoblast: A sophisticated fibroblast under central surveillance. Science. 2000;**289**:1504-1508

[23] Wise GE, King GJ. Mechanisms of tooth eruption and orthodontic tooth movement. Journal of Dental Research. 2008;**87**(5):414-434. DOI: 10.1177/154405910808700509

[24] Li Y, Jacox LA, Little SH, Ko C-C. Orthodontic tooth movement: The biology and clinical implications. Kaohsiung Journal of Medical Sciences. 2018;**34**:207-214

[25] Orthodontics: Current Principles and Techniques. 4th ed. Graber, Vanarsdall, Vig. Elsevier- Health Sciences Division

[26] Krishnan V, Davidovitch ZE. Cellular, molecular, and tissue-level reactions to orthodontic force. American Journal of Orthodontics and Dentofacial Orthopedics. 2006;**129**(4):469-4e1

[27] Ngan PW, Saito S, Saito M, Lanese R, Shanfeld J, Davidovitch Z. The interactive effects of mechanical stress and interleukin-1 beta on prostaglandin E and cyclic AMP production in human periodontal ligament fibroblasts in vitro: Comparison with cloned osteoblastic cells of mouse (MC3T3-E1). Archives of Oral Biology. 1990;**35**:717-725

[28] Shetty N, Patil AK, Ganeshkar SV, Hegde S. Comparison of the effects of ibuprofen and acetaminophen on PGE2 levels in the GCF during orthodontic tooth movement: A human study. Progress in Orthodontics. 2013;**14**:6

[29] Leiker BJ, Nanda RS, Currier G, Howes RI, Sinha PK. The effects of exogenous prostaglandins on orthodontic tooth movement in rats. American Journal of Orthodontics and Dentofacial Orthopedics. 1995;**108**:380-388

[30] Yamasaki K, Shibata Y, Imai S, Tani Y, Shibasaki Y, Fukuhara T. Clinical application of prostaglandin E1 (PGE1) upon orthodontic tooth movement. American Journal of Orthodontics. 1984;**85**:508-518

[31] Chung CJ, Baik H-S, Soma K. Bone formation and tooth movement are synergistically enhanced by administration of EP4 agonist. American Journal of Orthodontics and Dentofacial Orthopedics. 2007;**132**:427.e13-427.e20

[32] Yamasaki K, Miura F, Suda T. Prostaglandin as a mediator of bone resorption induced by experimental tooth movement in rats. Journal of Dental Research. 1980;**59**:1635-1642

[33] Kanzaki H, Chiba M, Takahashi I, Haruyama N, Nishimura M, Mitani H. Local OPG gene transfer to periodontal tissue inhibits orthodontic tooth movement. Journal of Dental Research. 2004;**83**(12):920-925. DOI: 10.1177/154405910408301206

[34] Tsichlaki A, Chin SY, Pandis N, Fleming PS. How long does treatment with fixed orthodontic appliances last? A systematic review. American Journal of Orthodontics and Dentofacial Orthopedics. 2016;**149**:308-318

[35] Miles P. Accelerated orthodontic treatment - what's the evidence? Australian Dental Journal. 2017;**62** (Suppl 1):63-70. DOI: 10.1111/adj.12477

[36] Wilcko WM, Wilcko T, Bouquot JE, Ferguson DJ. Rapid orthodontics with alveolar reshaping: Two case reports of decrowding. The International Journal of Periodontics & Restorative Dentistry. 2001;**21**:9-19

[37] Iino S, Sakoda S, Ito G, Nishimori T, Ikeda T, Miyawaki S. Acceleration of orthodontic tooth movement by alveolar corticotomy in the dog. American Journal of Orthodontics and Dentofacial Orthopedics. 2007;**131**(4):448-4e1

[38] Kole H. Surgical operations on the alveolar ridge to correct occlusal abnormalities. Oral Surgery, Oral Medicine, and Oral Pathology. 1959; **12**(5):515-529

[39] Düker J. Experimental animal research into segmental alveolar movement after corticotomy. Journal of Maxillofacial Surgery. 1975;**3**:81-84

[40] Suya H. Corticotomy in orthodontics. E. Hosl, A. Baldauf (Eds.), Mechanical and Biological Basis in Orthodontic Therapy, Huthig Buch Verlag, Heidelberg, Germany (1991), pp. 207-226

[41] Gellee T, Ouadi E, Ejeil A-L, Moreau N. Other interesting effects of alveolar corticotomies in orthodontics apart from the acceleration of tooth movement. Journal of Dentofacial Anomalies and Orthodontics. 2018;**21**:208

[42] Wang C-W, Yu S-H, Mandelaris GA, Wang H-L. Is periodontal phenotype modification therapy beneficial for patients receiving orthodontic treatment? An American Academy of Periodontology Best Evidence Review, Journal of Periodontology. 2019. DOI: 10.1002/JPER.19-0037

[43] Al-Jasser R, Al-Subaie M, Al-Jasser N, Al-Rasheed A. Rotational relapse of anterior teeth following orthodontic treatment and circumferential supracrestal fiberotomy. The Saudi Dental Journal. 2020;**32**(6): 293-299. DOI: 10.1016/j.sdentj.2019.10.003

[44] Hirschfeld J, Reichardt E, Sharma P, et al. Interest in orthodontic tooth alignment in adult patients affected by periodontitis: A questionnaire-based cross-sectional pilot study. Journal of Periodontology. 2019. DOI: 10.1002/JPER.18-0578

[45] Prato GPP, Chambrone L. Orthodontic treatment in periodontal patients: The use of periodontal gold standards to overcome the "grey zone". Journal of Periodontology. 2019. DOI: 10.1002/JPER.19-0306

[46] Lindhe J, Ericsson I. Trauma from occlusion: Periodontal tissues. In: Lang NP, Lindhe J, editors. Clinical Periodontology and Implant Dentistry. 6th ed. Oxford: John Wiley & Sons. 2015. pp. 313-324

[47] Wennström JL, Lindhe J, Sinclair F, Thilander B. Some periodontal tissue

reactions to orthodontic tooth movement in monkeys. Journal of Clinical Periodontology. 1987;**14**:121-129

[48] Polson A, Caton J, Polson AP, Nyman S, Novak J, Reed B. Periodontal response after tooth movement into intrabony defects. Journal of Periodontology. 1984;**55**:197-202

[49] Melsen B, Agerbaek N, Eriksen J, Terp S. New attachment through periodontal treatment and orthodontic intrusion. American Journal of Orthodontics and Dentofacial Orthopedics. 1988;**94**:104-116

[50] Melsen B. Tissue reaction to orthodontic tooth movement–a new paradigm. European Journal of Orthodontics. 2001;**23**:671-681

[51] Carvalho CV, Saraiva L, Bauer FPF, Kimura RY, Souto MLS, Bernardo CC, et al. Orthodontic treatment in patients with aggressive periodontitis. American Journal of Orthodontics and Dentofacial Orthopedics. 2018;**153**(4):P550-P557

Chapter 3

Current Methods for Acceleration of Orthodontic Tooth Movement

Mehmet Akin and Leyla Cime Akbaydogan

Abstract

The awareness of the society and, accordingly, the number of patients who need orthodontic treatment has increased gradually. Nowadays, the importance of the concept of time has focused the attention of researchers on the completion of orthodontic treatments in a shorter time. Heavy forces applied to shorten the treatment period in orthodontic treatments cause many undesirable conditions, such as root resorption, crushing of periodontal fibers, and formation of hyalinization tissue. Therefore, researchers are working on methods that will accelerate orthodontic tooth movement and shorten the treatment time. In this section, applications that accelerate orthodontic tooth movement will be discussed.

Keywords: tooth movement, piezocision, propel, vibration, corticotomy

1. Introduction

As a result of the awareness of the society and the increasing interest in esthetic appearance, the number of patients who want to receive orthodontic treatment, especially in adults, is increasing [1]. However, one of the biggest problems in orthodontic treatments is the length of the treatment period [2]. Increased caries risk [3, 4], external root resorption risk, [5, 6] and decreased patient cooperation [7] in long-term orthodontic treatments lower its success. For some patients, the long duration of orthodontic treatment may be the only reason for their refusal [8]. The fact that the concept of time has gained importance for both patients and physicians has led researchers to work on completing orthodontic treatment in a shorter time [9].

The methods used to accelerate tooth movement in orthodontic treatment are examined under three main titles as pharmacological and biological applications, mechanical-physical applications and surgical applications [10].

2. The methods used to accelerate tooth movement in orthodontic treatment

2.1 Pharmacological and biological applications

2.1.1 Prostaglandins

Prostaglandins, especially prostaglandin E2 (PGE2), are one of the most effective regulators of bone metabolism [11]. Since prostaglandins play a role in both bone destruction and bone formation, researchers have conducted many studies on the role of prostaglandins during tooth movement [11–14].

Yamasaki et al., in their clinical study, injected prostaglandin E1 (PGE1) submucosal into the distal canine tooth during canine distalization and reported that tooth movement occurred twice as fast. They stated that it is an effective and safe method that can be used to accelerate tooth movement without causing any side effects other than mild pain in patients [15].

Leiker et al., in an animal study examining the effects of PGE2 dose and the number of applications on orthodontic tooth movement, reported that there was no significant difference between a single dose and multiple applications; however, high doses and multiple injections may cause an increase in root resorption [12].

2.1.2 Corticosteroids

Also called steroids are a group of substances used as anti-inflammatory drugs for a wide range of conditions; its name was derived from an internal hormone produced by the adrenal cortex. Cortisone is the most famous type of this group that is used in the treatment of many inflammatory and autoimmune diseases such as rheumatoid arthritis, skin diseases, ulcerative colitis, adrenal insufficiency and asthma [16]. The effects of corticosteroid on the bone turnover were demonstrated in different studies, but the mechanism by which corticosteroids suppress the bone formation and increase bone resorption is still not really understood [17].

Ashcraft et al., in a study that included 16 New Zealand rabbits, in which they examined the effect of corticosteroids on tooth movement speed, stated that the speed of tooth movement was four times higher in the experimental group in which they gave cortisone acetate compared to the control group. In addition, in the histopathological examination of the bone sections they took, it was stated that the areas of bone resorption were higher in the experimental group than in the control group [18].

Ong et al. reported that there was no significant change in orthodontic tooth movement speed, but root resorption was less in their study on rabbits to which they applied prednisolone, a corticosteroid derivative [19].

2.1.3 Parathyroid hormone

The main task of the parathyroid hormone is to maintain the calcium balance in the body together with the hormones calcitonin and 1,25 dihydroxycholecalciferol. Parathyroid hormone accelerates bone remodeling by stimulating osteoclasts and osteoblasts [20].

Gianelly injected parathyroid hormone (PTH) locally into the distal mucosa of the upper left incisors of six rats and investigated its effect on tooth motility. As a result, he reported that the amount of tooth movement was higher in the PTH applied group [21].

Goldie and King reported in their study that in the group fed with a calcium-deficient diet, parathyroid hormone secretion increased and resulted in a decrease in bone density, resulting in increased tooth movement speed and less root resorption [22].

2.1.4 1,25-Hydroxyvitamin D

Another factor that is important in orthodontic tooth movement is 1,25 dihydroxycholecalciferol (1,25-DHCC), the active form of vitamin D, and is involved in calcium hemostasis. 1,25-DHCC stimulates bone deposition and inhibits PTH release. While it does not affect bone resorption at physiological doses, low doses stimulate the release of receptor activator nuclear kappa B ligand (RANKL) from osteoblasts, changing the receptor activator nuclear kappa B (RANK)/RANKL ratio and causing differentiation of osteoclasts. Thus, it takes part in the osteoclastic activity. It has also been shown to play a role in osteoblastic cell differentiation and bone mineralization in a dose-dependent manner in addition to its bone resorption function [14].

Collins and Sinclair examined the effects of injection of the active form of vitamin D on tooth movement in their study and reported that there was a 60% increase in tooth movement speed compared to the control group [23].

Takano-Yamamoto et al., in their study on rats, applied force to the maxillary first molar and additionally injected 1,25-dihydroxycholecalciferol locally every three days [24]. As a result, they reported that local injection of 1,25-dihydroxycholecalciferol with mechanical forces accelerated tooth movement, and the pause in tooth movement determined in the control group was not observed in the experimental group.

Kale et al., in their study evaluating the effects of locally applied 1,25-dihydroxycholecalciferol and PGE2 on orthodontic tooth movement using histological parameters, reported that both applications increased the speed of tooth movement, but the effects of the applications on the amount of tooth movement were similar [14].

2.1.5 Osteocalcin

Osteocalcin is a non-collagenous matrix protein that is abundant in bone tissue and functions as a negative regulator of mineral apposition and bone formation due to its high-binding strength with calcium and hydroxyapatite [25].

Hashimoto et al. injected local osteocalcin to the maxillary first molars of rats, while applying mesial motion with a spiral spring, and evaluated tooth movement histologically for a period of 10 days [26]. In their results, they determined that local application of osteocalcin accelerated tooth movement and explained this with the increase of osteoclast on the pressure side in the early period.

2.1.6 Nitric oxide

Nitric oxide is synthesized from arginine by the enzyme nitric oxide synthase. It is a short-lived molecule that plays a key role in the regulation of some functions of the nervous, defense, respiratory, circulatory, and reproductive systems [27]. Nitric oxide is also important in bone turnover and the regulation of pulpal blood flow [28].

Shirazi et al. injected L-arginine G-nitro-L-arginine methyl ester into experimental animals in their study. As a result, they reported increased bone remodeling and osteoclastic activity [28].

Akin et al., in their study, reported a significant increase in multinucleated osteoclasts, howship lacunae, vascularization and orthodontic tooth movement as a result of nitric oxide injection in rats [29].

2.1.7 Platelet rich plasma (PRP) and platelet rich fibrin (PRF)

Recently, there have been studies investigating the effect of PRP and PRF on orthodontic tooth movement speed. Studies have reported that these applications can accelerate orthodontic tooth movement [30–34].

In the last two decades, after a better understanding of the role of platelets in wound healing, the idea of using these cells for treatment has been proposed. The new autogenous product called PRP has been widely used in orthopedics, plastic surgery, and dentistry [35]. PRP is the plasma fraction obtained by centrifuging whole blood and containing a higher concentration of platelets than whole blood. It contains a high amount of platelets, growth factors, and coagulation factors in PRP [36].

After tooth extraction, resorptive remodeling of the alveolar bone usually occurs. This event is beneficial in accelerating tooth movement in patients with moderate crowding and undergoing fixed orthodontic treatment [37, 38].

In the literature, there are studies on the use of various bioactive grafts to increase the orthodontic tooth movement speed [39]. In orthodontic treatment, a sufficient amount of alveolar bone is required for successful orthodontic tooth movement during the closure of the extraction space. However, the application of different graft materials can promote bone formation. It has been reported that PRF has positive effects on bone healing, socket protection and acceleration of tooth movement [34].

In studies, it has been observed that PRP, which is applied at a high level, inhibits the division of bone cells and reduces bone density, and it is therefore thought that orthodontic tooth movement can be accelerated with this application [31, 40, 41]. Güleç et al., as a result of their experimental studies in which medium- and high-level PRP was injected into the mesial side of the first molar teeth of rats, showed that high-level PRP accelerated tooth movement by temporarily activating osteoclastic activity and that medium-level PRP applied at high level [31]. They reported that it accelerated tooth movement, although less than PRP. Rashid et al. reported in their study on dogs that local PRP injection can accelerate tooth movement without clinical and microscopic side effects [32].

Liou reported in their research on humans that submucosal PRP injection can increase the speed of tooth movement without surgical application and alveolar bone loss. In his clinical study, he reported that local submucosal PRP injection was 1.7 times faster in maxillary and mandibular leveling and this acceleration was PRP dose-dependent [30]. This PRP ratio (platelet count in PRP/platelet count in the blood) is <12.5. He stated that the ideal number of PRP platelets to be used to accelerate tooth movement should be 9.5–12.5 times the normal. On the other hand, PRP injection during en-masse retraction reduced alveolar bone loss by 71–77% on the pressure side, which is also dose-dependent. The optimal dose of PRP for optimal clinical performance is 11.0–12.5-folds, with submucosal injection of PRP accelerating orthodontic tooth movement and at the same time protecting the alveolar bone on the pressure side of orthodontic tooth movement. A single dose of PRP injection is effective for 5–6 months. It has been reported that the most effective period of PRP injection in accelerating tooth movement is the second half of the 4th month after the injection.

Tehranchi et al. in their study on humans, in eight patients who needed bilateral first premolar extraction, L-PRF was placed in the extraction socket on one side following a tooth extraction, and the opposite side constituted the control group. As a result of the study, tooth movement was found to be faster on the side where L-PRF was inserted into the extraction socket compared to the control side [34].

Nemtoi et al. reported that PRF placed in the extraction socket accelerates bone regeneration and tooth movement compared to the control side, and anterior and posterior teeth move faster toward the extraction cavity [33].

2.2 Physical/mechanical stimulation methods

2.2.1 Resonance vibration

In order to accelerate tooth movement, resonance or ultrasonic vibration applications are made. The application of vibration to accelerate tooth movement was first tried by Krishtab et al. [42]. Later, Ohmae et al. argued that ultrasonic vibration increases the speed of tooth movement, but they reported that ultrasonic vibration has a detrimental effect on the dental pulp [43].

Nishimura et al. showed in their study on rats that resonance vibration increases the speed of tooth movement and does not cause periodontal damage. They reported that the resonance vibration method was effective with the activation of RANK-RANKL in periodontal tissues [44].

In their study, Kau et al. had 14 patients undergoing fixed orthodontic treatment use a new commercial product, Acceledent™ (OrthoAccel Technologies, Inc., Bellaire, TX, USA) (**Figure 1**) for 20 minutes a day, in accordance with the manufacturer's recommendations [45]. They reported that there was an increase in tooth movement speed compared to the control group, which did not apply any acceleration method.

2.2.2 Direct electric current and electromagnetic stimulation

In animal studies investigating the effect of direct electric current on tooth movement, it has been reported that direct current is applied to the anode in the pressure regions and the cathode in the voltage regions, changing the bioelectric potential of the direct current and accelerating tooth movement. However, it has been reported that electrical current may have side effects such as ionic reactions causing damage to tissues and displacement of bone tissue with connective tissue [46].

Darendeliler et al. suggested that the static magnetic field accelerates tooth movement by shortening the pause period in which orthodontic tooth movement is not seen. It has been reported that the electromagnetic field affects the level of a group of enzymes responsible for the regulation of intracellular metabolism by changing the sodium-calcium exchange rate in the cell membrane, thereby increasing cellular proliferation [47]. By affecting the cellular activity in the periodontal space, it accelerates both osteoclastic and osteoblastic activities, and thus, the movement takes place in a shorter time in force-applied teeth. It has been reported that due to the stabilization of the rate of resorption due to increased bone formation, mobility in the teeth

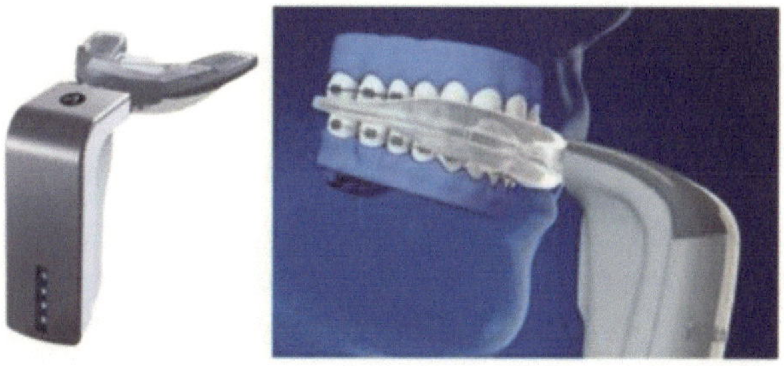

Figure 1.
Acceledent™.

decreases and pain is not observed in teeth exposed to chewing forces [48, 49]. In a study on the side effects of this method, it was reported that minor changes in blood chemistry may occur with a decrease in serum calcium level [47].

2.2.3 Low-level laser irradiation therapy

One of the techniques developed to accelerate tooth movement is low-dose laser application. Laser is a light source obtained by stimulating and amplifying radiation [50].

Laser application: It has been stated that it stimulates the proliferation of osteoclasts, osteoblasts, and fibroblasts and thus accelerates tooth movement by affecting bone remodeling [51]. Low-dose laser application activates the cytochrome C oxidase enzyme in electron transfer, causing an increase in adenosine triphosphate (ATP) in the cell, thus accelerating the tooth movement [52]. It has been reported that low-dose laser application accelerates tooth movement through RANK-RANKL, M-CSF, and the receptor of this factor [53].

In an animal study in which the effect of low-dose laser application on tooth movement speed was examined for the first time, 10 g orthodontic force was applied to the molar teeth of experimental animals for 12 days in three parts of the teeth (buccal, palatal, mesial) for a total of 9 minutes a day, 35.3 W/cm2 (54 Joule) Gallium aluminum arsenide (GaAlAr) diode laser with a wavelength of 830 nanometers (nm) was applied. As a result of histomorphometric and histological analyzes, it was reported that there was an increase in bone remodeling and a 1.3-fold acceleration in tooth movement with laser application [54].

Cruz et al. conducted the first clinical study on the effect of low-dose laser application on tooth movement and applied only mechanical activation on one side of the arch and laser with mechanical activation on the other side in 11 patients who were planned to undergo canine distalization [55]. After each force activation, GaAlAr semiconductor diode laser was applied at a power of 780 nm and a dose of 5 J/cm2 for 10 seconds. They showed that they could accelerate tooth movement by 34% when they applied four times a month over the mucosa from the buccal and palatal of the canine tooth to the cervical, middle and apical third of the root. They also found a significant reduction in patient discomfort and pain sensation.

Seifi et al. and Yamaguchi et al. reported that laser application did not cause any change in tooth movement speed [13, 56].

There have also been several studies showing contrasting results with low-level laser therapy. Therefore, more studies are needed to distinguish the optimum wavelength, optimum energy, and optimum duration.

3. Surgical methods

3.1 Corticotomy and osteotomy

Corticotomy and osteotomy are surgical techniques that have been used clinically for many years. Osteotomy a is surgical cut in the bone, including the cortical and trabecular bone [57, 58]. Corticotomy is incisions, cut and perforation procedures performed only in the cortical bone, not involving the medullary bone [51].

Corticotomy-assisted orthodontic tooth movement was first described by LC Bryan in 1893 [59]. However, corticotomy performed by Henrich Köle in 1959 to accelerate orthodontic tooth movement is an evolution in this regard [60]. Köle thought that the main resistance to tooth movement was the cortical bone and that tooth movement could be accelerated by disrupting the integrity and continuity of the cortical bone. Köle created "bone blocks" by making interradicular vertical corticotomy incisions on the buccal and palatal surface and subapical horizontal osteotomy incisions connecting these incisions in the buccopalatinal direction. He made the incisions only in the cortical bone without causing any damage to the cancellous bone. He reported that when high orthopedic forces are applied with adjustable screw appliances, major active tooth movement can be completed within 6–12 weeks [60].

The changes that occur in the bone after corticotomy was first described by Herald Frost as the Regional Acceleratory Phenomena (RAP) [61]. Based on this phenomenon, increasing the rate of tooth movement is not due to the decreasing bone resistance only but also the effects of the healing process on the rapidity of bone cell activation.

The most widely accepted technique today was put forward by Wilcko et al. [62, 63]. According to the results of their studies, they stated that tooth movement resulted from demineralization and remineralization in reversible osteopenia occurring in the alveolar bone during wound healing, in line with RAP, rather than bone block movement.

The Wilcko brothers introduced the technique called "accelerated osteogenic orthodontics"(AOO), in which they combined selective alveolar decortication, alveolar augmentation, and orthodontic tooth movement, later called "periodontally accelerated osteogenic orthodontics"(PAOO) or "Wilckodontics." The basic principle in this technique is to create a layer of bone of 1.5 mm or less on the root surface in the direction of intended tooth movement. Similar to techniques in which bone block is created, the flap is raised and vertical corticotomies are performed. Alternatively, horizontal corticotomies that do not descend into the medullary bone are performed under the roots of the teeth to be moved. Thus, it was stated that the vitality of the teeth was preserved. In order to accelerate healing, a bone graft was applied and RAP was modified. (**Figure 2**) As a result of the study, no periodontal problems, root resorption, luxation, and changes in alveolar bone height were found, and the duration of orthodontic treatment was reduced by 1/3 or 1/4 [62, 63].

The advantages of the technique are shortening the treatment period compared to conventional treatments, moving the teeth more, reducing hyalinization and root resorption due to the decrease in the pressure in the periodontal ligament, treating bone defects by grafting, and decreasing the recurrence rate by deteriorating tissue memory with corticotomies. The invasive surgical procedure, additional costs, risk of bone loss, and complications such as pain, edema and infection due to surgery are also disadvantages of the technique [62, 63].

The "rapid orthodontic treatment" technique developed by Chung is based on corticotomy and serial movement of the dentoalveolar segments with orthopedic forces [64]. The method is similar to the accelerated osteogenic orthodontic technique, but the difference of this technique is that the dentoalveolar segment is also moved along with the teeth [65].

3.1.1 Distracting the periodontal ligament

Liou and Huang, in their study, defined the technique as "distraction of the periodontal ligament," which is based on the formation of new bone due to the tension of the healing bone, by reducing bone resistance in principle similar to distraction

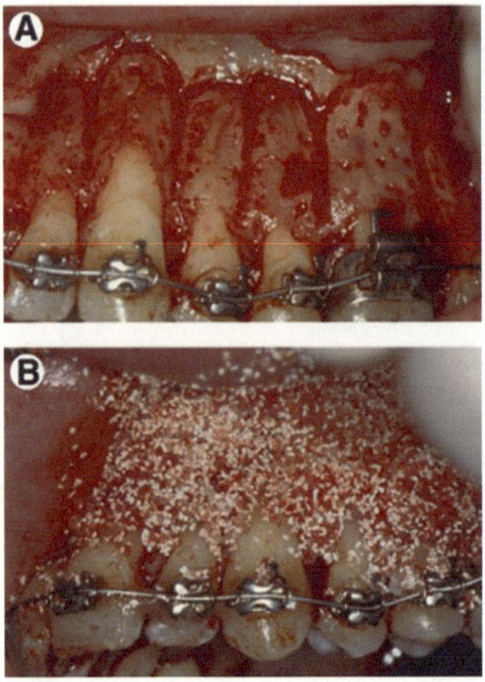

Figure 2.
Treatment of a 23 year-old male patient. A, Before treatment, anterior view. B, After treatment, total AOO treatment time 6 months 2 weeks,anterior view. Corticotomy and bone grafting (Wilcko 2009).

osteogenesis. The aim of this technique is to distalize in a short time, to prevent loss of anchorage in posterior teeth and resorption of canine teeth. In cases where they applied fixed treatment with first premolar extraction in this technique, the interseptal bone distal to the canine after extraction was vertically weakened with a drill [66]. Following the surgical procedures, a special tooth-supported intraoral distractors were placed and activated 0.5–1 mm per day. With this technique, the canines were moved 6.5 mm toward the extraction space in three weeks. It has been reported that this technique can accelerate tooth movement without causing serious root resorption, ankylosis and root fracture [51]. However, some conflicting results have been reported regarding the vitality of distalized canine teeth. Liou and Huang reported that 9 out of 26 teeth responded positively to the vitality test, while 7 out of 20 teeth responded positively to the vitality test after the sixth month of retraction, in the study by Sukurica et al. [66, 67]. Therefore, there are still uncertainties regarding this technique.

3.1.2 Dentoalveolar distraction

Dentoalveolar distraction differs from periodontal ligament distraction in that the tooth is moved together with the surrounding bone. Kişnişçi et al. presented this technique in order to shorten the duration of orthodontic treatment. In this technique, following the extraction of the first premolar tooth, the alveolar segment around the canine was mobilized and an intraoral distractor was placed and 0.8 mm of tooth movement per day was performed. Canine distalization was completed in 8–14 days. Researchers stated that there was no loss of anchorage, root resorption, ankylosis and discoloration in the first molar teeth [68, 69].

3.1.3 Micro-osteoperforation (MOP)

The method of creating holes in the alveolar bone to increase osteoclastic activity in order to accelerate orthodontic tooth movement is called "alveosynthesis." For this purpose, a disposable device called propel was designed by "propel orthodontics." It has been reported that microosteoperforations (MOPs) applied during canine distalization cause a significant increase in the amount of cytokines that increase osteoclast differentiation and number. It has been found that MOPs increase tooth movement 2–3 times compared to the control group during canine distalization. It was stated to be a comfortable and reliable method [70].

3.1.4 Piezocision

Corticotomy, which is one of the methods applied to accelerate orthodontic tooth movement, is an effective method, but it is a highly invasive method. Because it requires wide flap removal and bone surgery, which can cause discomfort and complications after surgery [71]. Vercellotti and Podesta, in their study, recommended the use of a piezosurgical blade in order to create safer and more precise corticotomies without causing osteonecrotic damage after flap removal in order to reduce surgical trauma and accelerate tooth movement [72]. Kim et al. applied the corticization method, which is a method that causes surgical damage to the bone without lifting the flap. They argued that this method increased the effect of BHF and accelerated tooth movement. However, due to the difficulty of accessing the periodontium and the surgical procedures, temporary dizziness was observed in the patients [73]. Most recently, Dibart et al. introduced the "piezoincision" technique, which is a new and minimally invasive method and performed without flap lifting [74].

As a result of a histological study, it has been shown that decortication with piezoincision has an effect similar to the BHF effect. In this study, it was shown histologically that transient osteopenia occurred and osteoclastic activity was stimulated in as little as one day. In addition, it has been determined that piezoincision application creates deeper demineralization areas and accordingly tooth movement is twice as fast [75] (**Figure 3**).

It has been reported that, depending on the difficulty of tooth movement and the bone morphology of the patient, the piezoincision procedure can be repeated 5–6 months later in order to reactivate the RAP [76].

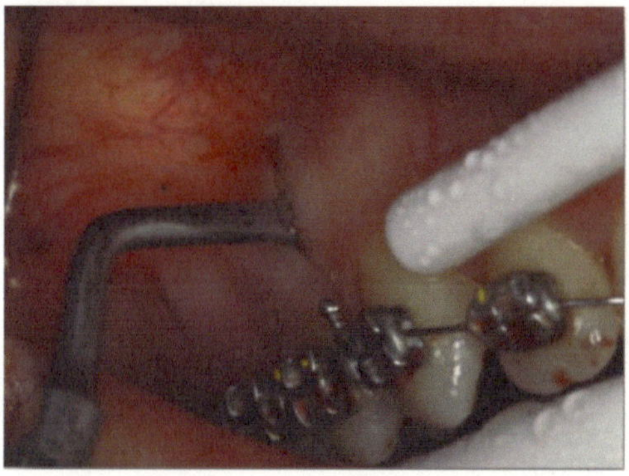

Figure 3.
RAP with piezocision. (Dibart 2015).

Aksakalli et al., in their study investigating the effect of piezoincision during canine distalization, reported that tooth movement speed increased, anchorage control was better in posterior teeth, and there was no transversal narrowing in the upper jaw. They also stated that periodontal health was not adversely affected [77]. It has been reported that the possibility of bacterial endocarditis should be considered in high-risk patients, since bacteremia may occur temporarily in patients with piezoincision [78].

The most important feature of piezoelectric surgery devices is that when they come into contact with soft tissue, the tissue can absorb vibrations and disperse them by converting them to a slight heat. In this case, the device cannot make the incision. When the physician realizes that the vibrations have stopped, he realizes that he is in contact with the soft tissue and stops the procedure. Even when you continue to force it in the same position, no rupture occurs in the vessels or nerves. In the worst case, the damage will usually be reversible. Due to this feature, it is possible to make precise incisions without damaging tissues such as nerves, vessels, and membranes [79]. One of the important advantages of the device is the cavitation phenomenon created by ultrasonic frequency. The cooling solution applied during the procedure takes the form of an aerosol and washes the treated area, clogs small vessels, and removes tissue residues and blood. In this way, it both reduces bleeding and provides a good viewing angle [80]. It is possible to make more precise incisions since macro-vibrations do not occur as in conventional techniques [81]. In addition, it is more comfortable for the patient as it produces less vibration and noise [82].

The vibrations created by the device and the shock waves that occur in the liquid environment act as a disinfectant and reduce the bacteria [83]. In another study, it was stated that the application of piezoincision may cause transient bacteremia and therefore the risk of bacterial endocarditis should be considered [78]. As a result of the examinations made on the bone fragments exposed during the surgical procedure, it was determined that the cells were alive and necrosis did not occur in the bone tissue [84]. It is more advantageous than conventional techniques in terms of wound healing and new bone formation, thanks to the reduction of the risk of necrosis and the ability to make precise incisions with micro-vibrations [72].

4. Conclusions

In the literature, there are many invasive and non-invasive methods that accelerate orthodontic tooth movement. More extensive studies should be done on this subject.

Conflict of interest

The authors declare no conflict of interest.

Acronyms and abbreviations

PGE2	prostaglandin E2
PGE1	prostaglandin E1
PTH	parathyroid hormone
1,25-DHCC	1,25 dihydroxycholecalciferol

RANK	receptor activator nuclear kappa B
RANKL	receptor activator nuclear kappa B ligand
PRP	platelet-rich Plasma
PRF	platelet-rich Fibrin
ATP	Adenosine triphosphate
GaAlAr	gallium aluminum arsenide
RAP	Regional acceleratory phenomena
MOP	micro-osteoperforation
AOO	accelerated osteogenic orthodontics
PAOO	periodontally accelerated osteogenic orthodontics

Author details

Mehmet Akin* and Leyla Cime Akbaydogan
Faculty of Dentistry, Alanya Alaaddin Keykubat University, Alanya, Turkey

*Address all correspondence to: mehmet.akin@alanya.edu.tr

References

[1] Cano J, Campo J, Bonilla E, Colmenero C. Corticotomy-assisted orthodontics. Journal of Clinical and Experimental Dentistry. 2012;**4**:54

[2] Fisher MA, Wenger RM, Hans MG. Pretreatment characteristics associated with orthodontic treatment duration. American Journal of Orthodontics and Dentofacial Orthopedics. 2010;**137**: 178-186

[3] Geiger AM, Gorelick L, Gwinnett AJ, Benson BJ. Reducing white spot lesions in orthodontic populations with fluoride rinsing. American Journal of Orthodontics and Dentofacial Orthopedics. 1992;**101**:403-407

[4] Bishara SE, Ostby AW. White spot lesions: formation, prevention, and treatment. In: Seminars in Orthodontics. US: Elsevier, WB Saunders; 2008. Vol. 14 pp. s 174-s 182

[5] Segal G, Schiffman P, Tuncay O. Meta analysis of the treatment-related factors of external apical root resorption. Orthodontics & Craniofacial Research. 2004;7:71-78

[6] Pandis N, Nasika M, Polychronopoulou A, Eliades T. External apical root resorption in patients treated with conventional and self-ligating brackets. American Journal of Orthodontics and Dentofacial Orthopedics. 2008;**134**:646-651

[7] Royko A, Denes Z, Razouk G. The relationship between the length of orthodontic treatment and patient compliance. Fogorvosi Szemle. 1999;**92**:79-86

[8] Lv T, Kang N, Wang C, Han X, Chen Y, Bai D. Biologic response of rapid tooth movement with periodontal ligament distraction. American Journal of Orthodontics and Dentofacial Orthopedics. 2009;**136**:401-411

[9] Genc G. The Effect of Application of Low Level Laser Therapy(LLLT) on Orthodontic Tooth Movement. Ankara: Hacettepe University; 2010

[10] Ren A, Lv T, Kang N, Zhao B, Chen Y, Bai D. Rapid orthodontic tooth movement aided by alveolar surgery in beagles. American Journal of Orthodontics and Dentofacial Orthopedics. 2007;131(2):160. e1-. 160.e10.

[11] Yamasaki K, Shibata Y, Fukuhara T. The effect of prostaglandins on experimental tooth movement in monkeys (Macaca fuscata). Journal of Dental Research. 1982;**61**(12): 1444-1446

[12] Leiker BJ, Nanda RS, Currier GF, Howes RI, Sinha PK. The effects of exogenous prostaglandins on orthodontic tooth movement in rats. American Journal of Orthodontics and Dentofacial Orthopedics. 1995;**108**(4): 380-388

[13] Seifi M, Shafeei HA, Daneshdoost S, Mir M. Effects of two types of low-level laser wave lengths (850 and 630 nm) on the orthodontic tooth movements in rabbits. Lasers in Medical Science. 2007;**22**(4):261-264

[14] Kale S, Il K, Atilla P, Asan E. Comparison of the effects of 1, 25 dihydroxycholecalciferol and prostaglandin E2 on orthodontic tooth movement. American Journal of Orthodontics and Dentofacial Orthopedics. 2004;**125**(5):607-614

[15] Yamasaki K, Shibata Y, Imai S, Tani Y, Shibasaki Y, Fukuhara T. Clinical application of prostaglandin E1 (PGE1) upon orthodontic tooth movement. American Journal of Orthodontics. 1984;**85**(6):508-518

[16] Walsh LJ, Wong CA, Pringle M, Tattersfield AE. Use of oral corticosteroids in the community and the prevention of secondary osteoporosis: A cross sectional study. British Medical Journal. 1996;**313**(7053):344-346

[17] Angeli A, Dovio A, Sartori ML, Masera RG, Ceoloni B, Prolo P, et al. Interactions between glucocorticoids and cytokines in the bone microenvironment. Annals of the New York Academy of Sciences. 2002;**966**(1):97-107

[18] Ashcraft MB, Southard KA, Tolley EA. The effect of corticosteroid-induced osteoporosis on orthodontic tooth movement. American Journal of Orthodontics and Dentofacial Orthopedics. 1992;**102**(4):310-319

[19] Ong CK, Walsh LJ, Harbrow D, Taverne AA, Symons AL. Orthodontic tooth movement in the prednisolone-treated rat. The Angle Orthodontist. 2000;**70**(2):118-125

[20] Shinoda Y, Kawaguchi H, Higashikawa A, Hirata M, Miura T, Saito T, et al. Mechanisms underlying catabolic and anabolic functions of parathyroid hormone on bone by combination of culture systems of mouse cells. Journal of Cellular Biochemistry. 2010;**109**:755-763

[21] Gianelly AA. Force-induced changes in the vascularity of the periodontal ligament. American Journal of Orthodontics. 1969;**55**(1):5-11

[22] Goldie RS, King GJ. Root resorption and tooth movement in orthodontically treated, calcium-deficient, and lactating rats. American Journal of Orthodontics. 1984;**85**(5):424-430

[23] Collins MK, Sinclair PM. The local use of vitamin D to increase the rate of orthodontic tooth movement. American Journal of Orthodontics and Dentofacial Orthopedics. 1988;**94**(4):278-284

[24] Takano-Yamamoto T, Kawakami M, Yamashiro T. Effect of age on the rate of tooth movement in combination with local use of 1, 25 (OH) 2D3 and mechanical force in the rat. Journal of Dental Research. 1992;**71**(8):1487-1492

[25] Tsao Y-T, Huang Y-J, Wu H-H, Liu Y-A, Liu Y-S, Lee OK. Osteocalcin mediates biomineralization during osteogenic maturation in human mesenchymal stromal cells. International Journal of Molecular Sciences. 2017;**18**(1):159. DOI: 10.3390/ijms18010159

[26] Hashimoto F, Kobayashi Y, Mataki S, Kobayashi K, Kato Y, Sakai H. Administration of osteocalcin accelerates orthodontic tooth movement induced by a closed coil spring in rats. The European Journal of Orthodontics. 2001;**23**(5):535-545

[27] Brennan P, Thomas G, Langdon J. The role of nitric oxide in oral diseases. Archives of Oral Biology. 2003;**48**(2):93-100.120

[28] Shirazi M, Nilforoushan D, Alghasi H, Dehpour A-R. The role of nitric oxide in orthodontic tooth movement in rats. The Angle Orthodontist. 2002;**72**(3):211-215

[29] Akin E, Gurton AU, Olmez H. Effects of nitric oxide in orthodontic tooth movement in rats. American Journal of Orthodontics and Dentofacial Orthopedics. 2004;**126**(5):608-614

[30] Liou EJ. The development of submucosal injection of platelet rich plasma for accelerating orthodontic tooth movement and preserving pressure side alveolar bone. APOS Trends in Orthodontics. 2016;**6**(1):5

[31] Gulec A, Bakkalbasi BÇ, Cumbul A, Uslu U, Alev B, Yarat A. Effects of local platelet-rich plasma injection on the rate of orthodontic tooth movement in a rat model: A histomorphometric study. American Journal of Orthodontics and Dentofacial Orthopedics. 2017;**151**(1): 92-104

[32] Rashid A, ElSharaby F, Nassef E, Mehanni S, Mostafa Y. Effect of platelet-rich plasma on orthodontic tooth movement in dogs. Orthodontics & Craniofacial Research. 2017;**20**(2): 102-110

[33] Nemtoi A, Sirghe A, Nemtoi A, Haba D. The Effect of a Plasma With Platelet-rich Fibrin in Bone Regeneration and on Rate of Orthodontic Tooth Movement in Adolescents. Revista de Chimie. 2018;**69**(12):3727-3730

[34] Tehranchi A, Behnia H, Pourdanesh F, Behnia P, Pinto N, Younessian F. The effect of autologous leukocyte platelet rich fibrin on the rate of orthodontic tooth movement: A prospective randomized clinical trial. European Journal of Dentistry. 2018;**12**(3):350

[35] Kocyigit I, Tunali M, Ozdemir H, Kartal Y, Suer B. Clinical application of second generation trombosite concentration. Cumhuriyet Dental Journal. 2012;**15**(3):279-287

[36] Paoloni J, De Vos RJ, Hamilton B, Murrell GA, Orchard J. Platelet-rich plasma treatment for ligament and tendon injuries. Clinical Journal of Sport Medicine. 2011;**21**(1):37-45

[37] Yuan X, Luo S, Shen G. Experimental study on selecting optimal time of orthodontic tooth movement into extraction sites. Hua xi kou qiang yi xue za zhi= Huaxi kouqiang yixue zazhi=. West China Journal of Stomatology. 2003;**21**(4):311-313

[38] Gurbuzer B, Pikdoken L, Tunali M, Urhan M, Kucukodaci Z, Ercan F. Scintigraphic evaluation of osteoblastic activity in extraction sockets treated with platelet-rich fibrin. Journal of Oral and Maxillofacial Surgery. 2010;**68**(5): 980-989

[39] M Dohan Ehrenfest D, Bielecki T, Jimbo R, Barbe G, Del Corso M, Inchingolo F, et al. Do the fibrin architecture and leukocyte content influence the growth factor release of platelet concentrates? An evidence-based answer comparing a pure platelet-rich plasma (P-PRP) gel and a leukocyte-and platelet-rich fibrin (L-PRF). Current Pharmaceutical Biotechnology. 2012;**13**(7):1145-1152

[40] Graziani F, Ivanovski S, Cei S, Ducci F, Tonetti M, Gabriele M. The in vitro effect of different PRP concentrations on osteoblasts and fibroblasts. Clinical Oral Implants Research. 2006;**17**(2):212-219

[41] Peerbooms JC, Colaris JW, Hakkert AA, Van Appeldorn M, Bruijn DJ, Den Oudsten BL, et al. No positive bone healing after using platelet rich plasma in a skeletal defect. An observational prospective cohort study. International Orthopaedics. 2012;**36**(10): 2113-2119

[42] Krishtab S, Doroshenko S, Liutik G. Use of vibratory action on the teeth to accelerate orthodontic treatment. Stomatologiia. 1986;**65**(3):61-63

[43] Ohmae M, Saito S, Morohashi T, Qu H, Seki K, Kurabayashi H.

Biomechanical acceleration of experimental tooth movement by ultrasonic vibration in vivo—part 1. Homo-directional application of ultrasonication to orthodontic force. Orthodontic Waves. 2001;**60**:201-212

[44] Nishimura M, Chiba M, Ohashi T, Sato M, Shimizu Y, Igarashi K, et al. Periodontal tissue activation by vibration: intermittent stimulation by resonance vibration accelerates experimental tooth movement in rats. American Journal of Orthodontics and Dentofacial Orthopedics. 2008;**133**(4):572-583

[45] Kau CH, Nguyen JT, English J. The clinical evaluation of a novel cyclical force generating device in orthodontics. Orthodontic Practice US. 2010;**1**(1): 10-15

[46] Davidovitch Z, Finkelson MD, Steigman S, Shanfeld JL, Montgomery PC, Korostoff E. Electric currents, bone remodeling, and orthodontic tooth movement: II. Increase in rate of tooth movement and periodontal cyclic nucleotide levels by combined force and electric current. American Journal of Orthodontics. 1980;**77**(1):33-47

[47] Darendeliler MA, Sinclair PM, Kusy RP. The effects of samarium-cobalt magnets and pulsed electromagnetic fields on tooth movement. American Journal of Orthodontics and Dentofacial Orthopedics. 1995;**107**(6):578-588

[48] Stark TM, Sinclair PM. Effect of pulsed electromagnetic fields on orthodontic tooth movement. American Journal of Orthodontics and Dentofacial Orthopedics. 1987;**91**(2):91-104

[49] Graber T. Magnets and impacted canines. In: Northcroft Memorial Lecture. British Society for the Study of Orthodontics: Manchester, UK; 1989

[50] Cernavin I, Pugatschew A, de Boer N, Tyas MJ. Laser applications in dentistry: a review of the literature. Australian Dental Journal. 1994;**39**(1): 28-32

[51] Nimeri G, Kau CH, Abou-Kheir NS, Corona R. Acceleration of tooth movement during orthodontic treatment-a frontier in orthodontics. Progress in Orthodontics. 2013;**14**(1):42

[52] Eells JT, Wong-Riley MT, VerHoeve J, Henry M, Buchman EV, Kane MP, et al. Mitochondrial signal transduction in accelerated wound and retinal healing by near-infrared light therapy. Mitochondrion. 2004;**4**(5-6): 559-567

[53] Fujita S, Yamaguchi M, Utsunomiya T, Yamamoto H, Kasai K. Low-energy laser stimulates tooth movement velocity via expression of RANK and RANKL. Orthodontics & Craniofacial Research. 2008;**11**(3): 143-155

[54] Kawasaki K, Shimizu N. Effects of low-energy laser irradiation on bone remodeling during experimental tooth movement in rats. Lasers in Surgery and Medicine: The Official Journal of the American Society for Laser Medicine and Surgery. 2000;**26**(3):282-291

[55] Cruz DR, Kohara EK, Ribeiro MS, Wetter NU. Effects of low-intensity laser therapy on the orthodontic movement velocity of human teeth: A preliminary study. Lasers in Surgery and 118 Medicine: The Official Journal of the American Society for Laser Medicine and. Surgery. 2004;**35**(2):117-120

[56] Yamaguchi M, Fujita S, Yoshida T, Oikawa K, Utsunomiya T, Yamamoto H, et al. Low-energy laser irradiation stimulates the tooth movement velocity

via expression of M-CSF and c-fms. Orthodontic Waves. 2007;**66**(4):139-148

[57] Lee W, Karapetyan G, Moats R, Yamashita D-D, Moon H-B, Ferguson D, et al. Corticotomy−/osteotomy-assisted tooth movement microCTs differ. Journal of Dental Research. 2008;**87**(9):861-867

[58] Wang L, Lee W, Lei D-l, Liu Y-p, Yamashita D-D, Yen SL-K. Tissue responses in corticotomy-and osteotomy-assisted tooth movements in rats: histology and immunostaining. American Journal of Orthodontics and Dentofacial Orthopedics. 2009;**136**(6): 770. e1-770.e11

[59] Sirisha K, Srinivas M, Ravindranath D. Wilckodontics-A Novel Synergy in Time to Save Time. Journal of Clinical and Diagnostic Research: JCDR. 2014;**8**(1):322

[60] Kole H. Surgical operations on the alveolar ridge to correct occlusal abnormalities. Oral Surgery, Oral Medicine. Oral Pathology. 1959;**12**(5): 515-529

[61] Frost HM. The regional acceleratory phenomenon: a review. Henry Ford Hospital Medical Journal. 1983;**31**(1): 3-9 Review

[62] Wilcko WM, Wilcko T, Bouquot JE, Ferguson DJ. Rapid orthodontics with alveolar reshaping: two case reports of decrowding. The International Journal of Periodontics & Restorative Dentistry. 2001;**21**(1):9-19

[63] Wilcko MT, Wilcko WM, Pulver JJ, Bissada NF, Bouquot JE. Accelerated Osteogenic Orthodontics Technique: A 1-Stage Surgically Facilitated Rapid Orthodontic Technique With Alveolar Augmentation. Journal of Oral and Maxillofacial Surgery. 2009;**67**(10): 2149-2159

[64] Chung K. Text Book of Speedy Orthodontics. Jeesung: J Seoul; 2001

[65] Chung K, Kim S, Kook Y. Speedy surgical orthodontic treatment with skeletal anchorage in adults. In: Distraction Osteogenesis of the Facial Bones. BC Decker: Hamilton, Ontario, Canada; 2006. pp. 167-186

[66] Liou EJ, Huang CS. Rapid canine retraction through distraction of the periodontal ligament. American Journal of Orthodontics and Dentofacial Orthopedics. 1998;**114**(4):372-382

[67] Sukurica Y, Karaman A, Gurel HG, Dolanmaz D. Rapid canine distalization through segmental alveolar distraction osteogenesis. The Angle Orthodontist. 2007;**77**(2):226-236

[68] Kisnisci RS, Iseri H, Tuz HH, Altug AT. Dentoalveolar distraction osteogenesis for rapid orthodontic canine retraction. Journal of Oral and Maxillofacial Surgery. 2002;**60**(4): 389-394

[69] Iseri H, Kisnisci R, Bzizi N, Tuz H. Rapid canine retraction and orthodontic treatment with dentoalveolar distraction osteogenesis. American Journal of Orthodontics and Dentofacial Orthopedics. 2005;**127**(5):533-541

[70] Alikhani M, Raptis M, Zoldan B, Sangsuwon C, Lee YB, Alyami B, et al. Effect of micro-osteoperforations on the rate of tooth movement. American Journal of Orthodontics and Dentofacial Orthopedics. 2013;**144**(5):639-648

[71] Keser EI, Dibart S. Sequential piezocision: a novel approach to accelerated orthodontic treatment. American Journal of Orthodontics and Dentofacial Orthopedics. 2013;**144**(6): 879-889

[72] Vercellotti T, Podesta A. Orthodontic microsurgery: a new surgically guided technique for dental movement. The International Journal of Periodontics & Restorative Dentistry. 2007;**27**:4

[73] Kim S-J, Park Y-G, Kang S-G. Effects of corticision on paradental remodeling in orthodontic tooth movement. The Angle Orthodontist. 2009;**79**(2):284-291

[74] Dibart S, Sebaoun J, Surmenian J. Piezocision: a minimally invasive, periodontally accelerated orthodontic tooth movement procedure. Compendium of Continuing Education in Dentistry (Jamesburg, NJ: 1995). 2009;**30**(6) 342-4, 6, 8-50

[75] Dibart S, Keser E, Nelson D. Piezocision™-assisted orthodontics: Past, present, and future. Seminars in Orthodontics. 2015; **21**(3):170-175

[76] Dibart S, Yee C, Surmenian J, Sebaoun JD, Baloul S, Goguet-Surmenian E, et al. Tissue response during Piezocision-assisted tooth movement: a histological study in rats. European Journal of Orthodontics. 2013;**36**(4):457-464

[77] Aksakalli S, Calik B, Kara B, Ezirganli S. Accelerated tooth movement with piezocision and its periodontal-transversal effects in patients with Class II malocclusion. The Angle Orthodontist. 2015;**86**(1):59-65

[78] Ileri Z, Akin M, Erdur EA, Dagi HT, Findik D. Bacteremia after piezocision. American Journal of Orthodontics and Dentofacial Orthopedics. 2014;**146**(4): 430-436

[79] Schaeren S, Jaquiéry C, Heberer M, Tolnay M, Vercellotti T, Martin I. Assessment of nerve damage using a novel ultrasonic device for bone cutting. Journal of Oral and Maxillofacial Surgery. 2008;**66**:593-596

[80] Torrella F, Pitarch J, Cabanes G, Anitua E. Ultrasonic ostectomy for the surgical approach of the maxillary sinus: a technical note. The International Journal of Oral & Maxillofacial Implants. 1998;**13**:1

[81] Pavlíková G, Foltán R, Horká M, Hanzelka T, Borunská H, Šedý J. Piezosurgery in oral and maxillofacial surgery. International Journal of Oral and Maxillofacial Surgery. 2011;**40**: 451-457

[82] Sohn D-S, Ahn M-R, Lee W-H, Yeo D-S, Lim S-Y. Piezoelectric osteotomy for intraoral harvesting of bone blocks. The International Journal of Periodontics & Restorative Dentistry. 2007;**27**:127

[83] Walsh LJ. Piezosurgery: an increasing role in dental hard tissue surgery. Australasian Dental Practice. 2007;**18**:52-56

[84] Robiony M, Polini F, Costa F, Zerman N, Politi M. Ultrasonic bone cutting for surgically assisted rapid maxillary expansion (SARME) under local anaesthesia. International Journal of Oral and Maxillofacial Surgery. 2007;**36**:267-269

Chapter 4

Short Root Anomaly in a Hispanic Population: Risk for Orthodontic Root Resorption

Tara Emerick, Maria Grace Viana and Carla A. Evans

Abstract

While the presentation of Short Root Anomaly (SRA) in Hispanic patients has been described previously, it is not known if this population is predisposed to increased orthodontic root resorption. This study evaluates the response of pre-existing short roots in Hispanic SRA patients to orthodontic treatment. Selected maxillary and mandibular teeth of 40 Hispanic SRA patients (19 male, 21 female) and 40 age and gender matched Caucasian patients (19 male, 21 female) with normal root length were evaluated for root resorption following comprehensive orthodontic treatment. The age range of the subjects was between 10 and 19 years. Relative root length was calculated before and after orthodontic treatment from digital panoramic radiographs. Overall, statistically significant root resorption occurred in the control group, but orthodontic root resorption was not significant in the Hispanic group ($p > 0.05$). When genders were separated, Hispanic females did experience a mild degree of root resorption in the upper incisors while resorption in Hispanic males was not significant. Caucasian females experienced greater root resorption than Caucasian males. Hispanic SRA patients may be safely treated with comprehensive orthodontics and could be at no more risk of root resorption than Caucasian patients with normal initial root length.

Keywords: orthodontics, short root anomaly, root resorption, Hispanics

1. Introduction

There are two main causes of short dental roots: 1) disturbances during root development or 2) resorption of well-developed roots. Developmentally short-rooted permanent teeth can be genetic, known as short root anomaly (SRA) [1, 2], or exogenous, including irradiation of the head and neck and/or chemotherapy in childhood during tooth development [3]. Resorption of dental roots as a result of orthodontic treatment is termed Orthodontically Induced Inflammatory Root Resorption (OIIRR) and is believed to result from a combination of genetics, environmental, and mechanical factors. Puranik et al. [4] identified a population of Hispanic orthodontic patients presenting with SRA. Although the Hispanic population only comprises 17.8% of the U.S. population, it is the largest minority ethnicity with 57.5 million people and continues to grow [5].

In cases of pre-existing short root length (**Figure 1**), orthodontists should be aware if greater root resorption is anticipated as normal orthodontic treatment could sentence these teeth to exfoliation or extraction. Short dental roots may complicate dental treatment planning when considering anchorage or estimating the ability of a tooth to carry masticatory forces. Two recent publications proposed such potential hazards, but did not supply clinical evidence [6, 7]. This is the first study, to the authors' knowledge, that has investigated the response of dental roots to orthodontic treatment in a Hispanic SRA population.

Root resorption is a common side effect of orthodontic treatment and is estimated to occur in 73% of orthodontically treated cases [8]. Luckily, in the majority of cases, resorption is classified as mild to moderate [9] and is clinically insignificant. While some studies have found females to experience more resorption [10], others report that gender is unlikely to have an effect on root resorption [11].

Short-root anomaly (SRA) is a developmental phenomenon in which permanent teeth never reach their normal length and appear very short and blunted [2]. Lind [1] first described SRA in 1972 as "abnormally short roots of a characteristically plump shape affecting maxillary central incisors primarily." It is considered to be familial [1] and prior to Lind, SRA was commonly misdiagnosed as root resorption. Interestingly, multiple studies have suggested a primarily autosomal dominant inheritance pattern. In a recent study by Puranik et al. [4], SRA was found to occur more frequently in Latino individuals with the majority having localized SRA and the minority having generalized SRA, in which every tooth in the mouth is affected [4].

Some studies have found that patients with short or blunted roots prior to treatment, undergo significantly more root shortening during orthodontic treatment than patients with no dental anomaly [12–14], while others have found a minor or non-significant relationship between blunted roots and root resorption with orthodontic treatment [2, 15, 16] and still others report that blunted teeth experience less resorption than normal-shaped teeth [11].

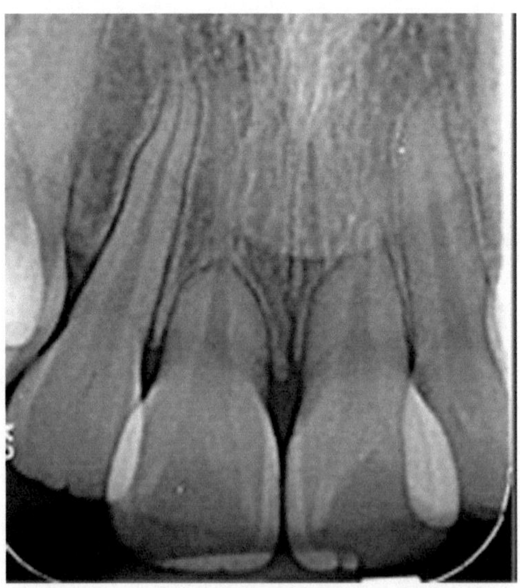

Figure 1.
Periapical radiograph showing an example of maxillary incisors in a Hispanic female subject with localized SRA before starting orthodontic treatment.

Some authors believe that this is due to a change in the position of the tooth's center of resistance, moving it more incisally. Studies that looked specifically at "pipette-shaped" roots, rather than blunted, consistently found greater root resorption [11]. Correlations have also been found between initial tooth length and the amount of resorption (i.e., a longer root was more likely to be resorbed with orthodontic treatment) [11, 17]. Mirabella and Artun [17] argued that teeth with longer roots require stronger orthodontic forces to move them; furthermore, the displacement of the root apex is greater during tipping and torquing movements of longer rooted teeth.

The objective of this study was to assess changes in root lengths that occur with orthodontic treatment by comparing: 1. pre-and post-treatment digital panoramic radiographs of Hispanic patients presenting with short dental root lengths; 2. the experience of Hispanic patients and Caucasian patients presenting with normal dental root lengths; and 3. gender differences within each ethnicity group.

2. Comparison of treatment outcomes

2.1 Material and methods

This was a retrospective study that included male and female Hispanic and Caucasian patients in a university orthodontic clinic. Dental records of 40 Hispanic SRA and 40 Caucasian patients were collected. In this clinic, most of the Hispanic patients are of Mexican heritage. The Hispanic group consisted of 19 male and 21 female adolescent patients and the Caucasian group consisted of 19 male and 21 female adolescent patients. The mean age of subjects was 14.7 + 1.91 years in the Caucasian group and 13.9 + 1.86 years in the Hispanic group. All pre-existing records were taken at the orthodontic clinic for comprehensive orthodontic treatment. All radiographs were taken in the Radiology Clinic. Panoramic radiographs were taken on a standard combined panoramic/cephalometric machine. All radiographs were consistent with the standard of care for all orthodontic patients in the clinic and included pre- and post-treatment panoramic radiographs. For every extraction case in the Hispanic group, an extraction case in the Caucasian group was included. All subjects were de-identified and assigned a coded number. Only the sex, ethnicity, and age in years and months at the start of treatment were retrieved from the patient chart. All subjects with developmental disorders or complicated medical histories were excluded. Individual teeth were excluded if 1) the apex was not closed, 2) the reference points were not clearly visible, 3) there was a history of dental trauma, root canal therapy, orthodontics, or an incisal or full-coverage restoration, 4) attrition or abrasion of the crown was present. In this study generalized and localized SRA patients were grouped together even though their pathogenesis may differ. IRB exemption was granted prior to data collection.

Root lengths were measured on maxillary and mandibular central and lateral incisors, and second premolars, from the apex to the midpoint of the cementoenamel junction (CEJ) on panoramic radiographs. The aforementioned teeth were selected because they are single-rooted teeth (with the exception of the variation in upper second premolar) and the root outline of these teeth can be more clearly visible on radiographs than multi-rooted teeth. Furthermore, SRA in a Mexican cohort most commonly occurred in maxillary central incisors and mandibular second premolars [4]. It is assumed that during orthodontic treatment, the crown length does not change. Therefore, the ratio between the root and crown length should reflect any changes in root length. Crown and root lengths were measured on panoramic radiographs using the Dolphin™ digital caliper (Dolphin Imaging 11.8, Chatsworth, CA).

The Lind method of relative root length calculation was used [1] in which the midpoint of the mesial and distal CEJ (median CEJ) is used to demarcate the transition from crown to root. Root length was measured from the median CEJ (point M) to the tip of the root (point R). Crown length was measured from point M to the incisal edge or tip (point I). Relative root length was calculated by dividing point M to point R length by point I to point M length [1]. Root length guidelines set by Holtta et al. [3] were used in the measurements of all panoramic radiographs.

Statistical analysis was done using IBM SPSS Statistics for Windows (version 22.0, IBM Corp., Armonk NY). Analyses were performed by the Explore function in SPSS to check the raw data distribution by Shapiro–Wilk Tests of Normality. Parametric tests were done based on the results that the majority of the variables showed normal distribution of the data. Student Paired Sample *t*-tests were used to assess the mean differences between pre and post measurements of all the variables in each of the Hispanic and Caucasian groups with the sample gender in consideration. Independent *t*-tests were done for the mean comparisons to all study variables between groups. All values were considered statistically significant for a value of $p<0.05$.

2.2 Results

The Caucasian group had a statistically significant differences between pre-orthodontic treatment and post-orthodontic treatment relative root lengths (**Table 1**). The post-orthodontic treatment relative root lengths (1.87 ± 0.30) were significantly less than the initial relative root lengths (2.10 ± 0.29), indicating root resorption

Group	Caucasian pre-orthodontic treatment Group (N = 40)		Caucasian post-orthodontic treatment Group (N = 40)		p-value
Tooth	Mean	S.D.	Mean	S.D.	
UR5	1.89	0.27	1.69	0.33	.005*
UR2	2.24	0.27	1.90	0.40	.000*
UR1	2.01	0.29	1.68	0.31	.000*
UL1	2.06	0.27	1.64	0.29	.000*
UL2	2.19	0.30	1.82	0.32	.000*
UL5	1.96	0.30	1.71	0.26	.000*
LL5	2.29	0.28	2.11	0.25	.000*
LL2	2.10	0.42	2.03	0.28	.387
LL1	2.09	0.28	2.06	0.24	.613
LR1	2.12	0.31	1.99	0.29	.048*
LR2	2.06	0.32	1.93	0.27	.038*
LR5	2.13	0.24	1.95	0.47	.026*

**Statistically significant at $p < 0.05$.*

Table 1.
Mean comparison of pre-orthodontic relative root lengths and post-orthodontic treatment relative root lengths in the Caucasian group.

from the orthodontic treatment in the Caucasian group. The only measurements that did not show statistical significance were the lower left lateral and lower left central incisors.

Overall, there was only a mild difference between Hispanic initial relative root lengths (1.57 ± 0.27) and Hispanic post-orthodontic treatment relative root lengths (1.55 ± 0.29) (**Table 2**). Significant root resorption was seen in five teeth: UR2, UR1, UL1, LR1 and LR2. Differences were also seen in the mandibular left second premolars which increased in relative root length after orthodontic treatment. Furthermore, the percentage decrease in relative root length was consistently higher in the Caucasian group (**Tables 1** and **2**).

Genders were separated and post-treatment relative root lengths were compared against pre-treatment relative root lengths in order to further evaluate any significant root resorption that occurred with orthodontic treatment. There was no difference in post-orthodontic treatment relative root length when sexes were compared within the Hispanic group. However, there was a difference between males and females in post-orthodontic treatment relative root length with Caucasian females (1.80 ± 0.28) experiencing a smaller post-orthodontic treatment relative root lengths than Caucasian males (1.95 ± 0.31). Statistically significant differences in post-orthodontic treatment relative root length were found in four teeth when Caucasian male and Caucasian female groups were compared (**Tables 3** and **4**). Specifically, the relative root lengths of UR1, UL1, LL2, and LL1 were found to be significantly less in the Caucasian female group than the Caucasian male group. Because there was no statistically significant gender difference in pre-orthodontic treatment root lengths in the Caucasian group, this finding suggests that Caucasian females experienced more root resorption from the orthodontic treatment than Caucasian males.

Group	Hispanic pre-orthodontic treatment Group		Hispanic post-orthodontic treatment Group		p-value
	(N = 40)		(N = 40)		
Tooth	Mean	S.D.	Mean	S.D.	
UR5	1.31	0.25	1.43	0.29	.009*
UR2	1.83	0.25	1.65	0.22	.002*
UR1	1.34	0.34	1.22	0.33	.009*
UL1	1.32	0.30	1.13	0.30	.000*
UL2	1.74	0.29	1.66	0.27	.070
UL5	1.31	0.20	1.50	0.35	.001*
LL5	1.56	0.34	1.68	0.38	.008*
LL2	1.83	0.20	1.82	0.20	.712
LL1	1.70	0.35	1.68	0.30	.581
LR1	1.72	0.23	1.64	0.24	.048*
LR2	1.78	0.27	1.68	0.18	.031*
LR5	1.52	0.25	1.54	0.41	.830

**Statistically significant at $p < 0.05$.*

Table 2.
Mean comparison of the pre-orthodontic relative root lengths and post-orthodontic treatment relative root lengths in the Hispanic group.

Group	CM pre-orthodontic treatment Group		CM post-orthodontic treatment Group		p-value
	(N = 40)		(N = 40)		
Tooth	**Mean**	**S.D.**	**Mean**	**S.D.**	
UR5	1.79	0.21	1.67	0.35	.252
UR2	2.31	0.30	1.99	0.41	.000*
UR1	2.01	0.29	1.79	0.36	.000*
UL1	2.07	0.31	1.75	0.33	.000*
UL2	2.24	0.30	1.91	0.37	.006*
UL5	1.89	0.33	1.78	0.26	.192
LL5	2.27	0.25	2.13	0.23	.036*
LL2	2.02	0.46	2.12	0.32	.432
LL1	2.01	0.24	2.13	0.24	.119
LR1	2.11	0.28	2.04	0.35	.387
LR2	1.99	0.31	2.01	0.30	.889
LR5	2.01	0.19	2.01	0.31	.937

Statistically significant at $p < 0.05$.

Table 3.
Mean comparison of pre-orthodontic relative root lengths and post-orthodontic treatment relative root lengths in the Caucasian male (CM) group.

Group	CF pre-orthodontic treatment Group		CF post-orthodontic treatment Group		p-value
	(N = 40)		(N = 40)		
Tooth	**Mean**	**S.D.**	**Mean**	**S.D.**	
UR5	2.00	0.28	1.71	0.32	.005*
UR2	2.17	0.24	1.82	0.39	.001*
UR1	2.01	0.29	1.58	0.23	.000*
UL1	2.04	0.24	1.55	0.21	.000*
UL2	2.15	0.30	1.74	0.26	.000*
UL5	2.02	0.27	1.64	0.24	.000*
LL5	2.31	0.31	2.09	0.28	.004*
LL2	2.18	0.36	1.93	0.21	.016*
LL1	2.16	0.29	1.99	0.22	.102
LR1	2.13	0.33	1.94	0.22	.077
LR2	2.11	0.32	1.86	0.24	.005*
LR5	2.24	0.23	1.91	0.57	.013*

Statistically significant at $p < 0.05$.

Table 4.
Mean comparison of pre-orthodontic relative root lengths and post-orthodontic treatment relative root lengths in the Caucasian female (CF) group.

In the Caucasian male group, significance was found in five teeth: UR2, UR1, UL1, UL2, LL5 (**Table 3**). In all five teeth, the final was smaller than the initial, indicating that these teeth did in fact experience statistically significant orthodontic root resorption.

Significance between pre and post-treatment relative root length was found for nearly every tooth in the Caucasian female group: UR5, UR2, UR1, UL1, UL2, UL5, LL5, LL2, LR2, LR5 (**Table 4**). All teeth showed decreased relative root lengths post-treatment, suggesting significant root resorption from the orthodontic treatment. The only teeth that did not show a significant difference between pre and post were the two lower central incisors: the post-treatment mean relative lengths for these teeth were still smaller than the pre-treatment.

When post-treatment relative root lengths were compared to pre-treatment root lengths in Hispanic males, three teeth showed a significant difference: UR5, UL5, and LL5 (**Table 5**). However, the mean relative root lengths showed that these root lengths increased in apparent length after treatment.

Significance was found for five teeth in the Hispanic Female group: UR2, UR1, UL1, UL5, LR2 (**Table 6**). While there does appear to be mild root resorption from orthodontic treatment in UR2, UR1, UL1, and LR2; the mean relative root length for UL5 is increased in the post group, suggesting an increase in relative root length with orthodontic treatment.

2.3 Discussion

There have been many claims that SRA predisposes patients to increased orthodontic root resorption, for example the study of Wang and Feng [6]. However, it is not

Group	HM pre-orthodontic treatment Group (N = 40)		HM post-orthodontic treatment Group (N = 40)		p-value
Tooth	Mean	S.D.	Mean	S.D	
UR5	1.31	0.27	1.49	0.24	.007*
UR2	1.87	0.21	1.72	0.18	.064
UR1	1.35	0.36	1.29	0.27	.444
UL1	1.36	0.33	1.24	0.26	.067
UL2	1.73	0.25	1.68	0.30	.445
UL5	1.36	0.18	1.54	0.28	.013*
LL5	1.52	0.34	1.73	0.44	.009*
LL2	1.78	0.22	1.78	0.19	1.000
LL1	1.68	0.38	1.65	0.32	.697
LR1	1.71	0.21	1.65	0.29	.276
LR2	1.69	0.20	1.66	0.20	.656
LR5	1.49	0.27	1.52	0.33	.728

**Statistically significant at $p < 0.05$.*

Table 5.
Mean comparison of pre-orthodontic relative root lengths and post-orthodontic treatment relative root lengths in the Hispanic male (HM) group.

Group	HF pre-orthodontic treatment Group (N = 40)		HF post-orthodontic treatment Group (N = 40)		p-value
Tooth	Mean	S.D.	Mean	S.D	
UR5	1.31	0.24	1.38	0.33	.305
UR2	1.78	0.29	1.58	0.24	.018*
UR1	1.34	0.34	1.18	0.36	.002*
UL1	1.28	0.28	1.05	0.30	.000*
UL2	1.74	0.33	1.64	0.24	.069
UL5	1.28	0.22	1.47	0.41	.018*
LL5	1.59	0.34	1.63	0.31	.392
LL2	1.89	0.16	1.86	0.21	.673
LL1	1.73	0.32	1.70	0.29	.709
LR1	1.72	0.26	1.64	0.19	.092
LR2	1.88	0.29	1.71	0.15	.013*
LR5	1.55	0.24	1.55	0.49	.962

**Statistically significant at $p < 0.05$.*

Table 6.
Mean comparison of pre-orthodontic relative root lengths and post-orthodontic treatment relative root lengths in the Hispanic female (HF) group.

known if this cohort indeed experiences a higher degree of orthodontic root resorption, or if they experience a similar degree of resorption to unaffected patients, but the appearance is more suggestive due to their pre-existing short roots. If a greater degree of relative root loss does occur, the orthodontic professional should be aware so that treatment complications can be anticipated when treating Hispanic SRA patients.

Post-orthodontic treatment relative root lengths were significantly smaller than the initial relative root lengths for the Caucasian group, indicating root resorption from the orthodontic treatment. Hispanic initial relative root lengths and Hispanic post-orthodontic treatment relative root lengths were similiar. Furthermore, the percentage decrease in relative root length was consistently higher in the Caucasian group, further supporting the finding that the Caucasian subjects experienced OIIRR while the Hispanic subjects had minimal, if any. Because the treating orthodontists in this study were aware of the pre-existing short roots in the Hispanic SRA group, it is likely that these patients were treated more conservatively, with lower forces, and with greater care. Studies have also speculated that shorter roots may experience less root resorption due to 1) shorter teeth requiring less force to move and 2) the root tip being displaced a shorter distance through the bone in second and third-order tipping motions [18, 19].

In the Caucasian male group, the maxillary incisors experienced statistically significant orthodontic root resorption. This finding agrees with the literature as the upper incisors are commonly the most affected teeth in orthodontic root resorption. However, in the Caucasian female group, root resorption was found in nearly every tooth measured and to a greater extent. There was no statistically significant root resorption found in the Hispanic male group. Conversely, statistically significant root resorption was found for four teeth in the Hispanic female group: UR2, UR1, UL1, and LR2 but the percentage decrease in relative root length was still mild in comparison to the degree of root resorption that both Caucasian groups (male and female) experienced. These findings that females experience greater OIIRR than males agree with other findings in the literature [10, 20].

Most teeth were bilaterally affected; however, resorption of the mandibular second premolar was the tooth that most commonly presented unilaterally. One of the limitations of this study was the assessment of closed apices in the SRA group. SRA roots are characterized by wide pulp chambers and truncated roots which is very similar in appearance to roots that are still undergoing development. Some of the second premolar measurements displayed slightly longer final root lengths than initial. Explanations for this finding are 1) some form of error in measurement, or 2) the second premolar root lengths were measured in the Hispanic group prior to cessation of root development.

Future studies are needed to complete a more detailed analysis regarding the nature of the genetic inheritance and prevalence of the SRA condition in the Hispanic population. In this study, Hispanic SRA patients were found to comprise approximately 2% of the total patient population treated in the university orthodontic clinic. A point of interest would include the geographic origins within Mexico and inheritance patterns of SRA Hispanic patients. Also, while there is much speculation regarding the etiology of SRA, the developmental process resulting in the SRA condition has yet to be determined. It is also not known whether the mechanism is the same across all subgroups of SRA.

3. Conclusions

The following conclusions were obtained from this study:

1. While OIIRR occurred in the Caucasian group, the Hispanic SRA group did not experience statistically significant root resorption from the orthodontic treatment when all teeth were combined. However, when individual teeth were evaluated, the Hispanic SRA group did experience OIIRR, but to a lesser degree than the Caucasian group.

2. Females were found to experience greater root resorption than males in both ethnicities. While Hispanic females experienced slightly greater root resorption in the upper incisors than Hispanic males, Caucasian females were found to experience much greater OIIRR than Caucasian males.

The observations of this study suggest that Hispanic SRA patients may be safely treated with comprehensive orthodontics and could be at no more risk of root resorption than Caucasian patients with normal pre-treatment root length. Clinicians are still advised to treat Hispanic SRA patients conservatively. Although more studies are needed, these findings can be considered when making educated treatment decisions for this specialized population of orthodontic patients. To the authors' knowledge, this is the first study to evaluate the response of Hispanic patients with SRA to orthodontic treatment.

Acknowledgements

The authors gratefully acknowledge substantive discussions with Drs. Chester Handelman and Ahmed Masoud.

Conflict of interest

The authors declare no conflict of interest.

Author details

Tara Emerick[1], Maria Grace Viana[2] and Carla A. Evans[3]*

1 Private Practice, Carmel, Indiana, USA

2 Department of Orthodontics, College of Dentistry, University of Illinois at Chicago, Chicago, IL, USA

3 Department of Orthodontics, Boston University, Boston, MA, USA

*Address all correspondence to: caevans@bu.edu

References

[1] Lind V. Short root anomaly. Scand J Dent Res 1972;80:85-93.

[2] Apajalahti S, Arte S, Pirinen S. Short root anomaly in families and its association with other dental anomalies. Eur J Oral Sci 1999;107:97-101.

[3] Holtta P, Nystrom M, Evalahti M, Alaluusua S. Root-crown ratios of permanent teeth in a healthy finnish population assessed from panoramic radiographs. Eur J Orthod 2004;26: 491-497.

[4] Puranik C, Hill A, Henderson Jeffries K, Harrell S, Taylor R, Frazier-Bowers S: Characterization of short root anomaly in a Mexican cohort – Heredity idiopathic root malformation. Orthod Craniofac Res 2015;18:62-70.

[5] US Census Bureau: census.gov/quickfacts/fact/table/US/PST045216. Accessed 18 Aug. 2017.

[6] Wang J, Feng JQ. Signaling pathways critical for tooth root formation. J Dent Res 2017;96:1221-1228.

[7] Dutra EH, Janakiraman N, Nanda R, Uribe FA. Targeted mechanics for treatment of patients with severe short-root anomaly. J Clin Orthod 2017; 51:279-289.

[8] Lupi J, Handelman C, Sadowsky C. Prevalence and severity of apical root resorption and alveolar bone loss in orthodontically treated adults. Am J Orthod Dentofacial Orthop 1996;109: 28-37.

[9] Levander E, Malmgren O, Stenback K. Apical root resorption during orthodontic treatment of patients with multiple aplasia: A study of maxillary incisors. Eur Orthod Soc 1998;20:427-434.

[10] Kjaer I. Morphological characteristics of dentitions developing excessive root resorption during orthodontic treatment. Eur J Orthod 1995;17:25-34.

[11] Sameshima G, Sinclair P. Predicting and preventing root resorption: Part I. diagnostic factors. Am J Orthod Dentofacial Orthop 2001;119:505-510.

[12] Thongudomporn U, Freer T. Anomalous dental morphology and root resorption during orthodontic treatment: A pilot study. Aust Orthod J 1998; 15:162-167.

[13] Newman W. Possible etiologic factors in external root resorption. Am J Orthod 1975;67:522-539.

[14] Valladares N, Rino N, de Paiva J. Orthodontic movement of teeth with short root anomaly: Should it be avoided, faced or ignored? Dent Press J Orthod 2013;18:72-85.

[15] Weltman B, Vig K, Fields H, Shanker S, Kaizar E. Root resorption associated with orthodontic tooth movement: A systematic review. Am J Orthod Dentofacial Orthop 2010;137: 462-476.

[16] Lee R, Artun J, Alonzo T. Are dental anomalies risk factors for apical root resorption in orthodontic patients? Am J Orthod Dentofacial Orthop 1999;116: 187-195.

[17] Mirabella A, Artun J. Risk factors for apical root resorption of maxillary anterior teeth in adult orthodontic patients. Am J Orthod Dentofacial Orthop 1995;108:48-55.

[18] Levander E, Malmgren O. Evaluation of the risk of root resorption during

orthodontic treatment. Eur J Orthod 1988; 10:30-38.

[19] Goldin B. Labial root torque: Effect on the maxilla and incisor root apex. Am J Orthod Dentofacial Orthop 1989;95:209-219.

[20] Newman WG. Possible etiologic factors in external root resorption. Am J Orthod 1975;67:522-539.

Section 2

Digitization and Workflow

Chapter 5

Finite Element Analysis in Orthodontics

Nandakishore Rajgopal

Abstract

One of the governing ideologies in orthodontics is gradually imposing remodeling, which involves progressive and irreversible bone deformations using specific force systems on the teeth. Bone remodeling results in the movement of the teeth into new positions, with two tissues having a major influence along with it: the periodontal ligament and the alveolar bone. There is a definite connection between the mechanical, biological and physiological reactions to the orthodontic forces. The development of the Finite Element Analysis and administration of this new age computer-aided method in orthodontics applies to this chapter. Finite Element Analysis is a computational procedure to calculate the stress in an element, which can show a model solution. The FEM analyses the biomechanical effects of various treatment modalities and calculates the deformation and the stress distribution in the bodies exposed to the external forces. The ideology behind this particular chapter is to introduce this scientific approach to the orthodontist and to reinforce the effects and advantages to the ones who are already aware of the same. In this chapter there is a detail discussion and explanation systematically on Finite element analysis method and its application strictly in and around orthodontics without much deviation from the subject.

Keywords: FEM, Nodes, Voxels, PDL, Orthodontic tooth movement (OTM)

1. Introduction

Orthodontics is the specialty of dentistry which in brief deals with correcting the malaligned teeth with the application of force delivery system, which includes wires, brackets, elastics etc. It is just one branch of dentistry which is deeply interlinked with the engineering branch of mechanics. Application of force and its resultant effects are the key stones in orthodontics, hence the fundamentals of physics also applies to the physics such as the Newtonian physics. The intention of the Orthodontist is to make betterment in function and esthetics. The treatment is just not limited it and has intentions to correct things like a tooth implanted to the alveolar bone can lead to caries or other paraodontal infections or affect the oral hygeine), esthetics (of the dentition or the face), or prosthetic (orthodontic treatment preceding a prosthetic replacement/missing tooth or teeth) [1].

An Orthodontic treatment might be carried out with evidence based system or by a clinical experience or by a acquiring knowledge and experience from a postgraduate curriculum or even via specific trainings and hands on programmes. Orthodontics is a spectacular as well as brain buzzer branch in dentistry where the work undertaken by an orthodontist could be considered as solving a puzzle, when he or she treats each case. It is associated with logical reasoning and through knowledge about the basics of biomechanics and even common sense. Turner et al. in 1956 introduced Finite element analysis (FEA). From then it has been used in different sectors such as in building aircrafts to dams to bridges etc. The usage of computer software's for the stressful calculations are used in order to find the stress and its distribution within a body for a given load. It also sketches the displacement of the body before and after the application of the load as well [2]. It could be a different dimensional opening for the chapter readers who are not familiar as well as to reinforce the knowledge for the readers who are already aware of this topic, so the chapter is designed to extremely simplify the concept of FEM and to integrate it with orthodontics from the very basic levels [2].

The Finite Element Method was introduced in orthodontics as a powerful tool for analyzing the biomechanical effects of various treatment modalities and is an approximation method to represent both the deformation and the 3Dstress distribution in bodies that are exposed to stress. The Finite Element Method is used to study the stresses and strains in engineering, it can be used to evaluate the biomechanical component such as displacement, strains and stresses induced in living structures from various external forces, the biomechanical response of the bone to external forces are quite complex. The FEM analyses the biomechanical effects of various treatment modalities and calculates the deformation and the stress distribution in the bodies exposed to the external forces. It should also be understood that the stress and strain in living tissues are thought to be key factors in biologic change, it is important to understand that stress and strain to understand its relationship to bone remodeling, the belief is such that the pattern of the stress will affect the localized proliferation of cells and growth activities [3]. The chapter is discussed from the fundamentals of FEM and further notes its usage in dentistry and particularly in orthodontics, followed by stepwise procedure explanations in detail.

The chapter further takes a road from its aspects such as construction of the models, which is the soul step in the FEM, with the help of scans such as the CT scans and FEM's credibility is in question due to the complexity and accuracy of the model seems to represent from truth and reality in the oral cavity [4].

Many new concepts and terminologies are being introduced and explained to its best in this chapter. Keeping in mind that many of readers, being from a medical academic background, including Orthodontists and clinicians hesitate to understand and relate the formulas and equations which are quite natural, a few vital equations are presented with ease. Further the chapter goes in detail to bone remodeling concepts and the brief explanations of individual components of the dental organ and its reaction to force and the chapter sinks with the concepts of FEM and orthodontics in the body. Towards the end the advantages as well as the limitations of FEM is discussed with some insight. This chapter is well supported with scientific literature evidence for the assertion it implies and it credits each and every scientist for their contributions and valuable time in life they have devoted for the good of the mankind.

2. Utility of finite element analysis

Orthodontics is periodically changing from an opinion-based practice to an evidence-based practice. Currently, it is necessary to have a scientific approach for any treatment modality and the evidence of tissue response to it [5]. Finite element analysis (FEA) has the ability of being applicable to solids of irregular geometry that contain heterogeneous material properties. It is therefore suited to evaluate the structural behavior of teeth. The use of FEM is wide seen in dentistry and in the field of orthodontics in the field of research in topics such as the geometry of the tooth, materials used, prosthetics etc. In the field of orthodontics, it's used to find the stress values or its distributions in appliances used in orthodontics etc. FEA could be wisely used to estimate the stress and strain patterns within the tooth structure, Periodontal Ligament (PDL) and the bone which is subjected to tooth movement by the means of orthodontics [6].

The forces to single-tooth system can also be modeled with the FEA with ease. The centre of resistance (C_R) of the tooth lowers and creates an altered stress pattern which is seen in the root as there is an experience of alveolar bone loss. The same effect could be experienced when there is an alteration of root length. The biomechanical properties of PDL are not the same for adult and adolescents respectively [7].

3. Road to finite element analysis

The principal of FEM is based on the division of a complex structure into smaller sub sections called as elements, in which the physical properties such as modulus of elasticity are applied to indicate the object response against an external stimulus which could be even an orthodontic force. It is said to be finite element analysis since, the elements are finite in count and the nodal points are the blocks which builds the model, which in turn connects to attribute to the formation of element [8]. A meshwork is considered to be a degenerated material which is subjected to modeling. There is an absolute control in the degree of simplification with this method which is an advantage to the FEM [9]. FEA techniques are potential to replace the stereo lithographic models for the presurgical planning. Every finite element is based on an assumed-shape function which expresses an internal displacement as a function of nodal displacement. Which means a certain element may give accurate answer for a particular type and location of support and loading but can give inaccurate answers for another type and location [10].

4. Steps in finite element analysis

1. The geometric model construction
2. The geometric model to a Finite element analysis model conversion
3. Data representation of the material properties
4. The boundary condition defining
5. Application of the load
6. Solution to the linear algebraic equation system.
7. Analyzing the results [10].

Basic Steps in Finite Element Method for any solution corresponds to the steps involved in finite element to analyze a structure.

4.1 The geometrical model construction

It is the first requirement for the analysis of the geometrical model. These can be created either in analysis software or the model can be created also in any CAD software and can be imported to the analysis software. The model has to be saved with extension *.iges or *.igs or *.sat to achieve this. The usage of a computed tomography image (fig ct img) can be done to serve as a geometrical model.

4.2 Discretization process

Discretization is a process of dividing the domain or component into number of elements & nodes. For this purpose, an assumption is made that the elements are interconnected by nodes. The idea behind the process is to improve the accuracy of the results. The entire component is divided into number of elements, then the stress distribution in each element will be almost the actual results and the operator gets accurate plot of the stress distribution in a component.

4.3 Applying material properties

The mechanical properties such as young's modulus, Poisson's ratio etc., are defined to the component in this particular step. This is done to feed the values for calculation of the solution. These values mark the natural properties to the built up model so that it can behave and react in the same manner as that of a natural biologic body would, when subjected to external stimuli (stress). For the particular element, the property is to be defined. First of all the operator has to define the type of element. There are several types of elements available, which can be implemented to the domain component.

4.4 Defining boundary conditions and nature of problem

The boundary condition is chosen depending upon the mode of analysis such as structural, dynamic, thermal, fluid etc.

4.5 Application of load

After the application of boundary conditions, the discretized domain is applied to the known loads. The application of loads will depend upon the geometry of the component used. The nodes are applied with loads. Different types of loads will include Forces or Moments, pressure, gravity. - For structural problems- Gravity, radiation, convection and temperature for thermal problems.

4.6 Solution or results

The results can be obtained instantly as well as in the most accurate manner. It will consist of model images which represent levels of stress by various colors signifying different stress for different colors respectively, which can be directly read from a color chart (provided below the image). The results can be further tabulated and subjected to analysis.

5. Computed tomography (CT) and extraction of morphological parameters from CT scans

Computed Tomography or C.T is cross-sectional image of an object from either transmission or reflection data collected by illuminating (by any kind of penetrating radiation) the object from many different directions or angles. Frankly speaking, tomographic imaging deals with the reconstruction of an image from its projections. The technique constitutes of irradiating a section of a sample from a number of positional angles and then the intensity of the transmitted or reflected radiation is measured. For example, the projections symbolize the X-rays attenuation within a body, the bodies' radioactive nucleoids decay as in the case of emission tomography, or the variation seen in refractive index in an ultrasonic tomography (USG).

When the X-ray is considered, the projections consist of line integrals of the attenuation coefficient. This attenuation of photons (tiny particles that constitute an electromagnetic radiation) are due to either being absorbed by the atoms of the material, or being scattered away from their original paths of travel. Photoelectric absorption involves an X-ray photon imparting all its energy to a tightly bound inner electron in an atom. The images are 2D maps of the distribution of the attenuation coefficient of the X-rays. By stacking the obtained 2D images, we can reconstruct 3D images. The attenuation coefficient is measured in Hounsfield Units (HU) [11].

This macroscopic response of the trabecular bone is closely related to the underlying microstructure. It is beyond scope of this book to describe in details the geometry and spatial arrangement of the trabeculae and its advised to refer standard textbooks for the same, The volume fraction which is considered one among the major parameter in characterization of microstructure of cellular materials geometrically, gives no much clue about the orientation as well as the organization of the above said microstructures. The material microstructure is modeled using tensors of higher rank which mimics the architecture of the microstructure and is the most common method adapted for the same. Fabric tensors are needed as a quantitative measure of the microstructural architecture, to serve as positive definite. The principal axes of a tensor whose principal axes coincide with the principal microstructural direction and its eigenvalues are proportional to the microstructure distribution with respect to its principal direction. It is a must thing to include the parameters which can define those orientations. Hence it

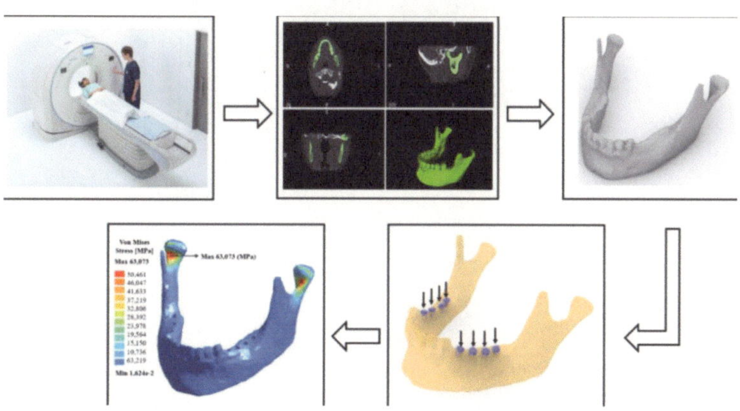

Figure 1.
Conversion of CT scan into a finite element model.

requires acquiring a 3D representation of the bone first using tomography. It is then a morphological analysis used to describe the microstructure (**Figure 1**) [12].

6. Generation of finite element model

Three primary considerations in the development of the three-dimensional finite element tooth model are to be considered; which includes the tooth and other periodontal geometry, properties of different materials and as well as the configuration of the load applied. In a given tooth geometry and structures of the periodontium and its associated geometry, one can say nodes simply as points that occupies the corners of the elements which meet each other; further the boundary conditions are well defined at all peripheral occupying nodes. A specific material property is assigned to individual elements. Location of the centre of resistance and centre of rotation of the modeled tooth will be deeply affected by the modeling of the root as a symmetric parabolic structure or as a real tooth, as well as root conicity, buccopalatal vs. mesiodistal bone levels and bone insertion [11].

The problem with three-dimensional models is that the geometrical input needs to be generated. The bone structure replicated with a CT scan is preferred as the geometrical input data which should be generated for the 3-D model, which is considered as one among the problems. It is suggested to convert the CT image voxel to eight node hexahedral; but the possibility of numerous element creations in model and the unwanted change in the model's external shape is the pay for this. In order to exempt the outer rough surfaces, it's better to model the external geometrical contours. After these steps, automatically a mesh is produced out as the result of the software. Material properties are assigned to each element of the model, once the generation of the mesh is done (**Figure 2**).

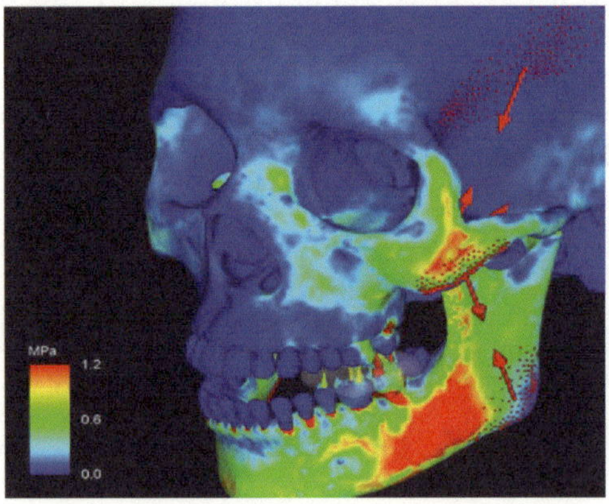

Figure 2.
FEA carried out on a modeled human skull.

7. Morphological analysis

Morphological analysis provides the tools to extract morphological parameters of an object. The actual values of the parameters extracted depend on the object as well as the quality of the object representation. Better way to say is voxel size affects the 3D images and pixel size would affect the 2D images. Higher the resolution better is the analysis quality. TV, BV, Tb.Th, and MIL are the four respective parameters of morphology which are taken into account.

7.1 Tissue (or total) volume TV

TV does quantification of the volume in total at the region of interest (ROI). If bone is to be considered, the entire trabecular bone and the total volume of its pores along could be considered as the term 'tissue'. It is a simple task to calculate TV, just by taking the product of the total number of voxels at the region of interest and the volume of a single voxel. The usage of 2-D images could be an option to obtain the volume. The volume is computed by assuming the cut thickness to be same as the pixel's side length measurement.

7.2 Bone volume BV

By multiplying the number of voxels in the solid objects, one can find out this parameter and it's the representation of the 3-D object's volume in total. Bone volume (BV) will therefore be interpreted as the solid phase volume.

7.3 Trabecular thickness (Tb. Th)

It is the thickness of the rods of the cellular solid [13].

7.4 BV/TV

The important parameter is the ratio of the two previous parameters.

8. Distribution of trabecular thickness (Tb.Th)

It is the thickness of trabeculae and its associated distribution.

Locally when it comes to thickness specifically at a point within a state of body is said to be the biggest sphere which consoles the spot, the spot is not needed to be the centre of the body but within the surface of the object which is considered as a solid [14]. To calculate (Tb.Th), the idea of structuring the body of the object is carried out, where the trabecular midline is used [15].

9. Fundementals in non linear computation method

The mechanics which is an engineering branch is the soul element in the field of (**Figure 2**) biomechanics; one can never understand biomechanics without understanding the fundamentals of mechanics. Mechanics deals with forces and the response of the object or body, whereas bio means study of living organisms, so the application of the forces and its response to the forces in living bodies are dealt in biomechanics. The hierarchical arrangement in organisms starts from sub atoms ending in organized living body. With the help of quantum mechanics, we can study at the cell or atomic levels and Continuum mechanics could be used in the higher levels such as the organ levels [16].

9.1 Finite strains associated with a body in its kinetics

The Continuum Mechanics is the ideology where volume $_{V(t)}$ is the amount of matter contained by a body in the respective space at a given time T and the surface area of the body could be symbolized as $S_{(t)}$. Further when we look the reader must understand that the body undergoes change in dimension from its initial orientation for the respective boundary definition after a stress is being applied to the body. The fact is such that, the irrelevance of working with the same body with and without stress because of the obvious above said reason of reasonable transition in shape of the body from initial and final state of the body before and after applying stress. It is mandatory for the above said reasons a thorough understanding of the basis of kinematics is required [17].

10. The FEM

Coming to the FEM we must strictly adhere to the principles of kinematics. The chapter is never complete without discussing few important equations in FEM, where shape functions (N) and the displacement of the nodes (q), which we are not certain about could attribute the displacement fields shape and could be equated as follows;

$$\mathrm{U(x)=N(x)q} \tag{1}$$

In Eq. (1) the nodal values (q) are determined by the method of calculating the equation which is already in a state of equilibrium via formulation which is made incrementally [18].

$$\delta\mathbf{q}\underbrace{\left[\mathbf{M}\ddot{\mathbf{q}}+\mathrm{Fint}-\mathbf{Fext}\right]}_{\mathbf{F}^{oe}}=0 \quad \forall\delta\mathbf{q} \tag{2}$$

In Eq. (2) q represents the nodal accelerations, M the mass matrix and Fint and Fext the (nodal consistent) internal and external forces respectively

$$\begin{aligned}
M &= \int_{V(t)} \rho N^{\top} N dV \\
F_{\text{int}} &= \int_{V(t)} B^{\top} \alpha d\,\mathrm{V} \\
\mathbf{F}ert &= \int_{V(t)} \rho \mathbf{N}^{\top} \mathbf{b} dV + \int_{S(t)} \mathbf{N}^{\top} t dS
\end{aligned} \tag{3}$$

In Eq. (3) B = ∇NT and t represents the traction on the surface.

$$\frac{\left\|\mathbf{F}^{oe}\right\|}{\mathbf{F}_{\mathrm{aXt}}} < \mathrm{prec} \tag{4}$$

In Eq. (4) Foe denotes the residual or remaining forces and it's not equal to zero. Prec is a user defined precision. The equilibrium equations are iteratively solved using Newton–Raphson method. Starting from a trial nodal displacement is given as, q0 (several possibilities to evaluate such a trial [19].

Field exist but will not be treated in this work), the displacement field is iteratively updated in such a way that:

$$\Delta q = -KT - 1\text{Foe}$$

$$\text{qi} + 1 = \text{qi} + \Delta\text{q} \tag{5}$$

Eq. (5) denotes KT = d Foe/dq, which is considered to be called as the tangent stiffness matrix.

The tangent stiffness matrix will be resolved into its parts as well as the shape. The shape aspect of this depends on the shape functions used in FEM [20].

By use of linearization of the small stress values with its corresponding strain values this can be obtained. Intergration tool is used to discrete the matrix of material stiffness [21].

11. Biomechanics of bone remodeling in orthodontics models in orthodontics

Within the field of dentistry and to its related field, mathematical models are used for research and treatment planning. The tendencies in mathematical models (either numerical FE models or analytical models) for tooth movement and in particular the constitutive models used for dental tissues. Many contributions exist focusing on implant related problems, which are not our interest. The forces alone are only considered and it's not about the means of force delivery system which may also include the brackets are to be considered in here [22].

11.1 The gingiva

The mechanism which is responsible for the asymmetrical behavior of the tooth when rotated around its main axis is at times assumed to be in the gingival tissue which is a complex fibrous structure that envelops the entire dental arch and it provides an additional anchorage to the teeth, tends to contract. This creates force acting on the different proximal teeth, which in turn produce an internal momentum and asymmetries. The gingiva has a viscous nature due to its composition of collagen. We do not consider or value much the mechanical activity of the gingiva during tooth movement in Finite element studies [23].

11.2 The dental components

11.2.1 Enamel

It is the hard as well as a brittle substance probably seen in the human body, which is composed of mainly inorganic materials. Enamel could be categorized as an elastic material which is linear in nature [24].

11.2.2 Cementum

Very few studies focus on characterizing the cementum, either mechanically or histologically. The group of Darendelier provides a comprehensive body of work on the physical characteristics of cementum.

11.2.3 The dentin

The Dentin is reinforced by radial microscopic tubules. These tubules are filled with fluid and this gives the dentin a viscoelastic character. Since the mid-1970's, studies shows its viscoelastic property and this is a supporting evidence.

Dentin is also looked as a non-homogeneous and anisotropic material in various recent experimental model studies.

11.2.4 Pulp

When there literature is reviewed, barely any studies are done to characterize the properties of the neither dental pulp nor acknowledges its existence [25].

The crown of the tooth is modeled as one material with 19 GPA modulus of elasticity, without even considering the 2 components of the crown (enamel, dentin) independently shows young's modulus of 80 and 18 GPA respectively. The Poisson's ratio is, regardless of the proposed study, taken as 0.3 [26].

11.2.5 The periodontal ligament (PDL)

The periodontium is a structure which constitutes the cementum, the PDL fibers and the alveolar complex. The PDL constitutes the tissues which are loose connective type. It is innervated as well as vascularized. It holds the teeth to the bone and compensates the wearing of the crown structure of the tooth at points in contact or the incisal/occlusal portion of the tooth. The functions of the PDL include the regulation of mastication as well because of the associated sensory nerve fiber innervations. It works well as an attached cushion between tooth and the alveolar bone, as well as act as a shock absorber. The load applied to the teeth during the functions like chewing and clenching is transmitted to the respective jaw bones through the PDL fibers [27].

Many studies on PDL take bilinear elastic nature of it; one can also find many studies which speak or valuate the anisotropy of the fibers of the PDL. There are advantages when it's done so, as it provides more accurate and validity of the stress calculation for a better eccentricity of the movements of the teeth [28]. But studies talk about the PDL and its non- linear nature which is stated by the properties like Poisson's ratio and the modulus of elasticity (Young's) (**Figure 3**).

A Young's modulus around 0.1 MPa is most likely to represent best of the linear part of the PDL's mechanical behavior. Bilinear elastic models are also found and are defined with three values which are tangential modulus, Young's modulus and a limit value of about 7% strains in tension tests. Last but never the least, Cattaneo et al., Verna et al. introduced a multi-linear model, different in tension and in compression [29].

Many researchers consider the PDL as a hyper elastic material (Mooney-Rivlin material with, for Natali et al., reinforced fibers, expressed in an Ogden-type formulation) and estimated strain which corresponds well with the in vivo experimental data by Parfitt.

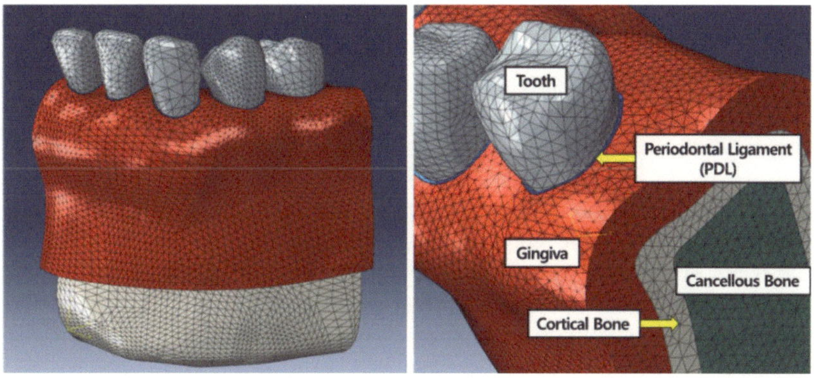

Figure 3.
Mesh model after assigning the charecteristic material properties of each constituent of dento-alveolar complex independently.

Models proposed by various other researchers, accounts for a time dependency through the use of viscoelastic models using up to four time-constants. These models are either generalized as Maxwell models [30].

There are instances where the periodontal ligament is believed to be composed of fibers which are arranged in linear nature [31]. The poroelastic model allows considering a time-dependent behavior through the fluid flow inside a porous matrix.

12. Orthodontic tooth movement (OTM) models

12.1 Initial tooth movement

The finite element (FE) method is used in orthopedic biomechanics since the early 1970's to evaluate and analyze and study the patterns of stress in the calcified tissues (bones). From then, this analytical tool of the modern era is being used in the field of Orthodontics as well. It very evident to find the use of FEM in the field of prosthodontics, implantology etc. as well to analyze the stress, the stress pattern and to optimize or go with the design of the appliances, to study the materialistic properties of the appliance as well as the reactions of the bone to it. We currently use for biomechanics in the field of orthodontics as well [32].

It is a wise decision to use the non-linear behavior of the periodontal ligament to study the wider aspects of tooth movements [33]. The initial design of models in Finite element methods FE models were 2 Dor axi symmetric models and now it's no more used since it's a 3-D era. The FEM can definitely analyze the stress and its patterns and can analyze the biomechanics and can determine the final position of the teeth from its initial positions [34]. Early models in the field of orthodontics were mainly directed to study the initial movement of the tooth in its socket (no bone remodeling included) following the implementation of a system of forces and moments by means of braces or fixed orthodontic appliances. Most current studies still follow the same principle, using geometry and a system of forces which is more complex. Within the initial tooth movement models, mainly fully linear elastic homogeneous isotropic models were used. How so ever, models with non uneven bone density is also used where modulus of elasticity is taken into account. Orthotropic behavior of the bone and the anisotropic nature of PDL also exist [35]. Studies consider the periodontal ligament to be elastic. All these could be applied to the posterior teeth, multi rooted and of different forms of roots as well [36].

12.2 Long-term tooth movement

The tooth movement due to bone resorption and apposition which obeys the pressure tension theory is not obeyed by the teeth initially and the early tooth movement is just the effect of the PDL fibers which instigate the tooth movement initially. After an initial tooth movement under the applied pressure the tooth tries to stay in that position and tries to attain stability in the newly moved position [37]. FEA models at times usually involve an update of displacement (in addition to that due to external forces) or of forces based on an empirical bone remodeling law: The stimulus for remodeling is either the strain energy density, strain dependent or stress dependent remodeling algorithms obey the laws of mathematical tools such as the integration under the limit of time. The FEM analyses the forces and the associated tooth movement with it in the model and it all obeys the laws of equilibrium from its initial to final position under the stipulated time.

13. Dento-facial orthopedics modeling

Since the early 1980's, finite element models of maxillary and mandible were used. The model is built with elements which is comparable or represents the bone structure and symbolizing its properties. The magnitude of the force levels applied by appliance like brackets or others like head gears or the expansion appliance etc. is taken into consideration. As a part of modeling the movement of the jaw, a great effort is made to characterize the temporomandibular joint (TMJ). In most cases, the type of materials used for the bone is linear elastic in nature. It is considered that cortical bone is distinguishable from trabecular bone. However, the presence/absence of teeth in the cranio-facial models is variable in nature. As for the models of the TMJ, the cartilage and the disks are modeled either as linear elastic materials or as hyper elastic ones. It can be also found out that the models include muscle activation of the jaw, either performing an inverse dynamic analysis to compute the activity of the large amount of muscles in the face, or modeling a given number of muscles, often by applying a spring model to describe the muscular forces. Finally, one can also find models of the facial bones and skull by analyzing the response to external orthopedic systems [38].

14. Bone remodeling models

In addition to growth of the skeleton and resorption of fractures, which are of temporary in nature, the structure of bone is, stabilized by the action of osteoclast and osteoblast and its metabolism is a total different interest of subject which is to be discussed, which in turn is beyond the scope of this chapter. Through understanding of the remodeling process of the bone should be understood by an orthodontist to get an idea of how the teeth move in the maxilla or mandible during tooth movement. The Roux hypothesis claims the whole remodeling procedure is a self-organized procedure where the stiffness of the bone is achieved after a force is applied and stress is developed within the bone, the bone trabaculae obeys the Wolff's law and last but not the least the bone reacts upon itself for load application. It is equally important to understand the Frost model of the bone which is stated as the mechanostat theory where is notes that if the stress range exceeds the limit, there is a chance of formation of a new bone, but if the same stress is lesser to the optimal value there is a bone loss associated to it as well. Both these goes hand in hand which creates a balance. The theory sounds simple for the readers but it's simply an effective one and a tricky one when equations are derived from it mathematically and used for computing. Earlier the bone in a bone model was technically considered to be a poroelastic media which is pooled by a liquid. Later models have proposed the universal mechanical nature of a living substances, here the depth of biological activity is considered, where as there is also another model which does not propose the depth of remodeling within the bone (Phenomenological model) [39].

15. FEM in orthodontic tooth movement

Now coming to the soul of this reading, the reader must understand the real fact initially that the FEM is a theoretical study concept and does not stand alone debates of scientific evidence based ideology without the gold standard of clinical trials. FEM deals with material properties and parameters, further the geometrical aspects are even being considered. The complete system with its constituent initial force, dimension of the body, stress developed is drastically different with respect to its final state. It is logical to think that it's inevitable without mathematical formulations and definite numerical values one cannot calculate or predict the final position of the tooth from its initial one [40].

Before the application of the FEM, there were several other methods which were implemented to carry out the stress strain relations and its calculations over the PDL, but due to the complex nature of it the end results achieved or obtained stayed insignificant. When the sequence of reactive force developed after an implementation of load is checked, the root suffers the most, followed by the PDL and the alveolar bone the least (due to its higher density). These findings are due to the different mechanical properties of each structure: such as the tooth, periodontal ligament and alveolar bone. The stress applied on the bone is the active factor in the new configuration arrangement of the bone. There is a significant association of the PDL in the remodeling procedure of the bone due to its viscous nature and the storage of energy within it due to the same nature.

The stresses are of different types such as the longitudinal stress, compressive stress, or the shear stress depending on the type of the force and its line of action over the body, so it's mandatory to specify it. There is always a chance for a tooth or teeth to undergo a combination of the above said stresses in various directions as well. When comparison is done among the types of tooth movements against each other, the tipping, extrusion and intrusion result in the greatest stress at the root apex. For extrusion and intrusion, the stress concentration is mainly at the apex of the root. Stresses at the root apex after intrusive tooth movement is seen but the distribution is different when compared to other types of tooth movement. When a vertical force is applied on the buccal surface of the tooth, some torque may be expected due to the relationship between the point of application of force and the centre of resistance of the tooth. In such cases, labial and lingual portion of the apical region of the root experiences way higher reactive forces to the applied tension.

After analyzing different FEM studies in orthodontics, studies show the stress distribution patterns are more in the crest of the alveolar bone, when compared to the periodontal ligament nor the crown or the root of the tooth. When the tipping forces where studied, it showed more or less the same feature of the stress distribution over the crest of alveolar bone. The tooth and the bone suffer greatest stress at the cervical level and the PDL at the apex.

The forces in rotation create the only difference of all the situations, where the apical stress is comparatively lesser. The FEM depends on the model and the property of the material assigned and boundary conditions, any change or errors creeping in these aspects will affect the foreseeing of the results. The type of the force delivered by each system is never the same, so there is change in the results. To get these right results the proper implementation of the force system and its understanding is inevitable. After all this there are other instances to point out like, up to 50% or more of the applied force can dissipate as friction in an edgewise bracket system; which can significantly affect the stress produced at the PDL of the tooth [41].

16. Limitations of finite element analysis

As with any theoretical model of a biological system, there are some limitations which need to be considered. A thorough reading and interpretation of this chapter would give the insight of the limitation of the FEM and it's not much to emphasis on the same. But then as said before any errors in modeling or material property assignment or the boundary conditions application, even wrong forces applied to wrong formulation, will earn the wrong results. It's a sophisticated and computer dependent or programme dependent analysis, so at most care should be taken during the modeling stages and the prior stages before the final run for the results to feed the correct input data for the expected outcome or results. It is highly difficult or impossible to be frank to replicate the exact living substance into mechanical models till date due to its complex nature [42]. The major limitation which you would have never guessed all through this chapter is that the cost of the FEM study. It should be highlighted that the FEM does not come with a reasonable price currently in many countries and it's used more for the research purposes. It's not a question to ask if FEM is considered in building bridges or dams or aircrafts but definitely when comes to field of dentistry or orthodontics, to use FEM for every single patient is never feasible.

17. Conclusion

The main fundamental in orthodontics is the movement of teeth or tooth within bones, which in other words means the movement of solid (tooth) in another solid (jaw bones bone) which is the toughest movement of all mediums and it's a slow process which consumes time. If we are smart enough to estimate the final position of the teeth form its initial one, it's like predicting the end result without the trial and error methods or without any unwanted disturbances which even if occurs could be foreseen and a right component of force. This ideology actually saves time and the pain to both the clinician as well as for the patient. The mechanical and biological/physiological reactions to orthodontic forces by the PDL and the alveolar bone are closely linked with each other. This coupling can be treated in biomechanical models, focusing on the mechanics and considering the phenomenological aspects of the biology. As a tool to describe the mechanics of orthodontic tooth movement due to remodeling, the Finite Element Method (FEM) can be definitely utilized. The FEM is an advanced engineering tool that has shown fruitful benefits in the field of dentistry, dental and biomedical research and as well as orthodontics. It is a highly precise technique which can expose various key research points in the research field.

It is a very big question to ask that have we discovered or implemented the complete aspect of the FEM and is it been used in our field. There are still researches going on. Clinically proved studies are rechecked with the software and after a series of studies, the FEM can be implemented in different cases to predict the results. Every person is unique, hence the bone density, the model etc. So definitely just one FEM study cannot predict all the results from that single result obtained from the unique model of a person. Running an FEM study for independently from person to person is also unique according to the author, which is not emphasized much in any of the literature ever before.

Acknowledgements

This humble chapter would be incomplete without words of gratitude to all those who have been a part of its existence. I would like to thank, Almighty and my parents and all my beloved ones, **Dr.Basil Joseph, MDS, Orthodontics, India** my beloved senior and friend, for his motivation and guidance till date.

Conflict of interest

The author declares no conflict of interest.

Notes/thanks/other declarations

I sincerely thank **Dr. Deena Dayalan**, professor, Dept. of Orthodontics and Dentofacial Orthopedics, SRMKDC, Chennai, Tamilnadu, India, for his keen support and motivation throughout my career.

Also, from the bottom of my heart I thank **Dr. Anil Kumar**, Reader, Dept. of Orthodontics and Dentofacial Orthopedics, AJIDS, Mangalore, Karnataka, India, for constantly guiding me in my postgraduate curriculum and for the support he offers me.

Appendix and nomenclature

*iges	The Initial Graphics Exchange Specification
*sat	Standard ACIS Text
HU	unit used in computed tomography (CT) (Dimension less unit)
E	Modulus of elasticity (Gpa)
S	Stress (Mpa)

Author details

Nandakishore Rajgopal
A.J. Institute of Dental Sciences, Mangalore, India

*Address all correspondence to: nandaku007@yahoo.com

References

[1] Abu, A. R., Rashid, K., and Voyiadjis, G. Z. A finite strain plastic-damage model for high velocity impact using combined viscosity and gradient localization limiters: Part I-theoretical formulation. International Journal of DamageMechanics, 2006; 15(4):293.

[2] Adachi, T., Tsubota, K., Tomita, Y., and Hollister, S. J. Trabecular surface remodeling simulation for cancellous bone usingmicrostructural voxel finite elementmodels. Journal of Biomechanical Engineering, 2001: 123(5):403-409.

[3] Anshul Chaudhry, Maninder S. Sidhu, Girish Chaudhary, Seema Grover, Nimisha Chaudhry, and Ashutosh Kaushik. Evaluation of stress changes in the mandible with a fixed functional appliance: A finite element study. Am J Orthod Dentofacial Orthop 2015; 147: 226-34

[4] Adachi, T., Kameo, Y., and Hojo,M. Trabecular bone remodelling simulation considering osteocytic response to fluid-induced shear stress. Philosophical Transactions of the Royal Society A: Mathematical, Physical and Engineering Sciences, 2010: 368(1920):2669

[5] Sarmah A, Mathur AK, Gupta V, Pai VS, Nandini S. Finite element analysis of dental implant as orthodontic anchorage. J Contemp Dent Pract. 2011;12:259-64.

[6] Akhtar, R.,Daymond,M. R., Almer, J. D., andMummery, P.M. Elastic strains in antler trabecular bone determined by synchrotron X-ray diffraction. Acta Biomaterialia, 2008:4 (6):1677-1687.

[7] Ammar, H. H., Ngan, P., Crout, R. J., Mucino, V. H., and Mukdadi, O. M. Threedimensional modeling and finite element analysis in treatment planning for orthodontic tooth movement. American Journal of Orthodontics and Dentofacial Orthopedics, 2011:139(1): e59–e71

[8] Shaw AM, Sameshima GT, Vu HV. Mechanical stress generated by orthodontic forces on apical root cementum: a finite element model. Orthod Craniofacial Res. 2004;7(2): 98-107.

[9] Jones ML, Hickman J, Middleton J, Knox J, Volp C. A validated finite element method study of orthodontic tooth movement in the human subject. Am J Orthod. 2001;28(1):29-38.

[10] Bailon-Plaza, A. and Van Der Meulen, M. A mathematical framework to study the effects of growth factor influences on fracture healing. Journal of Theoretical Biology, 2001:212(2):191-209

[11] Aversa, R., Apicella, D., Perillo, L., Sorrentino, R., Zarone, F., Ferrari, M., and Apicella, A. Non-linear elastic three-dimensional finite element analysis on the effect of endocrown material rigidity on alveolar bone remodeling process. Dental Materials, 2009:25(5): 678-690

[12] Arola, D. and Reprogel, R. Effects of aging on the mechanical behavior of human dentin. Biomaterials, 2005:26(18): 4051-4061

[13] Bagge, M. A model of bone adaptation as an optimization process. Journal of Biomechanics, 2000:33(11): 1349-1357.

[14] Bailon-Plaza, A. and Van Der Meulen, M. A mathematical framework to study the effects of growth factor

influences on fracture healing. Journal of Theoretical Biology, 2001:212(2): 191-209.

[15] Baïotto, S. and Zidi, M. Un modèle viscoélastique de remodelage osseux : approche unidimensionnelle. Comptes Rendus deMécanique, 2004:332(8): pp. 633-638.

[16] Beaupré, G. S. and Hayes, W. C. Finite element analysis of a three-dimensional opencelledmodel for trabecular bone. Journal of biomechanical engineering, 1985:107:249.

[17] Beaupré, G. S., Orr, T. E., and Carter, D. R. An approach for time-dependent bone modeling and remodeling-theoretical development. Journal of Orthopedic Research, 1990:8 (5):651-661

[18] Cattaneo, P. M., Dalstra, M., and Melsen, B. The finite element method: a tool to study orthodontic toothmovement. Journal of Dental Research, 2005:84(5):428-433.

[19] Cattaneo, P.M., Dalstra,M., andMelsen, B. Strains in periodontal ligament and alveolar bone associated with orthodontic tooth movement analyzed by finite element. Orthodontics & Craniofacial Research, 2009:12(2): 120-128.

[20] Chan, E. and Darendeliler, M. A. Physical properties of root cementum: Part 7. Extent of root resorption under areas of compression and tension. American Journal of Orthodontics and Dentofacial Orthopedics, 2006:129(4): 504-510.

[21] Charlebois, M. Constitutive Law for Trabecular Bone in Large Strain Compression. PhD thesis, Technische Universitat Wien, Institute of Lightweight Design and Structural Biomechanics, 2008.

[22] Committee, A. I.H. ASMHandbook: Properties and selection, volume 2. ASMInternational, 1990.

[23] Cowin, S.C. Themechanical and stress adaptive properties of bone.Annals of Biomedical Engineering, 1983:11(3-4): 263-295.

[24] Cowin, S.C. Themechanical and stress adaptive properties of bone.Annals of Biomedical Engineering, 1983:11(3-4): 263-295.

[25] Cowin, S. C. Tissue growth and remodeling. Annual Reviews of Biomedical Engineering, 2004:6: 77-107.

[26] Cowin, S. C. andDoty, S. TissueMechanics. Springer Verlag, 2007. Ch. 11 : Bone tissue.

[27] Cowin, S. C. and Hegedus,D. Bone remodeling I: theory of adaptive elasticity. Journal of Elasticity, 1976:6(3):313-326.

[28] Cowin, S.C. and Nachlinger, R. Bone remodeling III: uniqueness and stability in adaptive elasticity theory. Journal of Elasticity, 1978:V8(3):285-295.

[29] Cowin, S. C. Wolff's law of trabecular architecture at remodelling equilibrium. Journal of Biomechanical Engineering, 1986:108(1):83-88.

[30] Cowin, S. C., Hart, R. T., Balser, J. R., and Kohn, D. H. Functional adaptation in long bones: establishing in vivo values for surface remodeling rate coefficients. Journal of Biomechanics, 1985:18(9): 665-684.

[31] Crigel, M.-H., Ballig and, M., and Heinen, E. Les bois de cerf : revue de literature scientifique. Annales deMédecine Vétérinaire, 2001:145(1): 25-38.

[32] Cronau,M., Ihlow, D., Kubein-Meesenburg, D., Fanghänel, J., Dathe,H., and Nägerl, H. Biomechanical features of the periodontium: an experimental pilot study in vivo. American Journal of Orthodontics and Dentofacial Orthopedics, 2006:129(5):599. e13– 599.e21.

[33] Currey, J. Strain rate dependence of themechanical properties of reindeer antler and the cumulative damage model of bone fracture. Journal of Biomechanics, 1989:22(5):469– 475.

[34] de Bien, C. Analyse de la relation entre les propriétésmécaniques et lamicrostructure de matériaux cellulaires : contribution au développement d'une méthodologie basée sur le suivimicrotomographique de tests de compression. Master's thesis (in French), Université de Liège, Faculté des Sciences Appliquées, Département de Chimie Appliquée, 2010.

[35] de Giorgi, M., Carofalo, A., Dattoma, V., Nobile, R., and Palano, F. Aluminiumfoams structuralmodelling. Computers & Structures, 2010:88(1-2): 25-35.

[36] del Pozo, R., Tanaka, E., Tanaka, M., Kato, M., Iwabe, T., Hirose, M., and Tanne, K. Influence of friction at articular surfaces of the temporomandibular joint on stresses in the articular disk: a theoretical approach with the finite element method. Angle Orthodontist, 2003:73(3):319-327.

[37] Desmorat, R. and Otin, S. Cross-identification isotropic/anisotropic damage and application to anisothermal structural failure. Engineering Fracture Mechanics, 2008:75(11): 3446-3463.

[38] Dizier, A. Caractérisation des effets de température dans la zone endommagée autour de tunnels de stockage de déchets nucléaires dans des roches argileuses. PhD thesis, Université de Liège - Faculté de Sciences Appliquées - ArgEnCo, 2011.

[39] Doblaré, M. and García, J.-M. Application of an anisotropic bone-remodellingmodel based on a damage-repair theory to the analysis of the proximal femur before and after total hip replacement. Journal of Biomechanics, 2001:34:1157-1170.

[40] Frost, H. Bone "mass" and the "mechanostat": a proposal. The anatomical record, 1987; 219 (1):1-9.

[41] Frost, H. Skeletal structural adaptations to mechanical usage (SATMU): 1. Redefining Wolff's law: the bone modeling problem. The Anatomical Record, 1990; 226(4): 403-413.

[42] Gal, J. A., Gallo, L. M., Palla, S., Murray, G., and Klineberg, I. Analysis of human mandibular mechanics based on screw theory and in vivo data. Journal of Biomechanics, 2004;37(9):1405-1412.

Chapter 6

Interdisciplinary Reverse Planning in Orthodontics

Guilherme Nakagawa dos Santos, Charles Lenzi de Araujo and Romeu Cassiano Pucci da Silva Ramos

Abstract

Most adult patient cases are multidisciplinary cases, so it's planning can become difficult when we need to connect many dentistry fields to achieve ideal results. The interdisciplinary reverse planning is a well-known topic for dental rehabilitation professionals, so this chapter will address the role of orthodontics in reverse digital planning, improving longevity, reducing biological impacts and helping to communicate with patients, other doctors and dental technicians. 3D CAD technology allows us to plan these complex cases before the patient starts treatment, this tool will be essential to orchestrate the exact moment to start orthodontic, prosthetic and/or surgical interventions, so the workflow becomes ordenate and the outcome will be aligned with aesthetics and functional aspects and in harmony with facial references.

Keywords: orthodontics, cad/cam, interdisciplinary, clear aligners, virtual setup

1. Introduction

Among some factors that significantly increase the demand for esthetic rehabilitative treatments in dental offices, we can observe the greater access of patients to information, as well as the constant development of new technologies and dental materials, which enable a treatment with greater quality and longevity, and a bigger media appeal in this digital age. Although the search for esthetics is a major complaint and the patient's desire should be pleased, it is imperative to think about the function and balance of stomatognathic structures. It is the professional's duty to establish clear goals that can be replicated with predictability and to outline goals to be achieved for the success of the treatment.

Unfortunately, it is common to come across more complex cases where the need for a planning of all the specialties involved is present, and aiming to address only the patient's complaint, some factors and primordial steps are ignored. Analogously, transcribing and visualizing the treatment plan becomes a little more difficult for professionals who, due to incompetence, imprudence or simply negligence, abstain from more detailed planning. In order to fulfill all requirements and have a holistic view of the case, the digital reverse planning is an indispensable tool.

2. Interdisciplinary digital reverse planning

When talking about different areas of dentistry, we must pay attention to this integration. A multidisciplinary case is one that requires more than one approach (periodontics, orthodontics, implantology, etc.). However, these areas must speak the same language, that is, the goal must be common and convergent. Therefore, we must have an interconnected approach, that is, an interdisciplinary one.

2.1 Examples

2.1.1 Case 1

A 29-year-old female patient came to the office complaining that she would like to improve her esthetics through dental veneers. Upon clinical examination and complementary imaging exams, it was observed that a central incisor would be condemned for presenting a fracture and dentoalveolar abscess, the adjacent lateral incisor was decayed, and there was a moderate tooth crowding, which would require greater compensatory prepping teeth for ceramic veneers, or even endodontic treatment if the prepping was greater (**Figure 1**). Thus, aiming at the best result with less esthetic and biological damage to the patient, the case would require tooth extraction 1.1, caries removal and restoration of tooth 1.2, orthodontic alignment, implant in the tooth extraction space 1.1, tooth whitening and veneers in the upper teeth, and prosthesis on implant 1.1. Given these fundamental steps, how to organize these steps? What procedure would be mandatory? How would the esthetic defect of the loss of the upper incisive be minimized? Extract before or after orthodontic treatment?

To answer these questions, the philosophy of digital reverse planning was used, through esthetic, functional concepts and facial references [1], referenced by the integration and overlapping of digital files from the imaging exams, so that the final result could be seen with the predictability and esthetics required by the patient. The traditional approach in orthodontics sometimes does not meet the patient's expectations

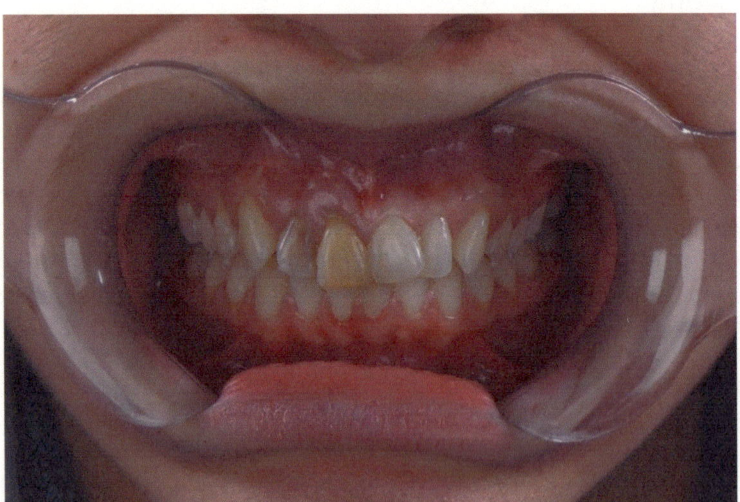

Figure 1.
First exam's intraoral picture.

regarding how long he will have compromised esthetics. The classic philosophy of planning in Orthodontics follows steps that make it difficult to immediately improve the patient's esthetics, always thinking about the diagnosis and long-term resolution. However, patients with esthetic problems suffer in relation to self-esteem and are in a hurry to remedy this type of problem. Therefore, solving the esthetic part, when possible without affecting the diagnosis of the case, should be shown to the patient.

Within a 3D planning software, the BDS Planning Center team performed a digital study [2] (**Figure 2**). As seen in the occlusal view (**Figure 3**), the need for greater prepping teeth 2.1 and 2.2 for the preparation of veneers is evident, and perhaps even the possibility of an endodontic treatment of the tooth 2.2. However, this study made it possible to visualize the needs of a multidisciplinary treatment, which facilitated decision-making by the patient and the professionals involved that the best conduct

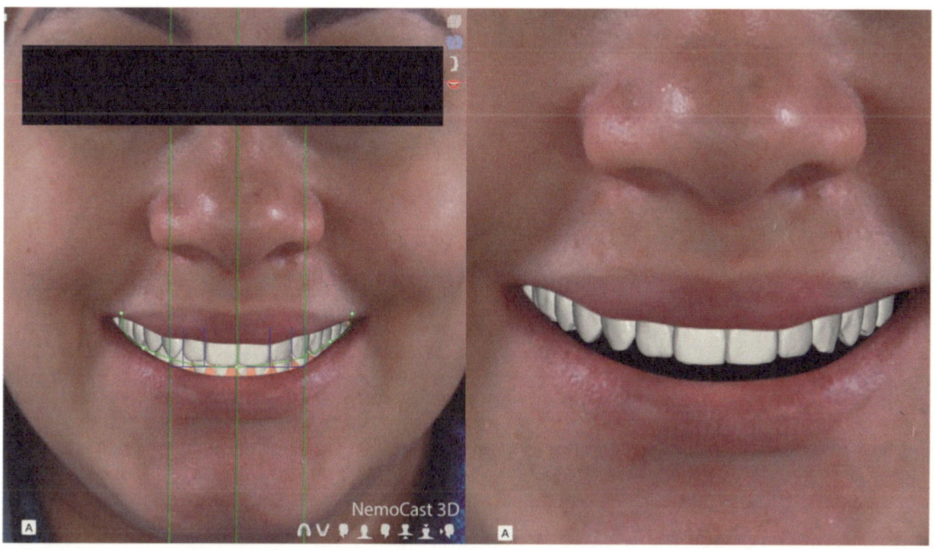

Figure 2.
Facially driven reverse digital planning showing the veneers.

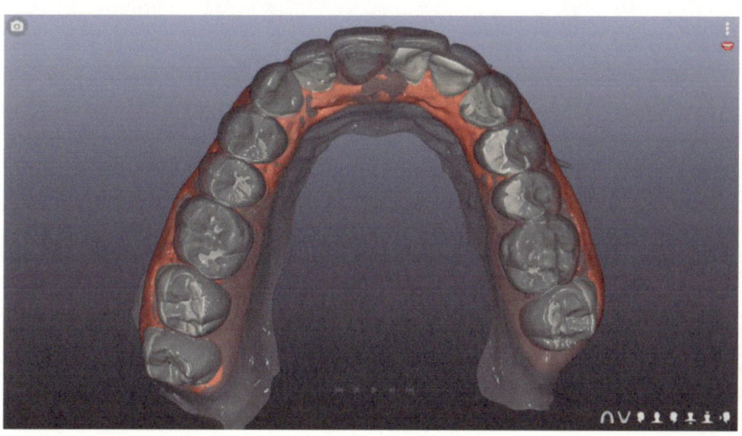

Figure 3.
Wax-up and initial models overlapping.

would be prior orthodontic treatment. After this orthodontic treatment plan was approved by the patient, she underwent tooth 11 extraction and a new intraoral scanning to proceed with the digital orthodontic setup, where this would be guided by the prior digital wax-up. (**Figures 4** and **5**).

We opted for a treatment with orthodontic aligners produced in-office to maintain an esthetic smile, with a pontic [3] on tooth 1.1, since this had a periradicular infection that prevented an immediate implant with a temporary one, thus as to be more predictable during orthodontic movements, enabling a centralization of the teeth for diagnostic waxing. As the biomodels exported by the Nemocast software (Nemotec) had a healing area of tooth 2.1, reliefs were created in the meshes in this area using the Meshmixer software (**Figure 6**), to allow tissue repair without compression of the alveolar ridge by the clear aligners. With the meshes already edited, the models were printed, and the orthodontic aligners were produced (**Figure 7**).

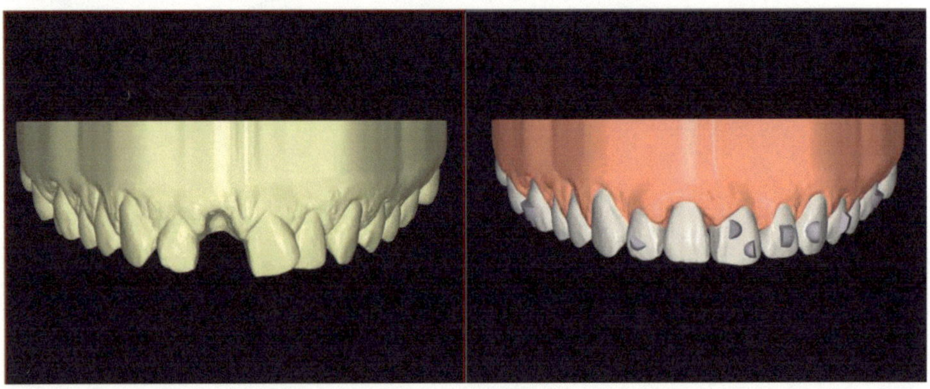

Figure 4.
Post extraction initial model and orthodontic setup.

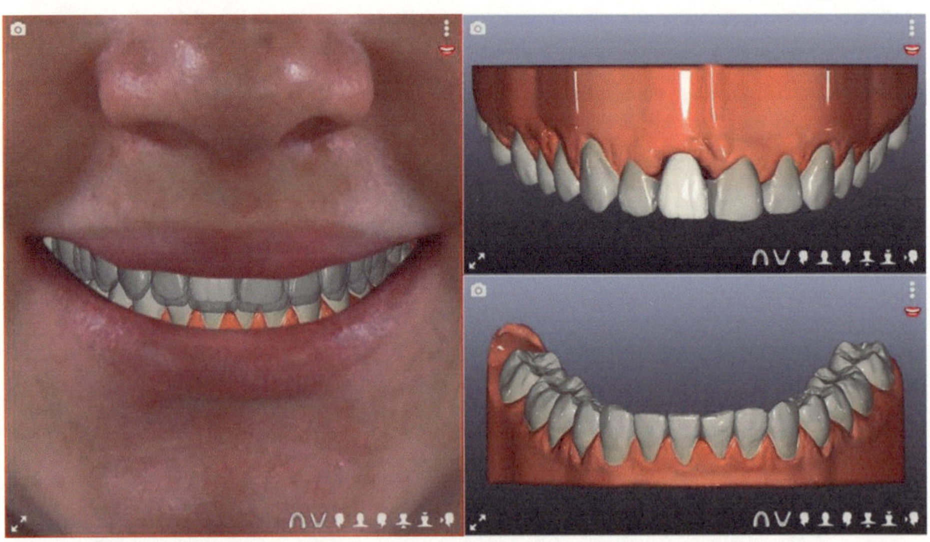

Figure 5.
Wax-up guided orthodontic setup.

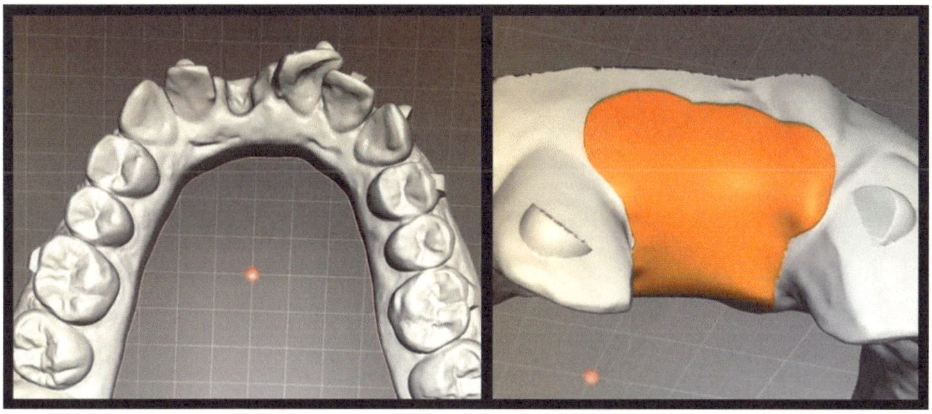

Figure 6.
3D mesh relief in Meshmixer software.

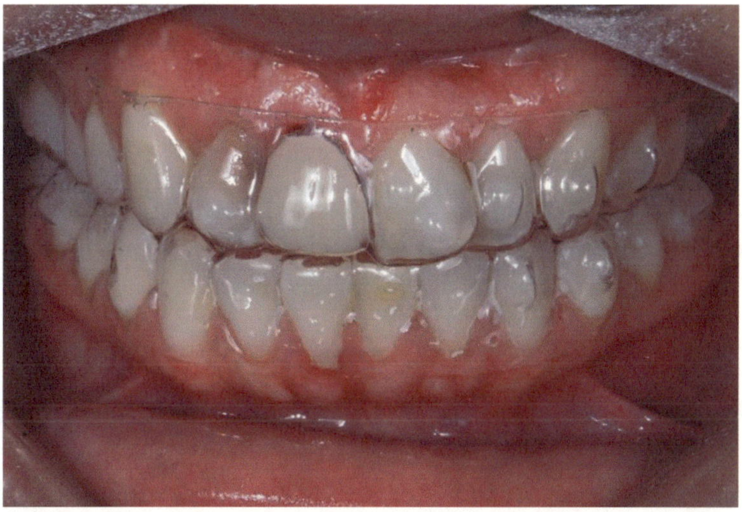

Figure 7.
Clear aligners with pontic on extraction space of tooth 1.1.

The treatment was carried out with a protocol of biweekly changes, where 15 aligners were needed for the upper arch and 8 for the lower arch, in a total of 8 months of treatment, considering the staging for greater predictability of the programmed movements. At the end of the last stage, the patient underwent a new intraoral scan, where this was superimposed on the wax-up study that served as a guide. (**Figure 8**). As verified in the overlapping models [4], the dental position obtained orthodontically was consistent with the planned one, with no need for touch-ups and alterations to the waxing study. Finally, the patient went on to implant the central incisive and subsequently perform the dental veneers as already established by the digital reverse planning, which proved to be effective and reproducible, especially because orthodontic treatment was performed using transparent aligners.

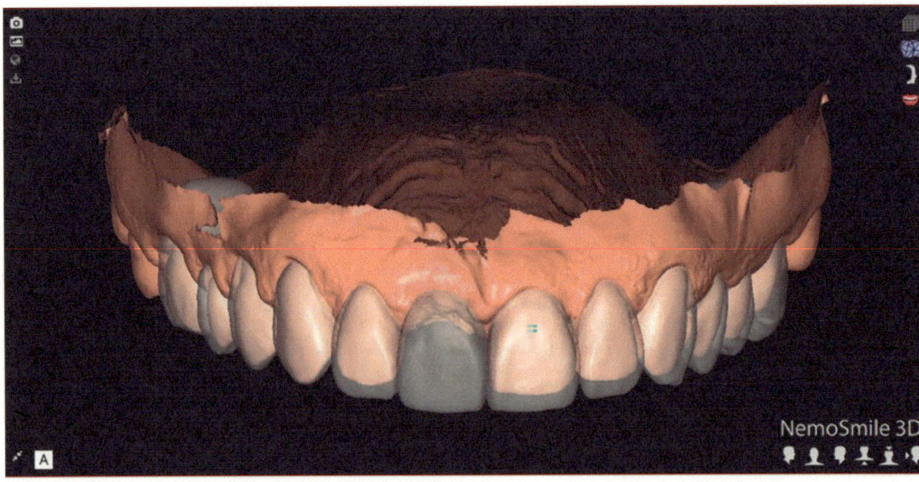

Figure 8.
Wax-up and final treatment scanning's models overlapping.

2.1.2 Case 2

Mesofacial patient, convex profile, good esthetic exposure of the smile with an inclined occlusal plane and angulation of the anterior teeth (**Figure 9**). Upper and lower tooth crowding, lower midline deviation of 2 mm to the right, caused by prolonged retention of tooth 75 with absence of its successor (tooth 35).

In view of the expectations of the results of the orthodontic treatment and the esthetic expectations of the patient, who did not accept having space for the extraction of the primary tooth, a reverse planning was carried out with an approach to installing the implant prior to orthodontic treatment. In this context, comfort and

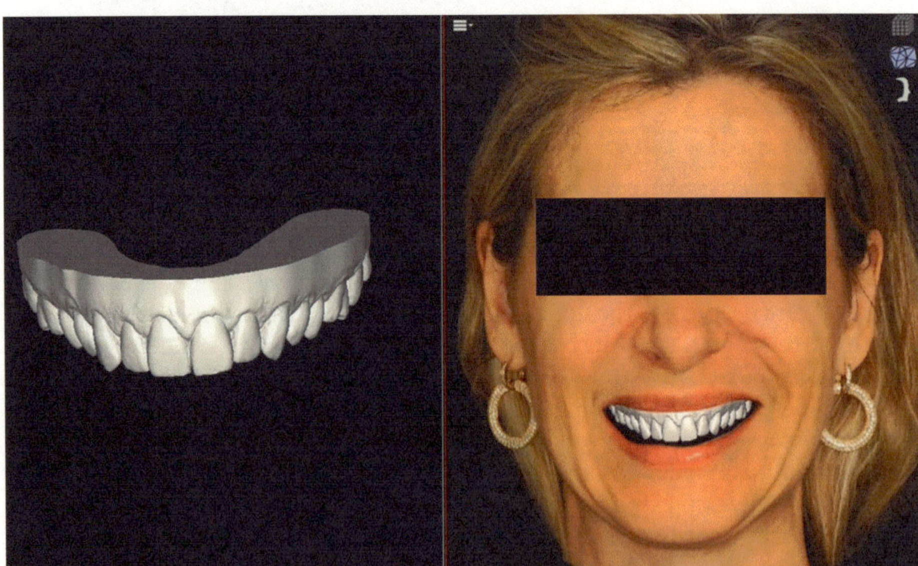

Figure 9.
Initial aspect.

safety are provided for the patient with preservation of esthetics in the area to be rehabilitated. Furthermore, the option of replacing a provisional retained in the appliance or in teeth, which may suffer constant fractures, especially located in the premolars or molars, subject to constant masticatory forces, it was decided to perform this implant in advance.

In the Nemocast software, virtual orthodontic correction was performed, guided by the face and its references, with extraction of tooth 75 (**Figure 10**). With the prediction obtained by the virtual setup of the final position of the teeth, the waxing of the crown of the 35 with the respective implant was planned (**Figure 11**). For

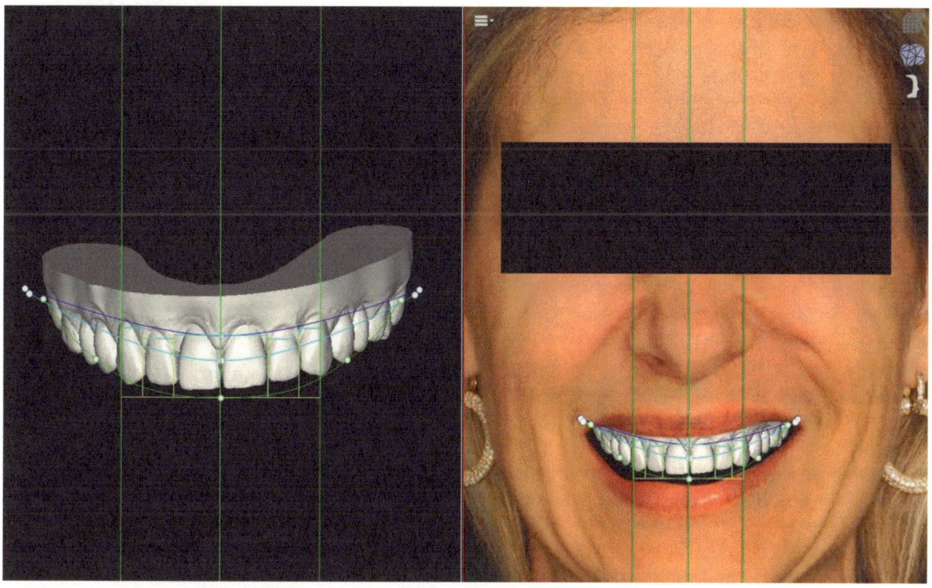

Figure 10.
Facially driven orthodontic setup.

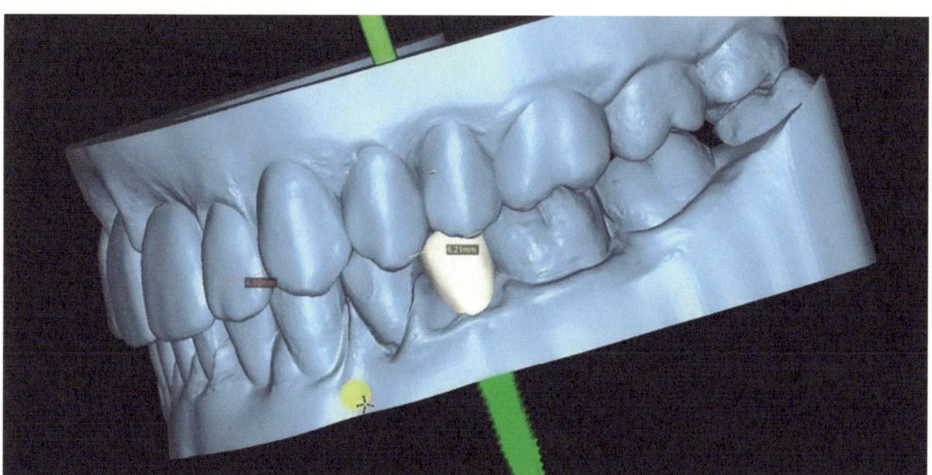

Figure 11.
Implant positioned based by orthodontic digital setup.

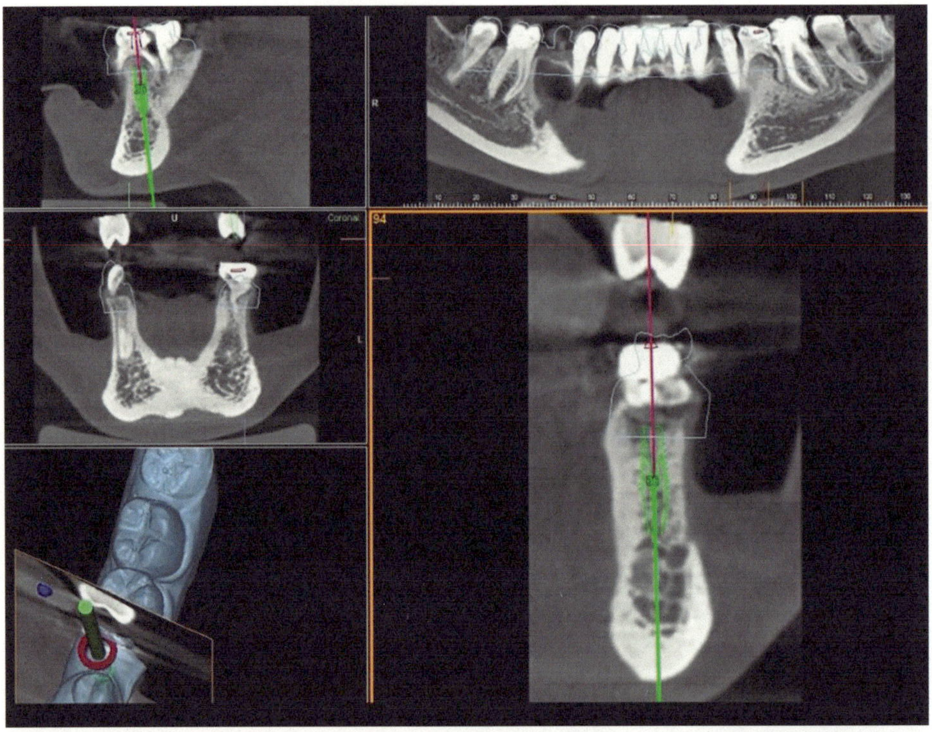

Figure 12.
CBCT and orthodontic setup model's overlapping to plan the ideal position of the implant.

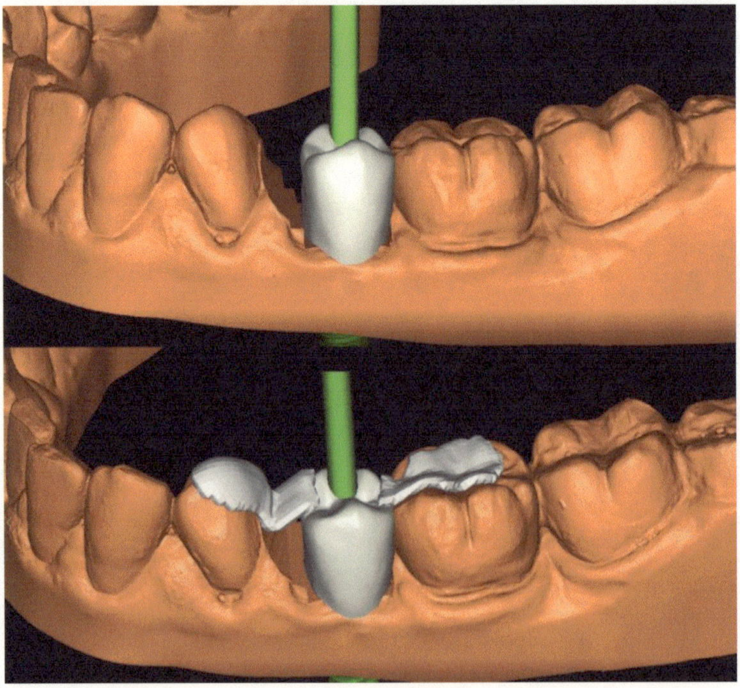

Figure 13.
Implant guide on the initial model. Tooth 75 was virtually extracted.

optimal placement of the implant, the STL model obtained from the orthodontic setup was overlaid with the CBCT DICOM file (**Figure 12**). About this project, there was the possibility of making a surgical guide for the installation of the implant, guided by the principles of ideal occlusion proposed by Angle in the 6 keys of occlusion (**Figure 13**) [5].

After planning (**Figure 14**) at the same surgical time, tooth 75 was extracted and tooth 35 was implanted guided, before the beginning of the orthodontic treatment.

In addition to the esthetic and functional gain with the anticipated surgery, the implant served as an absolute anchorage for the distalization of anterior teeth with midline correction and mesialization of the posterior teeth, guiding them to their positions predicted in the setup (**Figure 15**). With this mechanics, it is possible to establish the exact amount of movement of the adjacent teeth, having as the limit the dental contacts with this crown, minimizing the risk of loss of excessive anchorage or distalization less than necessary.

The remainder of the orthodontic sequence is not relevant to the purpose of the chapter, but rather the predictability and multiple functions of digital reverse

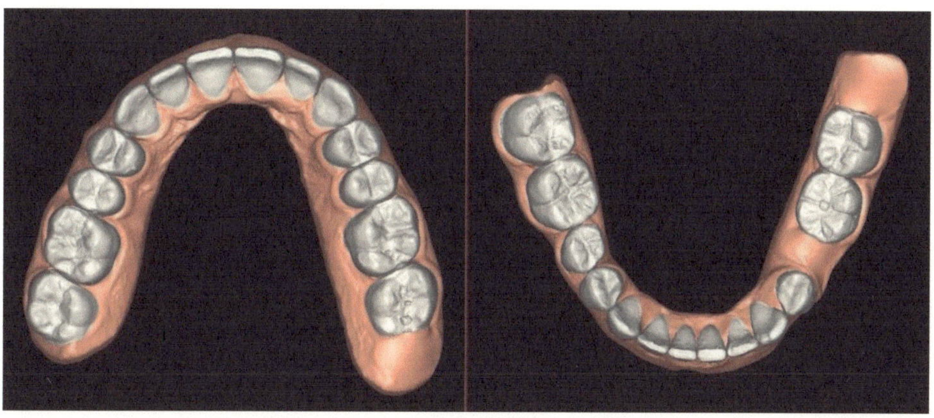

Figure 14.
Ideal digital orthodontic setup planned with virtual extraction of tooth 75.

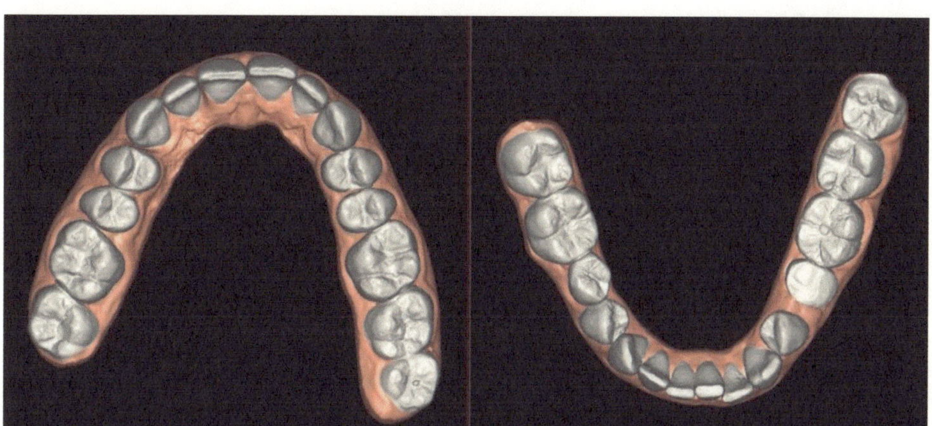

Figure 15.
Implant and crown installed new intraoral scan.

planning in orthodontics. It is noteworthy that performing the implant previously was essential to the success of the project for the acceptance of treatment and patient satisfaction.

3. Conclusion

As shown in the examples, digital reverse planning is a very important tool for the treatment of interdisciplinary cases, as it aims at better communication with the patient and among the professionals involved. The role of orthodontics in reverse planning is to orchestrate the progress of the clinical sequence, as dental rehabilitative planning often depends on the outcome of orthodontic treatment.

Acknowledgements

Special thanks to the Beyond Digital Solutions team for mastering the interdisciplinary virtual planning of the cases presented.

Author details

Guilherme Nakagawa dos Santos[1*], Charles Lenzi de Araujo[2]
and Romeu Cassiano Pucci da Silva Ramos[3]

1 UNOPAR, Londrina, Brazil

2 Tuiuti University, Curitiba, Brazil

3 Pontifical University Catholic of Paraná, Curitiba, Brazil

*Address all correspondence to: nksodontologia@hotmail.com

References

[1] Margossian P, Laborde G, Koubi S, Tardivo D, Magne P. Determination of Facial References for Esthetic Restorative Treatment. Int J Periodontics Restorative Dent. 2021;Jan-Feb;41(1):113-119. DOI: 10.11607/prd.4642. PMID: 33528459.

[2] León R, Torre M, Rubio A, Javier O. Digital tools and 3D printing technologies integrated into the workflow of restorative treatment: A clinical report. The Journal of Prosthetic Dentistry. 2018; 121.10.1016/j.prosdent. 2018.02.020.

[3] Vaid N, Revankar A, Vandekar M. I-Pontics for CAD/CAM Aligners. The Journal of Indian Orthodontic Society. 2013; 47(3):169-170 DOI:10.5005/ jp-journals-10021-1152.

[4] Anacleto M, Souki B. Superimposition of 3D maxillary digital modelos using opensource software. 2019; Dental Press J. Orthod 24(02); Mar-Apr.

[5] Andrews LF. The Six keys to normal occlusion. J Orthod. 1992 Sept;62(3): 296-309.

Chapter 7

Digital Workflow for Homemade Aligner

Dalal Elmoutawakkil and Nabil Hacib

Abstract

Advanced digital technology is rapidly changing the world, as well as transforming the dental profession. The adoption of digital technologies in dental offices allied with efficient processes and accurate high-strength materials are replacing conventional aligners workflows to improve overall patients' experiences and outcomes. Various digital devices such as 3D printers, intraoral and face scanners, cone-beam computed tomography (CBCT), software for computer 3D ortho setup, and 3D printing provide new potential alternatives to replace the traditional outsourced workflow for aligners. With this new technology, the entire process for bringing clear aligner production in-office can significantly reduce laboratory bills and increase patient case acceptance to provide high-quality and customized aligner therapy.

Keywords: digital workflow, orthodontics, aligner, thermoforming, 3D Printing, facial scan, planning software, homemade aligners

1. Introduction

The increasing esthetic need of patients for orthodontic devices has lead to the development of clear aligner therapy [1, 2]. Traditionally, orthodontists contract with an outside service to provide clear aligner treatments. Outsourcing to a provider has drawbacks for both the patient and the orthodontist. It can take over a month to produce and deliver an aligner set, and the provider requires a substantial service fee, cutting into potential profits.

Advancements in 3D printing technology, Intra-oral scanners, and 3D setup software improve the production of clear aligners. Nowadays, these solutions are widely available in private dental practices, allowing orthodontists in-house aligner production.

In-house 3D printing accelerates aligner turnaround, increases profitability, and improves patient satisfaction while offering complete workflow control.

In this chapter, we will suggest to orthodontists to centralize the production of aligners in the dental office by detailing the different stages of the production flow. Form acquiring extra-oral and intra-oral patient data and exploring necessary hardware and software for this acquisition. Until the production of the aligners, where we will discuss the equipment and materials mandatory for this production. Going through the planning, this section will detail the different software that an orthodontist can use for the 3D setup and the particularities of each of these softwares.

2. Materials and methods

The conventional clear aligner treatment is based on a complete outsourcing workflow, in this flow, the orthodontist will be restrained to check the setup proposal and request changes if he judges it necessary. To refer a case the orthodontist uploads the patient's data such as photos, X-rays, and digital dental impressions; then, he submits a prescription setup to aligner labs/companies. After a few days, the practitioner receives a setup proposition for review; the orthodontist evaluates the setup made by a technician and asks for some changes if necessary. Generally, there are 2 to 3 revisions with most aligner's laboratories before achieving a good treatment setup. This interaction between the orthodontist and the technician wastes time. Once the treatment setup has been approved, the orthodontist has to wait for the aligners to be fabricated and shipped to the office. Usually, the whole process takes 2–6 weeks.

In homemade clear aligner workflow, there are three main axes: data acquisition totally made by dental staff, planning of aligner setup, and aligner fabrication; these last two steps can be internalized in the dental office or outsourced to a third party. The outsourcing choice will depend on the time the orthodontist can allocate to planning, the cost/benefit ratio of acquiring software, and hardware and dental staff's ability to expand functions and competencies **Figure 1**.

2.1 Data acquisition

2.1.1 Digital model creation

The maxillary and mandibular digital working models and recording of the patient occlusion can be done directly on the patient by an intraoral scanner or by digitizing the analog impressions and/or plaster models with a desktop scanner or by a cone-beam computed tomography (CBCT).

Extraoral 3D scanners can be used to capture 3D images of both impressions and physical casts to acquire digital models. An optical scanner (OS) is an extra-oral digitization method that uses a white light that is cast on the plaster dental model. Later, the projected pattern is captured using a high-resolution camera, and a 3D image of the model is created. Dental labs often prefer optical digitizers, involving less acquisition time for scan construction [3, 4].

Digital measurements of tooth size, arch width, and Bolton tooth size discrepancy on digital models obtained from plaster dental model scanning and dental impression scanning showed high accuracy and reliability. No statistically significant differences

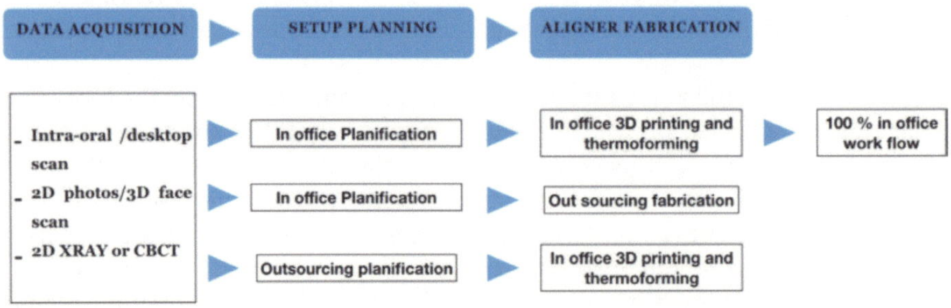

Figure 1.
Different Workflows for in-office aligners.

were noticed between direct measurements on the plaster models with a caliper and digital measurements on digital models obtained from plaster dental model scanning and dental impression scanning methods. Digital models can be alternative to plaster models with clinically acceptable accuracy and reliability of tooth size, arch width measurements, and Bolton analysis [5].

Intraoral scanner (IOS) is an alternative to OS for the digitization procedures of plaster dental models [3]. Various intraoral scanners are available in the market, with many different technologies, each with its own limitations, advantages, and costs [6]. The 3D scanning technologies depend on different physical principles and are defined in the subsequent classes [5]:

1. Laser triangulation 3D scanning technology uses either a laser line or a single laser point to scan across an object.

2. Structured light 3D scanning technology uses trigonometric triangulation.

3. Photogrammetry 3D scan scanning technology (photography) reconstructs 3D from 2D images.

4. Contact-based 3D scanning technology is based on the contact form of 3D data collection and uses a contact probe [7].

Advancements in the CBCT systems have made the digitization of plaster dental models possible [8]. Several CBCT manufacturers have started integrating extra cast digitization tools into their machines to simplify the workflow for data acquisition and surface extraction [3]. CBCT scans are acquired using a volume scan method instead of a surface scan method using a laser or LED source; therefore, CBCT scans are not affected by the angle of irradiation or the shape of the subject around the undercut area proximal contact. CBCT can even be used in cases of crowding without managing raw scanned data [9].

Digital model fabrication using scans of patient impressions obtained with CBCT in a dental office is another alternative method to create a model without an intraoral scanner or a desktop scanner and without directly irradiating the patient. If necessary, digital models and plaster models can be fabricated using a single impression [10].

2.1.2 3D Facial scan

The assessment and analysis of facial soft tissues are essential for orthodontic and maxillofacial diagnosis and treatment planning. In aligner therapy, using a two-dimensional (2D) digital photograph is a basic approach for facial structure assessment. However, this process has been progressively replaced by three-dimensional (3D) imaging. The 3D facial scan enables creating a virtual face that can be integrated with 3D models of the dentition obtained by intra-oral scanners and coupled with 3D radiographic images from CBCT for a 3D orthodontic set-up to achieve virtual patient [11].

There are two classifications of the scanning systems based on the type of equipment of the optical devices, namely stationary systems and portable/handled systems. In stationary systems, the optical devices are fixed on tripods or adjustable frames, while in handled/portable systems, the scanners are movable in real time around the target object [12].

Stationary facial scanning systems based on stereophotogrammetry technology were first introduced in dentistry [13]. Digital stereophotogrammetry captures 3D facial surface data using at least two cameras configured as a stereo pair. This procedure may be: passive or active. In active stereophotogrammetry, structured-light techniques are incorporated for higher resolution [14]. Because of the encumbrance, high cost of this technology, and their operating methods that require frequent calibration, hand-held scanning systems using laser or structured-light technology were developed [15].

Laser-based scanners function by projecting an eye-safe class 1 laser beam across a subject's face. The beam is scattered by the face and collected at a triangulation distance from the laser's origin. At the same time, Structured-light scanners (SLSs) generate 3D facial models by projecting a full structured light pattern (typically vertical stripes) onto a subject's face, recording deformations in this pattern produced by the face's morphology allow 3D face reconstruction [16].

Although most professional handheld scanners are considered acceptable in terms of their scan image quality, they are expensive and often require considerable training time to learn their complex scanning protocols [3, 9, 10]. Alternatively, 3D sensor cameras based on structured-light technology have been developed for smartphone and tablet devices [15]. Increasing interest is due to mobile devices' high portability, user-friendliness, cost-effectiveness, and popularity [17–19]. The advantages of smartphone face digitization include reducing time for scanning, image processing, technical learning [20, 21], and their high portability [22].

Motion artifacts were considered the primary source of error in the results of portable face-scanning systems [23–25], cautioning that the influence of involuntary facial movements has a more significant impact on mobile face-scan devices than stationary ones [11]. Prolonged scanning time and unstable movements of the scanners may magnify the motion artifacts caused by involuntary facial movements [25]. Therefore, using scanners that conduct a single and quick scan is recommended, mainly when the face scans are performed on children or people with special needs who struggle to stay immobile for a prolonged time [11, 25, 26].

2.1.2.1 3D dentofacial integration

The 3D dentofacial image integration is performed by matching the dental scans to the facial scans. Alignment of the two scans (facial scan and dental scan) can use teeth image only (TO), perioral area without marker (PN), or perioral area with markers (PM) [22].

For the 3D dentofacial integration using teeth images only, the teeth area visible on the facial scan images is used as a reference to match the facial scan with the intraoral scan **Figure 2** [27, 28].

The intraoral scan of the teeth area associated with the scan of perioral structures was proposed to enhance the accuracy of the dentofacial integration [29] **Figure 3**. This procedure aims to provide larger areas that can be used as a reference to coordinate the intraoral scan of the teeth with the 3D scan of the face. The effect of the perioral scan method on image matching depends on the use of artificial markers during the perioral scanning [22]. The absence of clear marks on the skin causes inaccuracy of the scan data obtained when capturing large areas of the perioral structures without the skin marker attachment by the intraoral scanner.

Artificial markers provide distinct references for similar adjacent areas so that they could help the image stitching process. Perioral scan with artificial skin markers significantly improved the accuracy of integration of dental model to the facial scan **Figure 4** [22].

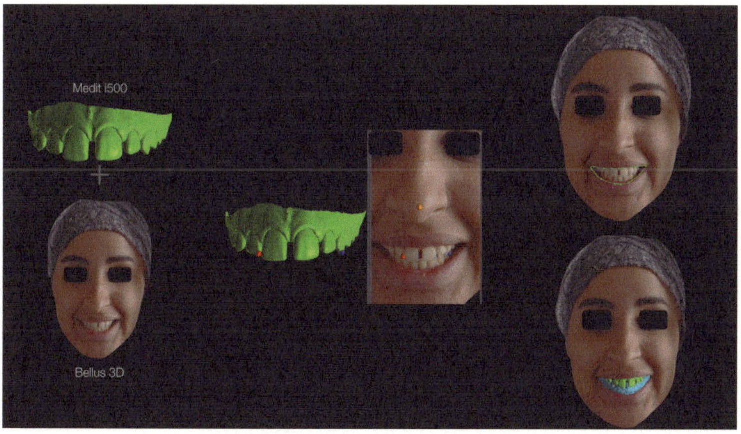

Figure 2.
Alignment of the two scans (facial scan and dental scan) using teeth image only (TO).

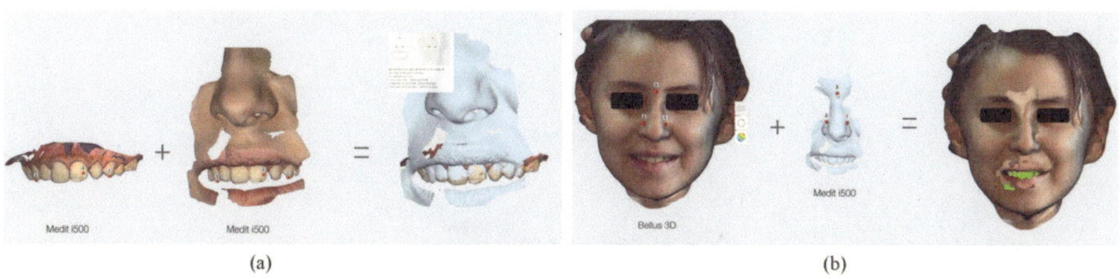

Figure 3.
Alignment of the two scans (facial scan and dental scan) using perioral area without marker (PN) The participant was scanned using Bellus 3D by rotating the head to the right and the left of the camera, following the manufacturer's instructions while maintaining the head at the camera's center. The scanning mode was set in high-definition (HD mode) in the scanning software. The intraoral and perioral anatomical structures were acquired using an intraoral optical scanner mediti500. The perioral structures, including the upper lip, philtrum, and nose, were obtained with the participant's anterior teeth in a broad smile position. a: The first step is matching perioral scan to intraoral scan; fixed mesh is intraoral scan. b: The second step is matching the 3D facial scan with the perioral scan previously aligned on the intraoral scan; the fixed mesh in this step is the perioral scan.

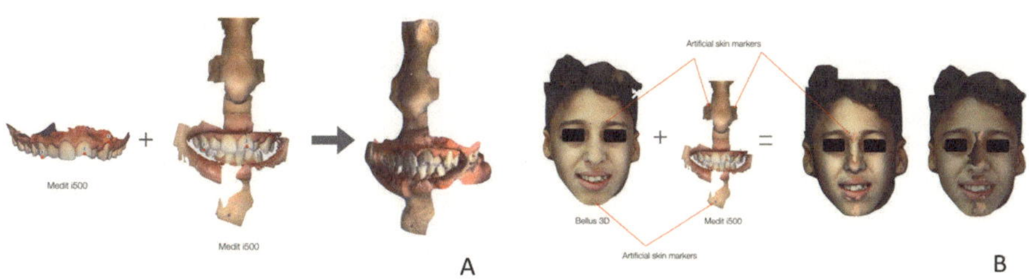

Figure 4.
The two scans (facial scan and dental scan) are aligned using perioral area with markers (PM). A: The first step is matching perioral scan to intraoral scan; fixed mesh is intraoral scan. B: The second step is matching the 3D facial scan with the perioral scan previously aligned on the intraoral scan; fixed mesh in this step is perioral scan. Artificial skin markers provide distinct references for the image stitching process.

2.1.3 3D X-ray: Cone-beam CT

Major planning solutions for aligners consider only the crown position, not the root shape. Complete tooth architecture information, including crown and root anatomies, would improve treatment planning and provide more predictable results [30].

2.1.3.1 Procedure

Dicom file is imported into 3D setup software; the orthodontist performs segmentation to have a 3D reconstruction of root morphology, then he stitches 3D segmented teeth to STL IOS model. Afterward, the orthodontist can adapt the position of the virtual tooth to segmented roots to have a correct pivot. Integrating 3D data from an optical scanner with volumetric data from CBCT imaging provides an optimal spatial reference for the most accurate hard and soft tissues models. **Figures 5** and **6**.

2.2 Digital treatment planning

Selecting software is the main concern for most clinicians to get started with homemade clear aligners. All 3D setup ortho planning software have typical workflow **Figure 7**. The software's options have comparable abilities at the core; however, some specific features add value and are determining when choosing a software. **Table 1** summarizes the different software available on the market with their respective options.

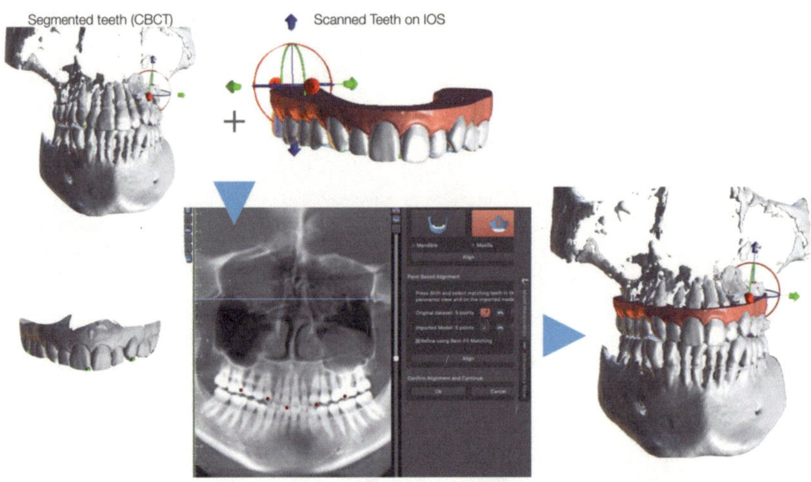

Figure 5.
Aligning 3D segmented Teeth (Roots & Crowns) to IOS Scanned teeth using teeth as references.

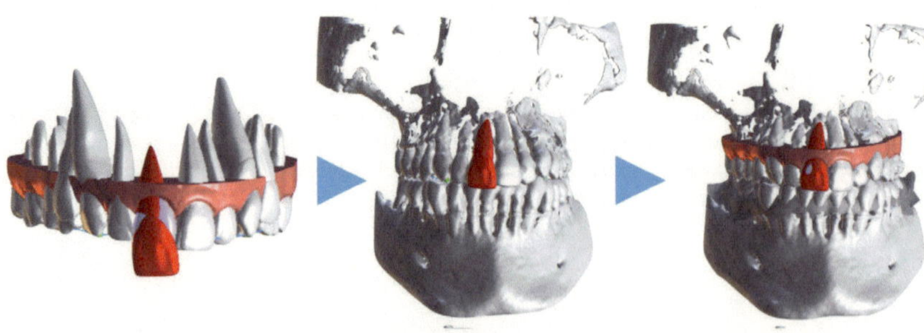

Figure 6.
Aligning virtual teeth of 3D setup software according to segmented roots (CBCT).

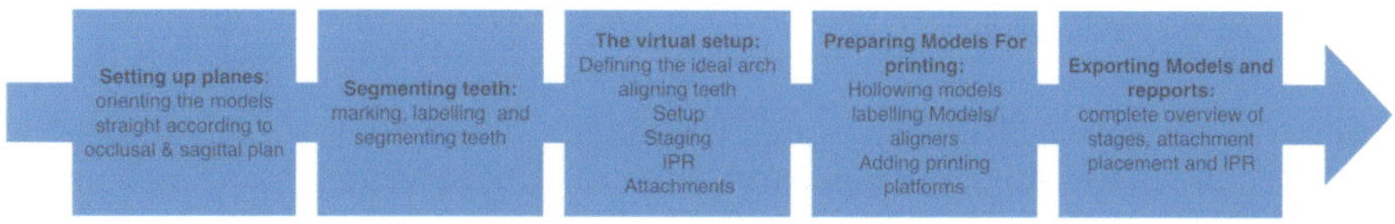

Figure 7.
Typical workflow for 3D ortho setup software.

	3shape		Sursmile	C+ model	Ulab	Ortup	BSB Ortho	ArchForm	SoftSmile
Grid overlay features	✓	✓	✓		✓	✓	✓	✓	✓
Automated Segmentation	✓	✓	✓	✓	✓	✓	✓	✓	✓
Individual or group movement of teeth	✓	✓	✓	✓	✓	✓	✓	✓	✓
Customize attachement size/ dimension	✓	✓	✓	✓	✓	✓	✓		✓
Auto place attachment					✓	✓	✓	✓	✓
IPR adjustment per contact		✓	✓	✓	✓	✓	✓	✓	✓
Staging IPR steps		✓	✓	✓	✓	✓			
Same day starts	✓		✓		✓			✓	✓
Automated set-up		✓	✓	✓	✓	✓	✓		
Print horizontal	✓	✓	✓	✓	✓	✓	✓	✓	✓
Print vertical: add platform				✓	✓		✓	✓	✓
Printing hollow				✓	✓		✓	✓	✓
Labels Models	✓	✓	✓	✓	✓	✓	✓	✓	✓
Aligners setps on models		✓		✓	✓		✓	✓	
Atomated aligner trimming for milling machine					✓		✓		
Predectibility and gradiant difficulty for tooth movement				✓					
License fee	✓	✓	✓		✓	✓		✓	✓
Fee per case/aligner exported				✓	✓		✓		
Directly print Aligner		✓					✓		
Pontic for extraction Cases			✓			✓			
Virtual root		✓				✓	✓		✓

Table 1.
Different software available on the market with their respective options.

2.2.1 Automatic segmentation

Almost all programs offer an automatic segmentation feature. Artificial intelligence (AI) algorithm finds the gingival border of each tooth. Using AI, the software will automatically segment and identify the teeth. Next, they will label the teeth and then automatically create a long axis, center groove line. If necessary, the software can manually adjust borders with an intuitive brush-editing feature, edit tooth labels, correct grooves, and adapt the long axis if needed [31, 32].

2.2.2 Realtime simulation

3D ortho setup software authorizes real-time simulation with features as intuitive alignment, enabling easily drag teeth to where they need to be, occlusal contact collision calculation, and IPR options. Also, 3D ortho setup software allows aligning the teeth to a customizable arch shape by adjusting the arch shape using the control points placed around it [33].

However, not all programs allow skeletal movements, evaluation of multiple treatment strategies, and creating treatment simulations for surgical, restorative, and extraction cases [34]. Plus, features relative to model capabilities as Bolton analysis on every model, automated measurements of tooth width, arch width are not available in all software.

The SoftSmile, Blueskyplan orthodontic, Deltaface, and Orth'up aligner software [31–36] create a 3D model of the orthodontic treatment plan, including a representation of teeth roots and movement of the lower jaw during the treatment. It creates optimized teeth movement and suggests, along with the knowledge and skill from the orthodontist, the exact number of aligners needed for reaching better results.

2.2.3 Advanced staging and sequencing

3D setup softwares make a staging proposal; the user feels the difference in the possibility of customizing this staging. BSB ortho, uLab, et ArchForm enable the orthodontist to select the teeth to move first, achieving sequential distalization and establishing the order of teeth movements [32–35].

2.2.4 Attachments

Adding an attachment is a standard option in 3D setup software. Some softwares stand out by features such as automatic attachment placement depending on the tooth movement or customized attachment with adjustable attachment size and gingival tilt to control tooth movement [35–37].

2.2.5 Ready to print models

From finishing the treatment plan to starting a print, much valuable time is lost on preparing printable.STL. All softweares allow STL export, but some make the entire manufacturing process smooth, intuitive, and straightforward.

Blueskyplan ortho, Archform and ULab automatically prepare models for 3D printing: in few clicks, all models are made hollow, and a bar for vertical printing without support is attached to them [35–37]. Usually technicians spend 5–7 minutes on the preparation of each model, but with BlueSkyPlan Ortho 2 minutes are spent on preparing the whole case's models. Features like hollowing models and vertical printing with optimized tilt make the virtual setup process smooth, quick and convenient, saving resin and printing time [35].

Labelling models is a standard feature that enables adding letters and numbers on models to identify patients and orthodontists. Nevertheless, special labelling such as auto labelling imprints onto the aligner is specific to only some software like BSB ortho, Archform, and Ulab [35–37].

2.2.6 Automatic pontics for concealing gaps and missing teeth

Developed especially for extractions cases, this functionality is not available in all software. On Archform, and ORTH'UP softweare [33, 37], teeth can be extracted at any stage during treatment planning. The two software allow clinicians to place a pontic that will change dimension as the space is closed. The pontic can have the same form as the extracted tooth, a mirror of the tooth on the other side, or a tooth selected from a library [37]. With SureSmile, either gaps are opened for an implant or closed after an extraction; once a space is bigger than 3 mm, a virtual tooth is added to fill the gap [34]. Efficient and fast, this functionality allows significant time-saving in the preparation of cases for the dental assistant.; avoiding manual waxing on printed models before thermoforming aligners [33].

2.2.7 Variable trim line

With BSB ortho, doctors can freely choose the trim line design; individualized positioning bases are added to the aligner to be trimmed in a high-precision automated laser cutting machine [35]. The Aligner Trim curve will be generated automatically based on the parameters "Curve Shape" and "Trim Margin" in Preferences. Both parameters can be adjusted as well and regenerate directly on the orthodontics panel. The export of the curve will be available in the last step for the automatic trimming of the aligners in the milling machines [35]. ORTH'UP software offers the possibility of calculating the aligner boundary at each step of the treatment plan and converts it into a 3D marking on the printed model. This visual reference makes cutting the aligners by the dental assistant faster and much more precise [33].

2.3 3D Printing

The dental sector has been undergoing radical change for many years, thanks to the digital dentistry movement. Additive manufacturing, in particular, has enabled the dental industry to expand its use of digital technologies. Indeed, the dental sector is a promising market for 3D printing technology because it responds to the issue of customized items.

3D printing is now easily approachable for orthodontists; 3d printing for orthodontics reduces production time and costs, and its potential is still growing [38].

2.3.1 Fused deposition modeling (FDM) 3D printing

Fused Deposition Modeling (FDM) 3D printing consists of creating several layers by injecting a molten plastic filament through a heated extruder. Any material that can be injected through a heated nozzle at melting temperature is printable by this technology. It comes in a long filament with a 1.75 to 3 mm diameter wound in a 500 g or 1 kg coil. Polylactic acid (PLA), Acrylonitrile butadiene styrene (ABS), and GreenTech pro are the most suitable materials for orthodontic models. Their prices vary from 20 to 40 euros [39].

PLA is a fully biodegradable polymer by industrial composting. It is obtained from the fermentation of starch, beet, corn, or sugar cane. It has the advantage of not giving off toxic fumes during printing. However, its glass transition temperature is around 60°, which limits its use under thermal stress, which goes against the thermoforming of aligners [39, 40]. PLA is generally used in 3D printing due to its very affordable price also in dental 3D printing to make dental models. New reinforced forms are proposed to endure mechanical and thermal stresses. (Pla Ultra, PLA-X3,) [40, 41].

Acrylonitrile butadiene styrene (ABS) is a thermoplastic polymer with excellent mechanical and thermal resistance. It is very affordable and is easily recycled by steaming [42, 43].

GreenTech pro is a 100% biodegradable biopolymer (DIN EN ISO 14855), made from organic, CO2 neutral, and environmentally friendly materials. The FDA has approved it for food contact. It has a mechanical and thermal superior resistance to ABS and PLA, ideal for dental models subject to thermoforming constraints [44].

2.3.2 Stereolithography 3D printing

Stereolithography 3D Printing (SLA) is the most widely used technology in dentistry, both for its precision and well-finished surface. For the same layer thickness, the surface roughness is far well finished compared to FDM. Stereolithography (SLA) is an additive manufacturing process that refers to the Vat Photopolymerization family. In SLA, an object is formed by selectively curing a polymer resin layer-by-layer using an ultraviolet (UV) laser beam [45, 46].

UV light can be a simple micrometers laser beam that will sweep the entire layer, point by point, just like a colored pencil that colors a 2D drawing to follow the same way on the next layer [45]. UV light projection can also be a light projection of an entire layer by a DLP projector (Direct Light Processing), resulting in a single-shot polymerization of the entire layer. Compared to SLA, the DLP is definitely faster [45].

Among the leading manufacturers of 3D SLA printers, 3D Systems, is at the origin of this technology, but also more recent players like Asiga, which was the first to have launched the Direct Light Processing (DLP) 3D printers in 2011, and Formlabs, which initiated the introduction of in-office 3D printers to the dental practice through its FORM2 printer allowing 3D printing dental materials.

This technology uses 385 nm or 405 nm photopolymerizable resins depending on the wavelength of projected light. There are many resins dedicated to dental models which have the advantage over other resins of being very fast in printing and having a color that helps thermoforming control and good mechanical and thermal resistance.

2.3.2.1 Dental model resin

All resin manufacturers began to produce dedicated dental resins for both prosthodontic and orthodontic models. Compared to standard resins, those resins have faster print speed, are very precise, and have a significantly lower degree of shrinkage. Dental models resins have a beige color [47].

2.3.2.2 Dental long term (LT) ® clear resin

It is a class IIa long-term biocompatible resin for printing rigid splints, durable orthodontic appliances, and night guards. According to some preliminary studies, this resin may be suitable for clear aligner direct 3D printing because it has good geometric precision and comparable mechanical properties to the thermoformed aligners [48, 49].

2.3.2.3 Tera Harz TC-85

Graphy, a South Korean-based company of 3D printable photopolymer resins, has revealed a dental 3D printing material mark, Tera Harz, intending to overcome the constraints posed by other 3D printable resins used within the dental field.

Graphy's Tera Harz has obtained CE, FDA, and KFDA medical device certification and is available in clear (TC-85DAC) or white (TC-85DAW). The clear Tera Harz resin is fully transparent and has high durability agreed with orthodontic treatment device purposes. In comparison, the white Tera Harz material features esthetics alongside durability **Figure 8**.

2.3.2.4 Post treatment

Objects produced with 3D printing technologies usually need some degree of post-production treatment. This crucial step of the 3D printing workflow is known as post-processing. First, 3d printed models must be washed in isopropyl alcohol (IPA) or tripropylene glycol monomethyl ether (TPM). For optimal cleaning, users have to shake parts around in the solvent as well as soaked. Habitually, cleaning 3D Printed models requires two washes in IPA or TPM to be fully clean.

When an SLA part finishes printing, the polymerization reaction may not yet be completed. Wich means that parts have not reached their final material properties and may not function as expected, particularly tough parts under strain. Exposing the printed objects to light and heat, called post-curing, will help solidify its materials properties. A UV box post-treatment is usually required to achieve the light-curing process and maximize material strength.

Post-curing is not mandatory for standard resins. Other resin types require post-curing to achieve their optical-mechanical properties. Each material should be submitted to the curing process for a specific amount of time. Printed models should be cleaned and cured before removing supports [46].

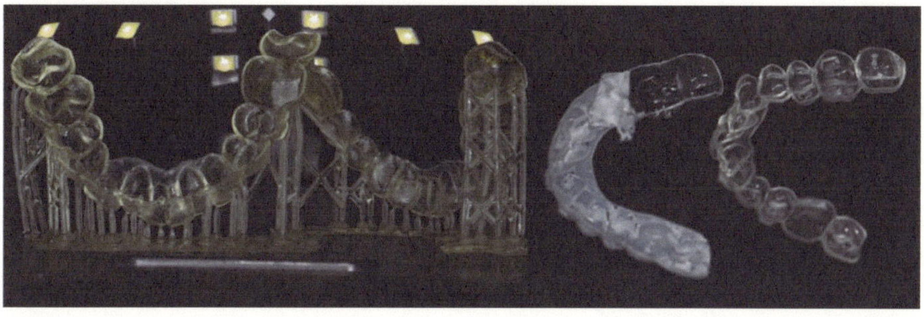

Figure 8.
Directly printed aligners with Tera Harz TC-85 resin (TC-85DAC) put, after post-treatment side by side with thermoformed aligner (Biolon 0,75 mm).

2.4 Thermoforming aligners

The first aligners developed by Align Technology corresponded to a single-layer rigid polyurethane produced from methylene diphenyl diisocyanate and 1,6-hexanediol. To enhance its mechanical proprieties and transparency Smart Track (Align Technology, 2012) developed a new thermoplastic polyurethane [50, 51]. The expansion in demand for clear aligners has commanded the development of additional thermoplastic materials for clear aligners by other entreprises, such as e.g. Invisalign, Duran, Biolon, Zendura, Erkodur, ClearCorrect, Erkoflex 95, Erkoloc pro, etc. [52, 53] **Table 2** summarizes the different sheets currently on the market [54].

The manhood of current aligner companies uses transformed polyethylene terephthalate glycol (PETG), although polypropylene, polycarbonate, thermoplastic polyurethanes, copolyester, and many other materials are also used [50].

The mechanical characteristics of dental polymers exhibit a myriad of influence factors, such as intrinsic factors (molecular and crystal structures, etc.) and extrinsic factors (temperature, humidity, etc.) [55, 56]. The used polymers are either amorphous or semi-crystalline. Low crystallinity of polymers typically means high flexibility, high elasticity, and adaptability to the tooth shape, but on the other side, they present low tensile strength, low chemical resistance, and stability [56]. From a clinical perspective, polymers with high flexibility and elasticity are more convenient for patients to insert or remove the aligners. Furthermore, they adjust better to the complexity of the tooth anatomy, attach perfectly to any surface. Correlated to aligners of rigid materials, they also guarantee continuity of force expression during the orthodontic treatment [56].

Product name	Component	Manufacturer
Zendura	Poly-Urethane (PU)	Bay materials
Zendura FLX.	Thermoplastic Polyurethane (TPU)	
Essix ace+	Copolyesther	Dentsplay
Essix c+	Polypropylene/ethylene/copolymer	Dentsplay
Clearaligner	Polyethylene terephthalate glycol (PETG)	Scheu Dental
Biolon	Polyethylene terephthalate glycol (PETG)	Dreve Dentamid gmbh)
Smilers	Polyethylene terephthalate glycol (PETG)	Biotech Dental
Smiletech	Polyethylene terephthalate glycol (PETG)	Ortodontica Italia srl
Taglus tuff	Polyethylene terephthalate glycol (PETG)	Allure Ortho
Clearcorrect	Zendura: POLY-URETAN (PU)	Strauman group brand
Duran	Polyethylene terephthalate glycol (PETG)	Scheu Dental
Track A	Polyethylene terephthalate glycol (PETG)	Forestadent
Track B	Polyethylene terephthalate glycol thermoplastic polyurethane (TPU/PET-G)	Forestadent
Erkodur-al	Copolyester	Erkodent gmbh

Table 2.
Different sheets currently on the market.

2.4.1 Thermoforming machines

Thermoforming consists of hot shaping thermoplastic products made of polymers. There are two types of thermoforming machines:

- Vacuum forming machines that operate on the principle of air depression. A draft takes place below the model to be thermoformed, thereby ensuring the plastic material's suction above. Example: Essix Machine®, Tray Vac®, Econo Vac®, Erkopress 240® [57].
- Pressure forming machines that generate pressurized air above the thermoplastic material to press it against the model. Steel granules partially coat the model limiting thermoforming to uncovered areas. Example: Ministar®, Erkoform® or Drufosmartscan® [57] **Figure 9**.

Vacuum forming machines are not recommended for making aligners because they are not accurate enough. The aligner must have a tight fit on the models to transfer that fit over the teeth and have the proper amount of force. For this purpose, pressure-forming machines are more adapted. These machines are usually already present in the dental office for making retainers, night guards, etc.

The selection of a forming machine will be made according to the compatibility of the machine to different brands of trays, the space allocated to thermoforming in the dental office, the Drufosmart® for example, takes up a little less space than the others because of its vertical forming design, or according to features that will facilitate and automate the task of dental assistants, such as the barcode reader where the materials setting are just scanned, or the possibility of thermoforming several models at the same time for mass production.

2.5 Tray trimming and polishing

After thermoforming, the aligner is first cut on the 3D printed model with large chisels; then, it is delicately removed to avoid permanent deformation on the aligner. The cutout is finished with curved scissors. Polishing the edges is done with polishers to avoid having sharp edges. Solutions for automated trimming exist on the market

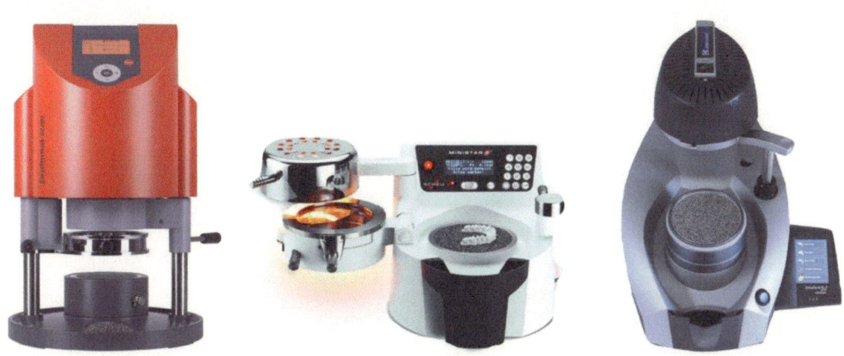

Figure 9.
Pressure forming machines for aligner's fabrication.

like Inlase for dental practices with an expanded production volume of aligners [58]. There are solutions for automated trimming on the market like iNLASE®, which is a laser trimming machine that automatically cuts thermoformed aligners in less than 15 seconds, without the need for manual cutting or polishing **Figure 10** [58].

2.5.1 Scalloped VS continuous curve

According to Cowley et al. [59], there are three designs for aligners at the gingival margin:

- A scalloped gingival margin design, along the gingival zenith, which is used by Invisalign and Orthocaps.
- A straight line gingival margin along the gingival zenith.
- A straight-line gingival margin above the gingival zenith (which is used by CA Clear Aligner) [59].

The difference between the techniques was remarkable. The straight cut 2 mm from the margins was about twice as retentive as the scalloped cut for clear aligners without engagers. For clear aligners with attachments, the straight cut 2 mm from the margins was over four times as retentive as the scalloped cut.

Cutting the aligners differently had more of an impact than supplementing or excluding attachments. Aligners are more comfortable with this technique because the aligners impinging on the unattached marginal gingiva is less risk. The edge of the aligner is covered further under patients' lips during everyday use; this should also slightly increase the discreetness of the aligners.

2.6 Packaging and delivery

Packaging and labelling is a step that is often overlooked in aligner fabrication. Standards bags with a zip-lock function can be easily found on the market and

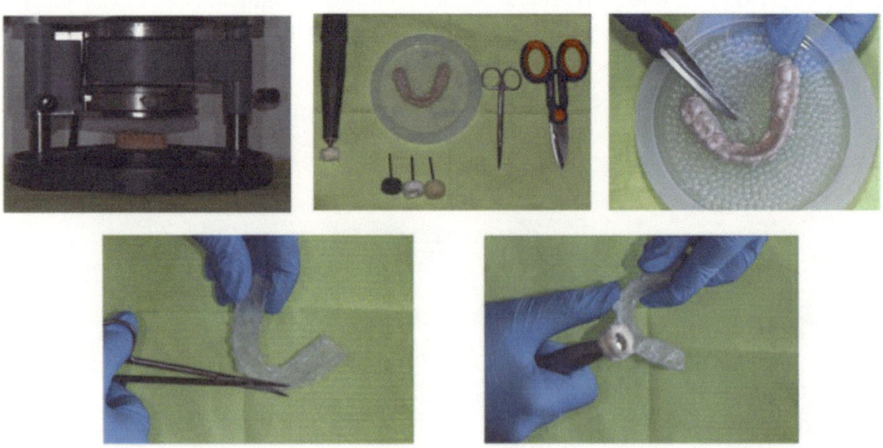

Figure 10.
In-office trimming of aligners.

handled for aligner packaging. Practitioners can easily utilize labels and print office logos and patient information. A bag or a box can be used to deliver the aligners to the patient; custom printed plastic bags are preferable to boxes. Besides being more cost-effective, custom printed bags take up less space and are easier to stock and deliver to the patient, particularly when only a few stages are required. From a branding perspective, practices with in-house aligner production should package the aligners in a way that promotes their office **Figure 11**.

2.7 Delegation

Delegation is a fundamental concept in management. It allows the practitioner to "optimize his diploma" by performing only acts or tasks which fall solely and specifically within his competence. On the other hand, it helps develop team motivation. Delegating tasks relating to new technologies such as 3D printing or digital impression helps to motivate and, above all, enhance dental assistant work.

For homemade aligners, 90% of the tasks can be delegated to a dental assistant. 10% of the remaining tasks concern planning of 3D setup, some steps of which can also be delegated. When outsourcing 3D setup, the whole production chain is delegated. **Table 3** shows the distribution of tasks relating to the homemade aligner.

The dental assistant must do all patient records. Indeed intraoral scanning, taking 2D or 3D X-rays, and face scanning all these tasks can be delegated to a well-trained dental assistant.

The dental assistant will import /export various STL/OBJ files either to prepare the 3D setup or to print the various stages. The dental assistant will also process data such as tooth segmentation, labelling, and nesting models on 3D printer software. The interoperability and intuitiveness of the software will allow the dental assistant to switch from one software to another seamlessly.

All tasks relating to 3D printing are delegable: removing models from building platforms, washing, drying, curing models, and removing supports. When choosing a 3D printer, the practitioner should consider user-friendly and intuitive 3D printing software that exports the models with the bases set at the correct angle. Likewise, selecting a 3D printer with features like calculating the amount of resin or filament needed for 3D printing to not run out of materials is crucial for overnight 3D printing. Samely when purchasing post-treatment hardware, the practitioner must choose automated systems for washing, drying, and curing models to make the task as efficient as possible for the assistant.

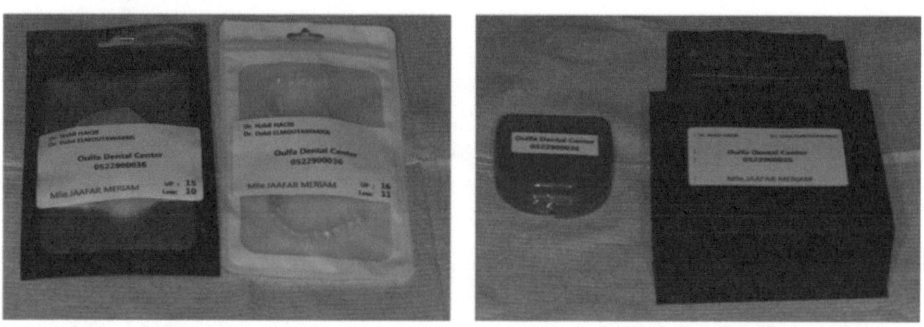

Figure 11.
Homemade packaging for aligners.

		Orthodontist	Dental assistant
Clinical work	Digital models		• Intra-oral scan • Closing model's holes • Exporting for set-up • Software/outsourcing
	2D X-Ray-CBCT		Taking 2D X-Ray/ CBCT
	Facial		2D photos 3DFacial scan
	Aligner's Initial insertion		Seats check
Laboratory work	Planning Software	• Aligning teeth • Choosing attachments • Staging	• Loading models in software • Marking teeth • Segmenting teeth • Pre-aligning teeth • Labeling models • Adding Platform • Exporting for 3D (hollowing models)
	3D printing		• Nesting models in 3D printer • Software
	Post processing		• Removing models • Washing & drying models • UV Curing models • Taking off platform /supports
	Aligner fabrication		• Thermoforming • Cutting/trimming • Polishing • Packaging

Table 3.
The distribution of tasks relating to the homemade aligner.

Aligner fabrication is a fully delegable task; the dental assistant must do the entire process, thermoforming, cutting, polishing, and packaging. Thus, the dental assistant performs the initial insertion of the appliance to check its fitting.

3. Results

Invisalign is the most common clear aligner option that is outsourced. The cost for Invisalign treatment is 575 $ for five aligners, 1199$ for 14 aligners cases, and 1779$ for full cases. For ClearCorrect, the price for five aligners is 395 $, 935$ for 14 aligners cases, and 1495$ for unlimited cases.

	Invisalign	Clear correct	In-office printing & thermoforming*	In-office fabrication out sourcing planning **
5 aligners	575 $	395$	72$	252$
10 aligners	925 $	695$	125$	305$
14 aligners	1199 $	935$	167$	347$
30 aligners	1779$	1495$	335$	515$
Revision	125$	95$	..	..

**5 $ fabrication cost per aligner and 20 $ software cost per case (2jaws) (10$ one jaw). Cost per aligner include materials cost/ printing cost and assistant's time to fabricate the aligner.*
***200$ for outsourcing planning (Labpronto).*

Table 4.
Comparison cost fee for different aligners systems.

When aligners are homemade, the cost for five aligners treatment turns around 70$. This includes printing, materials, assistant time to fabricate the aligner, and software fee. The cost per printed model is for resin models 1,75 $, and it depends on the brand of the resin and the use or not of supports while 3D printing. The cost per clear aligner sheet is 1,5$ (biolon 0,75 mm), and it also depends on the brand of the aligners sheet. In the USA dental assistant's average wage per hour is $ 25; for aligner fabrication, a dental assistant takes 5 minutes to make each clear aligner, so the cost per aligner for assistant time is roughly 2$. The total fabrication cost per aligner for homemade aligners is 5,25$. For an in-house clear aligner software, the fee per case is 20 $ for two arches (Bluesky plan ORTHO) and 10$ if only one arch is processed. If the orthodontist wants to outsource the planning, the cost for outsourcing planning is $ 200 (LabPronto). **Table 4** recapitulates the different costs according to the treatment options and the number of aligners.

4. Discussion

Orthodontic practices that integrate in-house aligners solution into their operation gain full control over the workflow eliminate outside lab fees, and achieve faster production turnaround time. Internalizing aligners manufacturing in the dental office reduces by at least half of the cost compared to commercial aligners suppliers **Table 4**.

Being able to reduce aligner fees for patients will increase profit line and case acceptance. Nowadays, direct to consumers companies propose clear aligners with competitive cost compared to conventional aligner treatment. Thus the do-it-yourself (DIY) aligners companies are trying to eliminate the orthodontist from the equation. With the homemade aligners the orthodontist can be competitive even with such companies.

In-office aligner's production allows complete management for the entire aligner-making process. Compared to a custom commercial aligners laboratory, this flow enables complete control over the treatment plan because planning is done by the orthodontist and gives particular options like having additional aligners/refinement or producing several aligners for the same step in different thicknesses for specific case's need.

Orthodontists have also control of the 3D printing process: by controlling materials, resolution, printing direction, models Hollowing, etc.. and managing aligner sheets materials in terms of composition, thickness, toxicity (Bisphenol A (BPA) free) [60], and the trim line, also being able to customize this factors for each specific clinic case. All these aspects have a significant impact on the efficiency of clear aligner therapy.

In-house aligner production authorizes faster processes for patients; Aligner production can begin as soon as the patient is ready to undergo oral scans. Practices can provide same-day or next-day starts service depending on the patient queue. In a same-day appointment, an orthodontist can take oral scans, plan out treatment, and print and form the first aligner stages before the patient leaves the office or within a few hours of the appointment. The expedited service provides optimal customer service and an immediate customer lock-in advantage.

4.1 Digital model creation

Digital models offer more advantages such as instant accessibility of 3D information without the need for the retrieval of plaster models from a storage area, reduced need for large areas for plaster model storing, and less time-consuming analysis [61]. With 3D digital models, clinicians can evaluate dental models in three-dimensional aspects and perform dental analysis in more detail. Interrelation between maxillary and mandibular arches can be better observed in occlusion on different scenes in 3D software [62]. Digital models also provide virtual treatment and virtual setup [63]. 3D models can be processed to analyze specific teeth and to estimate the axis or position of individual teeth, which provides a three-dimensional prediction of tooth movement by superimposing dental changes on stable reference structures [5].

Desktop Optical Scanning is a simple, fast, and straightforward procedure; models do not require a second scan due to the scan's lack of data or non-completion. Likewise, the OS procedure is an entirely delegable task. However, despite all the advantages, it is very cost-intensive and therefore unaffordable for many dental offices and labs, and for impression scanning procedures, the record of the patient's occlusion cannot be obtained [3].

Intraoral scanners introduce innovations in orthodontics such as monitoring dental movement through digital model superimposition aligners [64, 65], further customization of orthodontic appliances such as removable retainers [65], and last but not least, more accurate diagnosis, treatment planning and even simulation of possible orthodontic movement on appropriate software [66, 67]. Furthermore, scanning requires more chairside time, but it was found less unpleasant than the standard procedure of impression taking [68]; evidence exists that patients when asked which type of impression satisfy them more, choose digital due to patient-centered outcomes [69].

A systematic review [70, 71] of the accuracy of intraoral scans reported that inter- and intra-arch measurements from intraoral scans were more reliable and accurate in comparison to those from conventional impressions. Another systematic review in prosthodontics [72] reported that dental restorations fabricated using digital impressions exhibited a similar marginal fit to those fabricated using conventional impressions [73].

Many factors affect the accuracy of the IOS, such as [74, 75]:

1. Scanner: capacity to register details and its accuracy.

2. OperatorUser: scanning fundamentals and path's scanning.

3. Scanning area: the dimension of the scanning area, arch length, and surface irregularities.

4. Intraoral environmental factors: temperature, relative humidity, illumination, shiny, reflective, or transparent objects [7]. Solabrietta et al. denoted that the differences in accuracy between the scanners are rudimentary, and the characteristics that make everyday work easier and more pleasant for the doctor and the patient seem to be much more relevant [61].

After a conventional alginate impression, a median of 22 minutes is required for plaster modeling, including pouring and trimming. In Park JY, study [9], the digital models were obtained within 5 minutes after a rubber impression, with 14 seconds for the CBCT scan of the impression, 1 minute for CBCT file export, and 2 minutes for generating an STL file for each arch. In terms of efficiency, digital modeling using CBCT seems to be clinically feasible and is correlated to reduced laboratory time. No significant differences were found in most measurements between the cast scan models and CBCT digital models. CBCT may be suitable for use in clinical practice because of its advantages, including a reduced working time for digital model rendering [9]. For a dental professional who previously has a CBCT or an IOS device, the acquisition of another digitization system might seem redundant [3].

However, the 3D ortho setup is done on maxillary and mandibular 3D models in occlusion. Using a CBCT to digitalize dental arches is undoubtedly possible. However, the registration of the occlusion, which is indexing one model in relation to the other with this method, is not as intuitive as with an OS or IOS and will require additional CBCT scans of the models in occlusion and the passage through a third-party software to align, relate and index the models before importing them into the 3D setup software.

For Emara A, OS is the best choice for dental models' digitization. The CBCT, however, proved to be a highly precise option. Even if the tested IOS showed the lowest results in terms of accuracy, it is still a valid affordable option for model digitization, with results falling within the "clinically acceptable" range [3].

4.2 Facial scan

Facial scanner using a mobile device 3D sensor camera has been captivating much interest in recent years because it is highly portable and cost-effective and because of the popularity of mobile devices [14]. Smartphone- and tablet-compatible 3D facial scanners have been described to be a valuable tool for clinical use in prosthodontic treatment [12, 15–18]. However, the digital facial impression accuracy obtained with mobile device–compatible face scanners has not been investigated [15].

No significant difference was found between stationary and portable face-scanning systems concerning the accuracy of the resultant digital face models. Within the comparison of scanning methods, stereophotogrammetry, laser, and structured-light systems showed similar levels of accuracy in generating a digital face model [11].

The accuracy of mobile device–compatible face scanners in the 3D facial acquisition was not comparable to that of professional optical scanning systems, but it was still within the clinically acceptable range of <1.5 mm in dimensional deviation [15].

Amornvit et al. [76] and Liu et al. [77] reported that mobile device–compatible face scanners are comparable to professional 3D facial scanners when scanning simple and flat areas of the face such as the forehead cheeks, and chin. However, scanning accuracy was relatively low when mobile device–compatible face scanners were used to capture complex facial regions, such as the external ears, eyelids, nostrils, and teeth [76–79]. Higher inaccuracy was found in the facial areas with defects, depending on the depth of the defect [15, 20]. The teeth scan quality for the smartphone 3D face scan could be lower than that of the stereophotogrammetry because of the high sensibility to the depth of the smartphone facial scanner [16, 22].

The accuracy of the image integration using teeth images only principally relies on the spatial accuracy and the resolution of the captured anterior teeth image in the digital facial scan [28]. When only the teeth region was used for image matching between the facial scan and intraoral scan images, the alignement could be predisposed to error because of the image deformations of the 3D facial model at the mouth area due to the difficulties in scanning the complex structures of the teeth and the gingiva [22, 28].

The accuracy of virtual dentofacial combinations was mainly reliant on perioral scans and artificial skin markers. The most trivial midline deviation and frontal plan canting were found when the perioral image with artificial markers was used. In contrast, the highest divergences were found when the perioral image obtained without markers was employed for image alignment. Although stereophotogrammetry face scan generally showed higher accuracy of virtual dentofacial integration than the smartphone 3D depth camera face scan, the difference between the devices was not significant when the perioral scans were used as references for image matching.

4.3 Setup planning

Unique features make some software high valuable, when choosing software for homemade aligners, orthodontists should look for a program that includes the functionality of matching CBCT data to IOS data and the possibility of positioning the virtual roots of the 3D setup software according to 3D segmented teeth from CBCT. Accurate superimposition of the intraoral scan over the CBCT data would allow the orthodontist to clearly view a dimensionally true representation of a tooth and its root relative to the alveolar ridge [80, 81]. While the conventional virtual setup focuses on moving the crowns, the 3D digital model includes root positions, thus enabling a better outcome [82–84].

BSB ORTHO offers advanced options such as integration of CBCT and facial scan data, the superposition of these data with the 3D models is seamless with BSB ORTHO software, also import and export high definition models to have as little decimation as possible and achieve a good fitting of the aligner [35].

Archform, uLab, and 3Shape software create the same-day functionality without spending time creating a complete treatment set-up. This adds value for the clinician offering super-speed turnarounds and bringing instant orthodontics into their practices [84].

Carestream's Model+ software is a relative newcomer to the aligner software space; Carestream's Model+ software has a unique feature that only is within their software. Model+ allows the clinician to assess individual tooth movements and grade both case complexity and predictability of individual tooth movements [84].

ArchForm can be used across multiple computers and keep patient data in synchronization. For example, the orthodontist can start a design on the office computer and continue it on his laptop at home. Plus, the software keeps patients on track, turning around refinements in one day by instant adjusting treatments mid-course for faster treatment and more precise results [37].

ArchForm and ULab's AI-assisted software includes one-touch bracket removal features that make finishing bracket cases in aligners or preparing finishing retainers in advance easier by allowing easy removal of the brackets post-scanning [85].

Direct 3D printing of aligners is more innovative and is gradually gaining market share, especially with the emergence of more suitable resins. It is a breakthrough. Deltaface & BSB Ortho are the only two software on the market that offer this functionality; the rigidity of the aligner is set on that software by locally adjusting the thickness of the aligners. This technic offers many advantages, notably: better precision, saving of time by eliminating the steps of thermoforming, cutting, and polishing; it also allows a saving of resin by removing the need to print the models, which has an ecological virtue [31, 35].

Many software options require monthly subscription fees, pay-per-case export fees, or pay-by-aligner pricing, and it is crucial to select cost-effective and functional software for the office.

4.4 3D printing

FDM printer extrudes a resin that has been heated just beyond its melting point, placing it layer by layer. The heated material hardens immediately after being extruded, thus minimizing inaccuracies. Of the available materials, the most common are polylactic acid and acrylonitrile butadiene styrene (ABS). These often come on spools that can easily be replaced as needed. FDM 3D printing has the advantage of printing at a low cost and not needing post-processing, but it is relatively slow and less well finished than stereolithography. However, it offers relatively sufficient precision for orthodontic models because it easily makes dental models print with 100 to 50 microns accuracy with semi-professional 3D printers like the Ultimaker S5 and Raise3D E2. It is possible to recycle old ortho models through filament extrusion machines (for example: 3DEVO) to achieve almost zero production cost and ecological production [86].

Nanometric particles are emitted during ABS 3D printing process and are harmful if inhaled. To avoid the harmful inhalation of these particles, practitioners who want to integrate this technology in their practice area should use a fully enclosed 3D printing room equipped with a fume extractor-ultrafine particle emissions from desktop 3D printers [87]. Adding adherent agents on the printing bed is strongly recommended to limit the warping (Detachment of the part from the plate during printing) of the ABS [86].

Generally, there is no post-processing for FDM 3D printed dental models as they are generally horizontally printed and do not need any supports or printing platform. Despite being slow, this technology requires the minimum intervention from the operator because after detaching the model from the printing bed, models are prompt for thermoforming process.

In the aligner-manufacturing context, biocompatibility resin is not mandatory except in direct 3D printing aligners that will emerge soon. However, according to other authors, the Dental LT could be subject to an overall thickness inaccuracy compared to the designed file, leading to undesired movements [88]. In addition, 3D printing orientation and post-processing conditions; (exposure time to UV light and heat) could impact mechanical properties and biocompatibility of Dental LT resin [53, 89]. Further studies both in vitro and in vivo are needed based on these claims to test this resin and other direct aligner printable resins [90].

With the evolution of materials, the direct printing of aligners will take over the thermoforming process, save a considerable amount of models resin, streamline production, and reduce costs [91].

4.5 Thermoforming aligners

4.5.1 Influence of thermoforming

Ruy et al. examined the impact of thermoforming on the physical and mechanical properties of various thermoplastic materials for clear aligners (Duran, Essix A+, Essix ACE, and eCligner). They observed that the optical transparency, the tensile force, and the elastic modulus of the aligner materials decline after the thermoforming process, while water absorption was increased [92].

Moreover, they recommended evaluating these materials' durability after thermoforming to characterize their properties for their clinical application [92]. From a clinical perspective, the authors also proposed choosing the polymers depending on the treatment required, as some of them show a significant decrease in flexural strength after thermoforming and exhibit permanent deformation during treatment. On the other side, the application of large forces to the teeth can lead to absorption of the apical root [92].

Kwon et al. [51] assessed the force delivery properties of thermoplastic orthodontic materials. They found that the forces delivered by thin materials were more significant than those delivered by thick materials of the same brand [92].

4.5.2 Esthetic appearance

Transparency is evaluated to investigate the esthetic aspect of the materials. The transparency of materials decreased with an increase in their thickness. In addition, with decreased thickness after thermoforming, the transparency also decreased, which can be explained by the structural deformation of thermoplastic materials resulting in decreased transparency. Nevertheless, this transparency change did not compromise the esthetic appearance of clear aligners [92].

Many studies evaluate the stability of the materials after their average use of two weeks through the colorimetric alterations of aligners [93]. Bernard et al. affirm that there are foods that stain more than others (above all black tea) and that the Invisalign aligners (TPU) were more prone to pigmentation than the ClearCorrect (PU) or the Minor Tooth Movement devices (PET-G) after exposure to coffee or red wine. Black tea caused important stains on the surface of the three tested brands [93, 94].

4.5.3 Water absorption

Water absorption can negatively influence the mechanical properties of polymers leading to irreversible deterioration because water absorption is often appended to swelling and, thus, a deterioration of the polymers [95, 96]. Besides the deterioration effect, the swelling also leads to dimensional variations of the mouth devices, which affects the orthodontic forces [96]. Therefore, an ideal thermoplastic material for a clear aligner should have a low water absorption [54].

Tamburino et al. investigated the properties of materials for the thermoforming production of aligners. The materials used in their study were: Duran® (PETG, Sheu dental GmbH), Biolon (PETG, Dreve Dentamid GmbH) and Zendura®

(PU, Zendura Dental). Artificial saliva was used as an aging agent at a temperature of 37°C for 7 days [97]. The liquid absorption of Duran material is only almost half of the Zendura one. In addition to higher water uptake, the authors observed a decline of the mechanical properties of the Zendura that can be related to the mechanism of intramolecular bond destruction by water molecules [97].

Ryokawa et al. [8] reported that water absorption by both PETG and copolyester increased to 0.8 wt% in their 2-week experiment. In addition, water absorption by PETG differed depending on the type of thermoplastic material [55]. Zhang et al. [93] reported that water absorption increased when polyurethane was added to PETG during the development of new thermoplastic material for thermoformed aligners [92].

4.5.4 Mechanical properties

Tamburino et al. investigated the mechanical properties of the aligner materials Duran, Biolon, and Zendura in the as-delivered state, after thermoforming, and after storage in artificial saliva [97]. The authors found that the tensile yield stress of the Duran and Biolon materials only slightly changed after thermoforming (9% increase for Duran, 6% decrease for Biolon), while it decreased by one-third for the Zendura [54]. After exposure to artificial saliva, the tensile yield stress of the Duran material decrease back to it as-supplied strength, while the tensile yield stress of Biolon and Zendura materials slightly increase (to −3% respectively to −28%). Based on their finding, these authors propose to select a material for orthodontic devices after characterizing its mechanical properties after the corresponding manufacturing process and storage test in an intraoral simulation environment [54].

4.5.5 Elastic modulus

A higher elastic modulus is beneficial for aligners as it increases the force delivery capacity of the aligner under constant strain [98, 99]. Plus, materials with a higher elastic modulus can produce the same forces from thinner thickness [99]. The elastic modulus is proportional to the material stiffness. In their study [97], Tamburino et al. also examined the elastic modulus of the aligner materials Duran, Biolon, and Zendura in the as-delivered state, after thermoforming and after storage in artificial saliva. The elastic modulus of the Duran and Zendura materials increased by 11% respectively 17% after thermoforming, while the one of the Biolon material falls by 7%. Looking at the elastic modulus after artificial saliva exposure of the materials shows different behavior [100]. The elastic modulus of Biolon and Zendura material is relatively stable, while a significant decrease was observed for Duran. This decrease can be explained by water uptake happening during the storage in artificial saliva fluid [54].

5. Conclusions

Practice owners need to invest in material resources, but they also need to invest in education to help their team implement homemade aligner workflow. While 3D printing aligners in-house require that practices invest time and money, eliminating lab fees and the ability to provide same-day high-quality, consistent services justifies the investment by increasing profit margins, decreasing treatment timelines, and improving patient satisfaction. In-house production of aligners is the best option for practices that want more profitable and faster service. It just requires flexibility and an openness to learning new workflows that will carry the practice forward.

Conflict of interest

The authors declare no conflict of interest.

Author details

Dalal Elmoutawakkil* and Nabil Hacib
Independent Researchers

*Address all correspondence to: dr.elmoutawakkil@gmail.com

References

[1] Robertson L, Kaur H, Fagundes NCF, Romanyk D, Major P, Flores Mir C. Effectiveness of clear aligner therapy for orthodontic treatment: A systematic review. Orthod Craniofac Res. 2020 May;23(2):133-142. DOI: 10.1111/ocr.12353.

[2] Kassam SK, Stoops FR. Are clear aligners as effective as conventional fixed appliances? Evid Based Dent. 2020 Mar;21(1):30-31. DOI: 10.1038/s41432-020-0079-5.

[3] Emara A, Sharma N, Halbeisen FS, Msallem B, Thieringer FM. Comparative Evaluation of Digitization of Diagnostic Dental Cast (Plaster) Models Using Different Scanning Technologies. Dent J (Basel). 2020 Aug 2;8(3):79. DOI: 10.3390/dj8030079.

[4] Beuer, F.; Schweiger, J.; Edelho_, D. Digital dentistry: An overview of recent developments for CAD/CAM generated restorations. Br. Dent. J. 2008, 204, 505-511.

[5] Gül Amuk N, Karsli E, Kurt G. Comparison of dental measurements between conventional plaster models, digital models obtained by impression scanning and plaster model scanning. Int Orthod. 2019 Mar;17(1):151-158.

[6] Trebuoa P, 3D Scanning Technologies and the 3D Scanning Process, Aniwaa Pte. Ltd., France, 2019.

[7] Amornvit P, Sanohkan S, Peampring C. Studying the Optical 3D Accuracy of Intraoral Scans: An In Vitro Study. J Healthc Eng. 2020 Feb 14;2020:5739312. DOI: 10.1155/2020/5739312.

[8] Baumgaertel, S.; Palomo, M.; Palomo, L.; Hans, M.G. Reliability and accuracy of cone-beam computed tomography dental measurements. Am. J. Orthod. Dentofac. Orthop. 2009, 136, 19-28.

[9] Park JY, Kim D, Han SS, Yu HS, Cha JY. Three-dimensional comparison of 2 digital models obtained from cone-beam computed tomographic scans of polyvinyl siloxane impressions and plaster models. Imaging Sci Dent. 2019 Dec;49(4):257-263. DOI: 10.5624/isd.2019.49.4.257. Epub 2019 Dec 24.

[10] Lee SM, Hou Y, Cho JH, Hwang HS. Dimensional accuracy of digital dental models from cone-beam computed tomography scans of alginate impressions according to time elapsed after the impressions. Am J.

[11] Mai HN, Kim J, Choi YH, Lee DH. Accuracy of Portable Face-Scanning Devices for Obtaining Three-Dimensional Face Models: A Systematic Review and Meta-Analysis. Int J Environ Res Public Health. 2020 Dec 25;18(1):94. DOI: 10.3390/ijerph18010094.

[12] Volonghi, P.; Baronio, G.; Signoroni, A. 3D scanning and geometry processing techniques for customized hand orthotics: An experimental assessment. Virtual Phys. Prototyp. 2018, 13, 105-116.

[13] Gherlone, E.; Ferrini, F.; Crespi, R.; Gastaldi, G.; Capparé, P. Digital impressions for fabrication of definitive "all-on-four" restorations. Implant. Dent. 2015, 24, 125-129.

[14] Savoldelli C, Benat G, Castillo L, Chamorey E, Lutz JC. Accuracy, repeatability and reproducibility of a handheld three-dimensional facial imaging device: The Vectra H1. J Stomatol Oral Maxillofac Surg. 2019 Sep;120(4):289-296. DOI: 10.1016/j.jormas.2019.03.012. Epub 2019 Mar 25.

[15] Mai HN, Lee DH. Accuracy of Mobile Device-Compatible 3D Scanners for Facial Digitization: Systematic Review and Meta-Analysis. J Med Internet Res. 2020 Oct 23;22(10):e22228. DOI: 10.2196/22228.

[16] Petrides G, Clark JR, Low H, Lovell N, Eviston TJ. Three-dimensional scanners for soft-tissue facial assessment in clinical practice. J Plast Reconstr Aesthet Surg. 2021 Mar;74(3):605-614. DOI: 10.1016/j.bjps.2020.08.050. Epub 2020 Aug 25.

[17] Granata, S.; Giberti, L.; Vigolo, P.; Stellini, E.; Di Fiore, A. Incorporating a facial scanner into the digital workflow: A dental technique. J. Prosthet. Dent. 2020, 123, 781-785.

[18] Hong, S.-J.; Noh, K. Setting the sagittal condylar inclination on a virtual articulator by using a facial and intraoral scan of the protrusive interocclusal position: A dental technique. J. Prosthet. Dent. 2020.

[19] Revilla-León, M.; Raney, L.; Piedra-Cascón, W.; Barrington, J.; Zandinejad, A.; Özcan, M. Digital workflow for an esthetic rehabilitation using a facial and intraoral scanner and an additive manufactured silicone index: A dental technique. J. Prosthet. Dent. 2020, 123, 564-570.

[20] Elbashti M, Sumita Y, Aswehlee A, Seelaus R. Smartphone application as a low-cost alternative for digitizing facial defects: is it accurate enough for clinical application? Int J Prosthodont 2019; 32(6):541-543. DOI: 10.11607/ijp.6347

[21] Liu, C.-H.; Lin, I.-C.; Lu, J.-J.; Cai, D.; Housbane, S.; Yano, T. A Smartphone App for Improving Clinical Photography in Emergency Departments: Comparative Study. JMIR mHealth uHealth 2019, 7, e14531.

[22] Mai HN, Lee DH. The Effect of Perioral Scan and Artificial Skin Markers on the Accuracy of Virtual Dentofacial Integration: Stereophotogrammetry Versus Smartphone Three-Dimensional Face-Scanning. Int J Environ Res Public Health. 2020;18(1):229. Published 2020 Dec 30. DOI:10.3390/ijerph18010229

[23] White, J.D.; Ortega-Castrillon, A.; Virgo, C.; Indencleef, K.; Hoskens, H.; Shriver, M.D.; Claes, P. Sources of variation in the 3dMDface and Vectra H1 3D facial imaging systems. Sci. Rep. 2020, 10, 4443.

[24] Gibelli, D.; Pucciarelli, V.; Cappella, A.; Dolci, C.; Sforza, C. Are portable stereophotogrammetric devices reliable in facial imaging? A validation study of VECTRA H1 device. J. Oral Maxillofac. Surg. 2018, 76, 1772 1784.

[25] Bakirman, T.; Gumusay, M.U.; Reis, H.C.; Selbesoglu, M.O.; Yosmaoglu, S.; Yaras, M.C.; Seker, D.Z.; Bayram, B. Comparison of low cost 3D structured light scanners for face modeling. Appl. Opt. 2017, 56, 985-992.

[26] Gibelli, D.; Dolci, C.; Cappella, A.; Sforza, C. Reliability of optical devices for three-dimensional facial anatomy description: A systematic review and meta-analysis. Int. J. Oral Maxillofac. Surg. 2020, 49, 1092-1106.

[27] Park, J.-M.; Oh, K.C.; Shim, J.-S. Integration of intraoral digital scans with a 3D facial scan for anterior tooth rehabilitation. J. Prosthet. Dent. 2019, 121, 394-397.

[28] Rangel, F.A.; Maal, T.J.; Bergé, S.J.; Van Vlijmen, O.J.; Plooij, J.M.; Schutyser, F.; Kuijpers-Jagtman, A.M. Integration of digital dental casts in 3-dimensional facial photographs. Am. J. Orthod. Dentofac. Orthop. 2008,134, 820-826.

[29] Russo, L.L.; Di Gioia, C.; Salamini, A.; Guida, L. Integrating intraoral, perioral, and facial scans into the design of digital dentures. J. Prosthet. Dent. 2020, 123, 584-588.

[30] Barone, S.; Paoli, A.; and Razionale, A.V.: Geometrical modeling of complete dental shapes by using panoramic X-ray, digital mouth data and anatomical templates, Comput. Med. Imaging Graph. 43:112-121, 2015.

[31] https://deltaface.com/fr/aligner-conception-gouttiere-dentaire-transparente/

[32] https://www.3shape.com/fr/software/clear-aligner-studio

[33] https://www.3d-totem.fr/orthup/

[34] https://www.suresmile.com/en-us/

[35] https://www.blueskyplan.com/orthodontic /

[36] https://softsmile.com/

[37] https://www.archform.co/software /.

[38] Bartkowiak T, Walkowiak-Śliziuk A. 3D printing technology in orthodontics – review of current applications. Journal of Stomatology. 2018;71(4):356-364. DOI:10.5114/jos.2018.83410.

[39] Tümer, E.H.; Erbil, H.Y. Extrusion-Based 3D Printing Applications of PLA Composites: A Review. Coatings 2021, 11, 390.

[40] https://imprimante-3d-volumic.com/prototypage-pla-ultra-la-matiere-ultime/

[41] https://www.3drepublika.com/wp-content/uploads/2018/02/PLA-X3.pdf

[42] https://www.3dnatives.com/plastique-abs-06062019

[43] https://www.sculpteo.com/fr/glossaire/abs-definition-fr/

[44] https://cdn-3d.niceshops.com/upload/file/201906-msds-greentecpro-en.pdf

[45] Huang, J.; Qin, Q.; Wang, J. A Review of Stereolithography: Processes and Systems. Processes 2020, 8, 1138. DOI.org/10.3390/pr8091138

[46] Haoyuan Quan. Ting Zhang. Hang Xu. Shen Luo. JunNie. XiaoqunZhu. Photo-curing 3D printing technique and its challenges. Bioactive Materials Volume 5, Issue 1, March 2020, Pages 110-115.

[47] https://dental-media.formlabs.com/datasheets/DentalModel-DataSheet.pdf

[48] Jindal, P.; Juneja, M.; Siena, F.L.; Bajaj, D.; Breedon, P. Mechanical and geometric properties of thermoformed and 3D printed clear dental aligners. Am. J. Orthod. Dentofacial. Orthop. 2019, 156, 694-701.

[49] Jindal, P; Worcester, F; Siena, FL;Forbes, C; Juneja, M; Breedon,P. Mechanical behavior of 3D printed vs. thermoformed clear dental aligner materials under non-linear compressive loading using FEM. Journal of the Mechanical Behavior of Biomedical Materials, Volume 112, 2020. DOI: org/10.1016/j.jmbbm.2020.104045.

[50] Lombardo L, Martines E, Mazzanti V, Arreghini A, Mollica F, Siciliani G. Stress relaxation properties of four orthodontic aligner materials: A 24-hour in vitro study. Angle Orthodontist. 2017; 87: 11-18.

[51] Kwon J-S, Lee Y-K, Lim B-S, Lim Y-K. Force delivery properties of thermoplastic orthodontic materials. American Journal Orthodontics and Dentofacial Orthopedics. 2008; 133: 228-234.

[52] Papadimitriou A, Mousoulea S, Gkantidis N, Kloukos D. Clinical effectiveness of Invisaligh orthodontic treatments: a systematic review. Progress in Orthodontics 2018; 19: 37.

[53] Schuster S, Eliades G, Zinelis S, Eliades T, Bradley G. Structural conformation and leaching from in vitro aged and retrieved Invisalign appliances. American Journal Orthodontics and Dentofacial Orthopedics. 2004; 126: 725-728.

[54] Hallmann L and GerngroB MD. Effect of Dental Thermoplastic Materials on the Clinical Effectiveness of Clear Aligner. Austin J Dent. 2021; 8(1): 1151.

[55] Ryokawa H, Miyazaki Y, Fujishima A, Miyazaki T, Maki K. The mechanical properties of dental thermoplastic materials in a simulated intraoral environment. Orthodontic Waves. 2006; 65: 64-71.

[56] Condo R, Pazzini L, Cerroni L, Pasquantonio G, Lagana G, Pecora A, et al. Mechanical properties of two generations of teeth aligners: change analysis during oral permanence. Dental Material Journal. 2018; 37: 835-842.

[57] Cellier PL. Les aligneurs orthodontiques: nouvel outil thérapeutique, utilization au cabinetet perspectives. Sciences du Vivant [q-bio]. 2019. ffdumas-02170054f.

[58] https://orthoin3d.com/inlase/

[59] Cowley DP, Mah J, O'Toole B. The effect of gingival-margin design on the retention of thermoformed aligners. J Clin Orthod. 2012 Nov;46(11):697-702; quiz 705.

[60] Martina S, Rongo R, Bucci R, Razionale AV, Valletta R, D′ Anto. In vitro cytoxicity of different thermoplastic materials for clear aligners. Angle Orthodontist. 2019; 89: 942-945.

[61] Jedliński M, Mazur M, Grocholewicz K, Janiszewska-Olszowska J. 3D Scanners in Orthodontics-Current Knowledge and Future Perspectives-A Systematic Review. Int J Environ Res Public Health. 2021;18(3):1121. Published 2021 Jan 27. DOI:10.3390/ijerph18031121

[62] Sousa MVS, Vasconcelos EC, Janson G, Garib D, Pinzan A. Accuracy and reproducibility of 3-dimensional digital model measurements. Am J Orthod Dentofacial Orthop 2012;142:269-273.

[63] Hajeer M, Millett D, Ayoub A, Siebert J. Current products and practices: applications of 3D imaging in orthodontics: part I. J Orthod 2004;31:62-70.

[64] Lee, R.J.; Pham, J.; Choy, M.; Weissheimer, A.; Dougherty, H.L., Jr.; Sameshima, G.T.; Tong, H. Monitoring of typodont root movement via crown superimposition of single cone-beam computed tomography and consecutive intraoral scans. Am. J. Orthod. Dentofac. Orthop. 2014, 145, 399-409.

[65] Kravitz, N.D.; Groth, C.; Jones, P.E.; Graham, J.W.; Redmond,W.R. Intraoral digital scanners. J. Clin. Orthod. 2014, 48, 337-347.

[66] Grünheid, T.; McCarthy, S.D.; Larson, B.E. Clinical use of a direct chairside oral scanner: An assessment of accuracy, time, and patient acceptance. Am. J. Orthod. Dentofac. Orthop. 2014, 146, 673-682.

[67] Mangano, F.; Gandolfi, A.; Luongo, G.; Logozzo, S. Intraoral scanners in dentistry: A review of the current literature. BMC Oral Health 2017, 17, 1-11.

[68] Wesemann, C.; Muallah, J.; Mah, J.; Bumann, A. Accuracy and efficiency of full-arch digitalization and 3D printing: A comparison between desktop model scanners, an intraoral scanner, a CBCT model scan, and stereolithographic 3D printing.

[69] Joda, T.; Brägger, U. Patient-centered outcomes comparing digital and conventional implant impression procedures: A randomized crossover trial. Clin. Oral Implant. Res. 2016, 27, e185–e189.

[70] Goracci C, Franchi L, Vichi A, Ferrari M. Accuracy, reliability, and efficiency of intraoral scanners for full-arch impressions: a systematic review of the clinical evidence. Eur J Orthod. 2016;38:422-428.

[71] Arag'on ML, Pontes LF, Bichara LM, Flores-Mir C, Normando D. Validity and reliability of intraoral scanners compared to conventional gypsum models measurements: a systematic review. Eur J Orthod. 2016;38:429-434.

[72] Chochlidakis KM, Papaspyridakos P, Geminiani A, Chen CJ, Feng IJ, Ercoli C. Digital versus conventional impressions for fixed prosthodontics: a systematic review and meta-analysis. J Prosthet Dent. 2016;116:184-190.

[73] Kang SJ, Kee YJ, Lee KC. Effect of the presence of orthodontic brackets on intraoral scans. Angle Orthod. 2021 Jan 1;91(1):98-104. DOI: 10.2319/040420-254.1.

[74] H.-N. Park, Y.-J. Lim, W.-J. Yi, J.-S. Han, and S.-P. Lee, "A comparison of the accuracy of intraoral scanners using an intraoral environment simulator," The Journal of Advanced Prosthodontics, vol. 10, no. 1, pp. 58-64, 2018.

[75] R. G. Nedelcu and A. S. K. Persson, "Scanning accuracy and precision in 4 intraoral scanners: an in vitro comparison based on 3-dimensional analysis," the Journal of Prosthetic Dentistry, vol. 112, no. 6, pp. 1461-1471, 2014.]:

[76] Amornvit P, Sanohkan S. The accuracy of digital face scans obtained from 3D Scanners: an in vitro study. Int J Environ Res Public Health 2019 Dec 12;16(24):5061 DOI: 10.3390/ijerph16245061.

[77] Liu C, Artopoulos A. Validation of a low-cost portable 3-dimensional face scanner. Imaging Sci Dent 2019 Mar; 49(1):35-43 DOI: 10.5624/isd.2019.49.1.35.

[78] Koban KC, Perko P, Etzel L, Li Z, Schenck TL, Giunta RE. Validation of two handheld devices against a non-portable three-dimensional surface scanner and assessment of potential use for intraoperative facial imaging. J Plast Reconstr Aesthet Surg 2020 Jan;73(1): 141-148. DOI: 10.1016/j.bjps.2019.07.008] [Medline: 31519501.

[79] Ross MT, Cruz R, Brooks-Richards TL, Hafner LM, Powell SK, Woodruff MA. Comparison of three-dimensional surface scanning techniques for capturing the external ear. Virtual and Physical Prototyping 2018 Jul 05;13(4):255-265. DOI: 10.1080/17452759.2018.1493803.

[80] Macchi, A.; Carrafiello, G.; Cacciafesta, V.; and Norcini, A.: Three-dimensional digital modeling and setup, Am. J. Orthod. 129:605-610, 2006.

[81] D'Alessandro AC, D'Antò V, Razionale AV, Allesandri-Bonetti G. Integrating CBCT and virtual models for root movement with clear aligners. J Clin Orthod. 2020 Mar;54(3):159-166.

[82] Zhang, X.J.; He, L.; Guo, H.M.; Tian, J.; Bai, Y.X.; and Li, S.: Integrated

three-dimensional digital assessment of accuracy of anterior tooth movement using clear aligners, Kor. J. Orthod. 45:275-281, 2015.

[83] Guo, H.; Zhou, J.; Bai, Y.; and Li, S.: A three-dimensional setup model with dental roots, J. Clin. Orthod. 45:209-216, 2011.

[84] Shotell M, DMD, MS. Overview of Software Options for In-Office Clear Aligners. Available from: https://learndentistry.com/software-options-for-in-office-clear-aligners/

[85] https://www.ulabsystems.com/udesign-6-0/

[86] https://www.hubs.com/knowledge-base/introduction-fdm-3d-printing/

[87] Stephens B, Azimi P, El Orch Z, Ramos T. Ultrafine particle emissions from desktop 3D printers. Atmospheric Environment 2013, 79, pp. 334-339.

[88] Jindal, P.; Juneja, M.; Bajaj, D.; Siena, F.L.; Breedon, P. Effects of post-curing conditions on mechanical properties of 3D printed. Clear dental aligners. Rapid. Prototyp. J. 2020, 26, 1337-1344.

[89] McCarty, M.C.; Chen, S.J.; English, J.D.; Kasper, F. Effect of print orientation and duration of ultraviolet curing on the dimensional accuracy of a 3-dimensionally printed orthodontic clear aligner design. Am. J. Orthod. Dentofac. Orthop. 2020, 158, 889-897.

[90] Tartaglia GM, Mapelli A, Maspero C, Santaniello T, Serafin M, Farronato M, Caprioglio A. Direct 3D Printing of Clear Orthodontic Aligners: Current State and Future Possibilities. Materials (Basel). 2021 Apr 5;14(7):1799. DOI: 10.3390/ma14071799.

[91] http://itgraphy.com/download/eng/TC-85DAC.pdf

[92] Ryu JH, Kwon JS, Jiang HB, Cha JY, Kim KM. Effects of thermoforming on the physical and mechanical properties of thermoplastic materials for transparent orthodontic aligners. Korean J Orthod 2018;48:316-325.

[93] Putrino A, Barbato E, Galluccio G. Clear Aligners: Between Evolution and Efficiency-A Scoping Review. Int J Environ Res Public Health. 2021 Mar 11;18(6):2870. DOI: 10.3390/ijerph18062870.

[94] Bernard G, Rompré P, Tavares JR, Montpetit A. Colorimetric and spectrophotometric measurements of orthodontic thermoplastic aligners exposed to various staining sources and cleaning methods. Head Face Med. 2020 Feb 18;16(1):2. DOI: 10.1186/s13005-020-00218-2.

[95] Zhang N, Bai Y, Ding X, Zhang Y. Preparation and characterization of thermoplastic materials for invisible orthodontic. Dental Materials Journal. 2011; 30: 954-059.

[96] Boubacri A, Elleuch K, Guermazi N, Ayedi HF. Investigations on hygrothermal aging of thermoplastic polyurethaane material. Materials and Design. 2009; 30: 3958-3965.

[97] Tamburrino F, D'Anto V, Bucci R, Alessandri-Bonett G, Barone S, Razionale AV. Mechanical properties of thermoplastic polymers for aligner manufacturing: in vitro study. Dentistry Journal. 2020; 8: 47.

[98] Lombardo L, Palone M, Longo M, Arveda N, Nacuchi M, Pascalis FD, et al. Micro CT X-ray comparison of aligner gap and thickness of six brands of

aligners: an in-vitro study. Progress in Orthodontics. 2020; 21: 12.

[99] Alexandropoulos A, Jabbari YSA, Zinelis S, Eliades T. Chemical and mechanical characteristics of contemporary thermoplastic orthodontic materials. Australian Orthodontic Journal. 2015; 31: 165-170.

[100] Papadopoulou AK, Cantele A, Polychronis G, Zinelis S, Eliades T. Changes in roughness and mechanical properties of Invisalign® appliances after oneand two-weeks use. Materials. 2019; 12: 2406.

Chapter 8

Surgical Digitally Guided Planning for the Mini-Screw Assisted Rapid Palatal Expansion (MARPE) and Suture Perforation: MARPE Guide

Cristiane Barros André, Bruno de Paula Machado Pasqua, José Rino Neto and Fábio Dupart Nascimento

Abstract

The surgical planning digitally guided for the mini-screw assisted rapid palatal expansion (MARPE) technique consists of a three-dimensional positioning of MARPE and its mini-implants by a nasomaxillary anatomic evaluation. This technique also includes the simulation of the perforation areas on the midpalatal and transpalatal sutures. This type of planning is performed by superimposing the patients' files (STL and DICOM). Correct positioning without colliding with the lateral tissues of the palate and the bicortical positioning of each mini-implant are important components of the case study. The MARPE device permits individualization of the height of the mini-implant rings in each region. To avoid incorrect insertion of the drill, the location of the midpalatal and transpalatal sutures was determined using digital planning. A positioning that avoids contact with important structures, such as the nasopalatine canal, while permitting bicortical drilling of the sutures is recommended. Then, a guide that reproduces MARPE positioning and another guide that reproduces the perforations are fabricated, providing exact reproducibility as performed virtually.

Keywords: orthodontic anchorage procedures, palatal expansion technique, skeletal anchorage, cone-beam computed tomography

1. Introduction

The mini-screw assisted rapid palatal expansion (MARPE) technique comprises rapid maxillary expansion (RME) in adult patients using a mini-implant-supported device, permitting orthopedic expansion with few side effects [1–3]. This procedure is well accepted by patients owing to its low cost and less invasiveness compared to surgically assisted RME [4].

To perform the MARPE technique, cone-beam computed tomography (CBCT) is essential as it allows a complete anatomical evaluation of the nasomaxillary complex region where the expander screw and mini-implants are placed [5]. Moreover, by assessing bone thickness from CBCT images, the amount of bicortical mini-implant thread insertion can be measured [6]. This is critical as the bicortical positioning of mini-implants permits wider distribution of expansion forces, avoiding the concentration of stress areas around the mini-implants, providing better skeletal effects [7, 8].

Therefore, an evaluation protocol using CBCT [9] was introduced to select the ideal region for the mini-implants. However, this technique does not consider all anatomical variations in each patient, and the lack of a guide that reproduces this planning in the patient's oral cavity is a matter of concern. Thus, André [6] described a technique that performs a careful evaluation of important anatomical structures, such as nasal septum deviation, maxillary sinus extension, the sinuosity of the sutures evaluated, and location of the incisive foramen and transpalatal suture. Although the planning is more comprehensive, there is still a lack of guidance for reproducibility in the oral cavity.

With the advent of digital flow technology, a new technique was introduced, not only for planning, but also to reproduce the virtual placement of the entire appliance, providing accuracy, reproducibility, and safety to the MARPE technique. This technique, called MARPE Guide, consists of a three-dimensional digital placement, which comprises the positioning of the mini-implants specific for MARPE, as well as the expander screw itself. To overcome the shortcomings of the previously described planning techniques, a guide is generated that reproduces this digital placement [5, 10–15].

By superimposing the intraoral digital scanning file (STL) and CBCT (DICOM), it is possible to choose the correct location accurately and safely for the placement of the mini-implants and expander screws. Additionally, the structures of the nasomaxillary complex in a three-dimensional form are individually evaluated (**Figure 1**). Thus, the

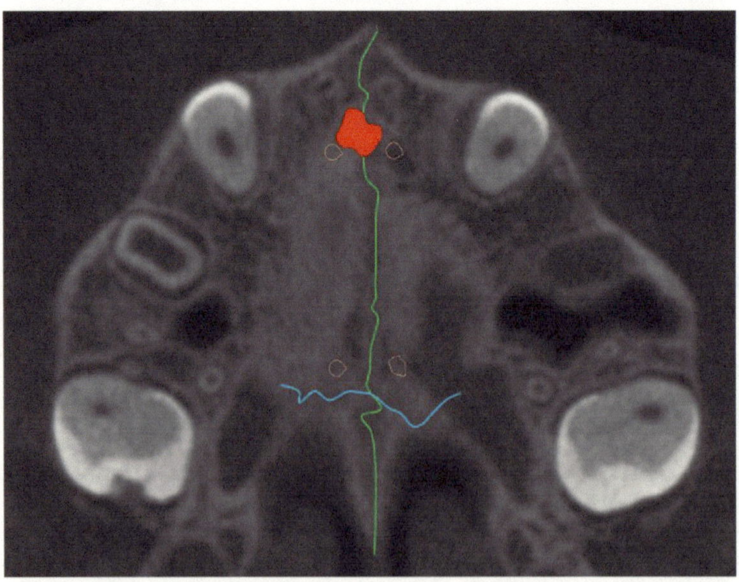

Figure 1.
The image of this case shows a MARPE complex positioning between the incisive foramen and transpalatal suture, not extending to the soft palate area. The midpalatal suture is observed in green, transpalatal suture is represented in blue, nasoapalatine duct is visualized in red, and mini-implants are presented in orange.

chances of failure are reduced using the MARPE guide, as it is possible to select the size and amount of mini-implant thread insertion of each mini-implant. Moreover, it permits accurate prediction of the mini-implant trajectory. Even in the most complex cases of anatomical variations, injury to important anatomical structures is avoided. This increases the safety of the technique, as well as the chances of success. For patients with severe transverse maxillary deficiency, increased palatal depth, or severe asymmetry, the MARPE Guide is associated with a MAEPE model called MARPE EX, developed in 2017 by Peclab (Peclab®, Belo Horizonte, Brazil). This device has an individualized mini-implant ring height, which permits positioning of the MARPE complex without colliding with the lateral palatal soft tissues. Height adjustment is performed according to the anatomy of each patient's palate, even in severe cases of transverse deficiency and maxillary asymmetry [16]. Among the physical characteristics of MARPE EX, the increased distance between the anterior and posterior mini-implant rings is observed, in search of a larger support area for the mini-implants. Regarding the tension exerted by this device on the skull, less tension on the supporting teeth was observed, as well as a wider tension distribution over the entire lateral lamina of the pterygoid process [16].

However, in complex cases of varying thickness of the maxilla and cases of advanced maturation of the midpalatal suture, even with virtual planning, these cases are limited. The increased interdigitation of the midpalatal suture is a strong resistance during RME. Therefore, Suzuki et al. [17] proposed the performance of corticoperforations in the region of the midpalatal suture during RME, to reduce the resistance by weakening the midpalatal suture, relying on the phenomenon of regional acceleration (corticoperforations). Although it appears to be an effective method, it is not a precise procedure as drilling is performed based on the palatal raphe (soft tissue), which does not always coincide with the midpalatal suture itself. Therefore, the Corticoperfuration Guide (Cortex guide) provides the most effective weakening of this suture, enabling guided drilling, performed precisely following its path, that may be sinuous, rectilinear, or curved. Another important and unmentioned factor is perforation along the transpalatal suture. Perforation in the more posterior region is of utmost importance, as the maxillary posterior region demonstrates greater resistance during RME [16, 18].

By adding this new technique of digital planning with the advantages of MARPE EX, treatments are anticipated to become safer, more accurate; thus, expanding the possibility of treatment for patients with severe transverse deficiency, maxillary asymmetry, and variations in the maxillary thickness. Thus, this book chapter proposes the presentation of the virtual MARPE placement as well as the guided corticoperforation technique (Cortex Guide).

2. Materials and methods

2.1 Anatomical evaluation and virtual placement

The analysis of the maturation of facial sutures is performed through the file in DICOM format. For the midpalatal suture, the analysis follows the method proposed by Angelieri et al. [19], where the operator must be calibrated to perform this technique with reproducibility [20]. This technique is critical as an auxiliary diagnostic method, as it provides information regarding the challenge and resistance during the separation of the midpalatal suture according to its maturation stage. Next, another suture, the zygomaticomaxillary suture, involved in RME is classified (established by Angelieri et al. [21]). This evaluation is performed by accessing the sagittal and coronal sections of the CT scan, and the suture is evaluated in a stage from A to E, where A is the earliest stage of maturation and E is the most advanced stage. The pterygopalatine suture was also evaluated, although there is no consolidated classification in the literature. When it is in an advanced stage of maturation, this suture is quite homogeneous compared to neighboring bone tissues, which is alarming to orthodontists as it suggests greater resistance to RME. Next, the location and shape of the transpalatal suture are analyzed. It is ideal to perform virtual placement of the mini-implants anteriorly to this suture (**Figure 1**); however, in many cases, owing to the positioning of the incisive foramen and reduced anteroposterior dimension of the maxilla, the most anterior virtual placement is not always feasible [5] (**Figure 2**).

In addition to the maturation stage, it is critical to verify the shape and aspect of these sutures as they can be straight, sinuous, or curvilinear. This can occur both horizontally and vertically (observed in coronal and axial sections). This verification is of total importance to perform the virtual placement without touching the sutures (**Figure 3**).

After suture analysis, the three-dimensional files (STL and DICOM, **Figure 4**) were superimposed [10–15]. As described in the literature [5], both files should be of good quality because they provide essential information, such as hard and soft tissue thickness, anatomical variations, and location and trajectory of the mini-implants. Failure to take this information into account may lead to complications and failure of the MARPE technique.

This procedure can be performed in any software that accepts the superimposition of the STL and CBCT files and also permits the importation of mini-implants and the MARPE expander screw-in STL format. This combination allows a three-dimensional

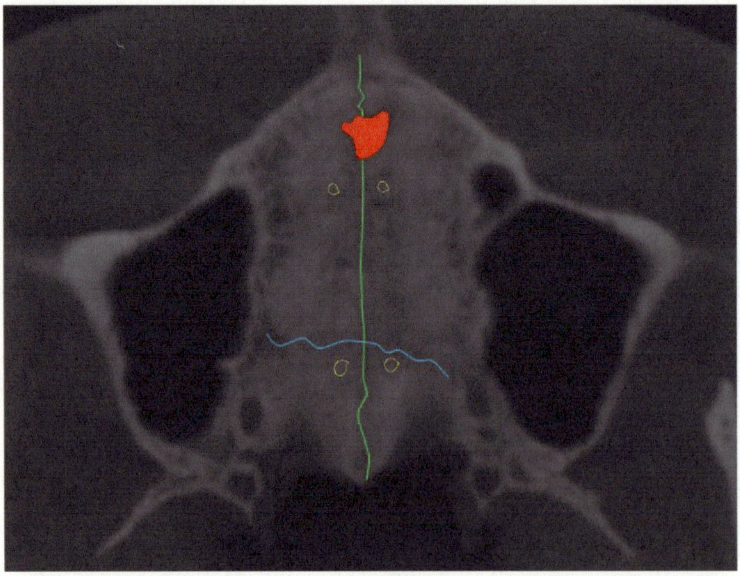

Figure 2.
In this case, the posterior mini-implants could not be placed anterior to the transpalatal suture due to the reduced sagittal size of the maxilla, and the variation in shape and size of the incisive foramen. The midpalatal suture is observed in green, the transpalatal suture is observed in blue, the nasopalatine duct is visualized in red, and mini-implants are presented in red.

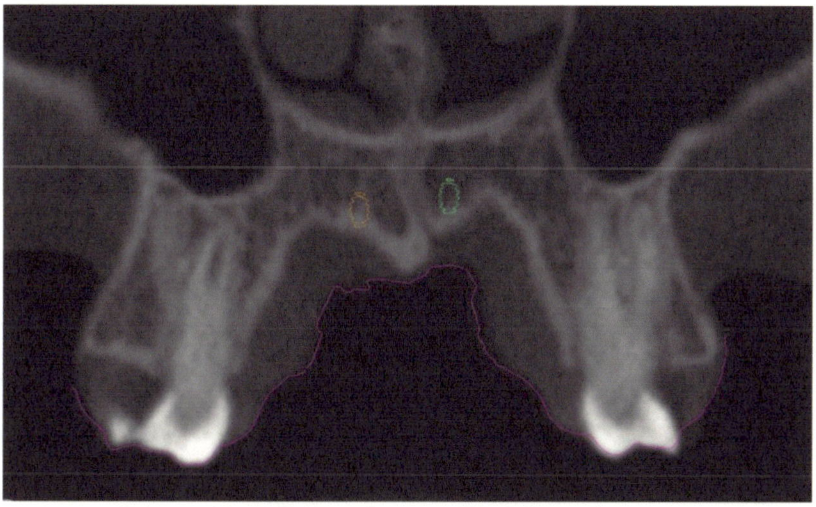

Figure 3.
Anterior mini-implants bordering a sinuous suture, without touching it.

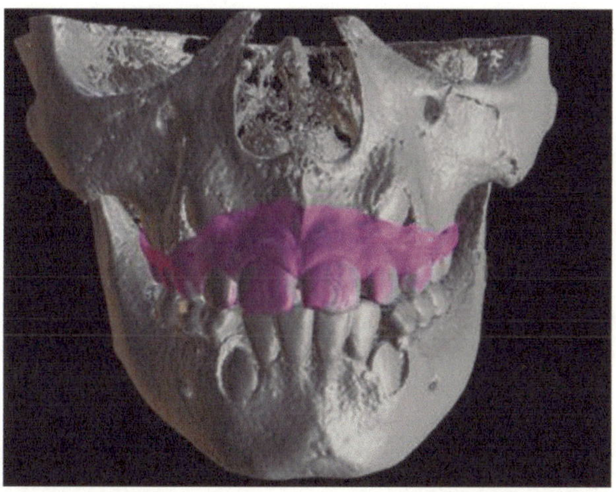

Figure 4.
Superimposition of the CBCT file (DICOM) and the digital file reproducing the teeth and the soft tissue of the upper dental arch (STL).

evaluation of the maxilla; therefore, the orthodontist can evaluate important aspects for the digital positioning of the MARPE device, as it permits simulation of the positioning in different regions.

The ideal region for the mini-implant insertion should contain sufficient bone to perform the expansion, advocating a bicortical positioning [7], as observed in **Figure 5A**. In cases of reduced bone thickness along the maxilla, it is currently feasible to add two more mini-implants to the device [22], as depicted in **Figure 5B**.

After the initial evaluation of the region with the most appropriate bone thickness, a complete anatomical evaluation is initiated, where the location of the midpalatal suture, transpalatal suture, and incisive foramen are first considered.

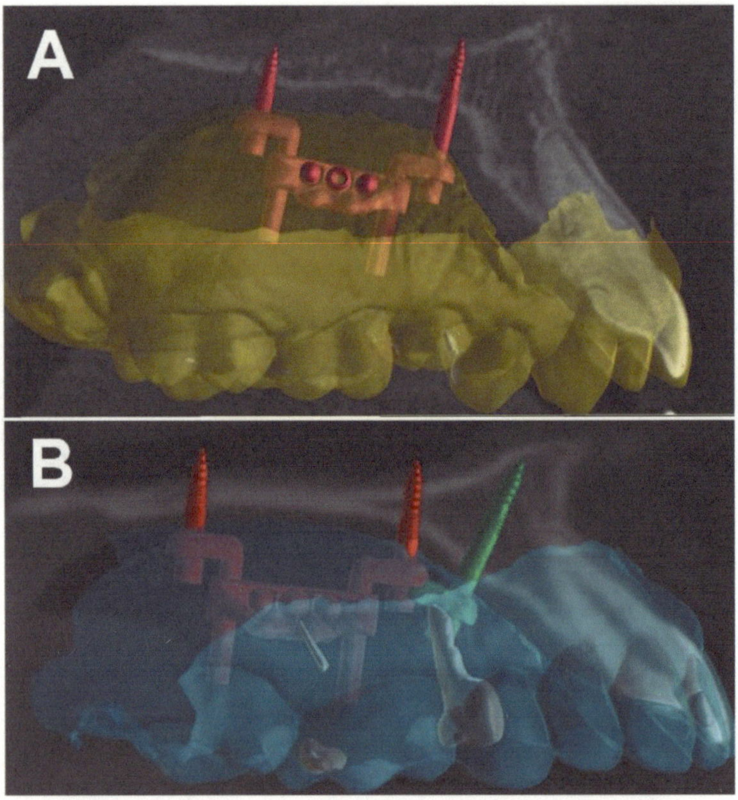

Figure 5.
(A) Bicortical insertion of mini-implants in a patient with good bone thickness. (B) Reduced bone thickness along the entire maxilla, requiring the placement of two additional mini-implants.

These three anatomical components plus adequate bone thickness are the key factors for positioning the EX expander screw and the four or six mini-implants. However, it is critical to observe the distance of this complex from the lateral mucosa to maintain soft tissue integrity during RME.

Anatomical variations are common and must be thoroughly observed when planning the MARPE digital placement such as deviated septum (**Figure 6**), maxillary sinus extension (**Figure 7**), impacted teeth (**Figure 8**), maxillary torus (**Figure 9**), palate depth, and maxillary reduced shape and size (**Figure 7**). For patients with V-shaped palate in the anterior region the digital planning requires a posterior displacement of the appliance for the mini-implant support rings to be well adapted, bicortical, and have an adequate amount of excess mini-implant thread.

Digital placement with MARPE EX permits not only to individualize the height of the mini-implant rings in each region (respecting the anatomy of each individual and a safe distance from the mucosa) but also to measure and place different mini-implant lengths, always preconizing a bicortical positioning [2, 14]. This positioning is verified in each section of the tomography (**Figure 10**) and in the three-dimensional reconstruction.

For more complex cases, such as bone volume variation, advanced age and advanced skeletal maturation, guided corticoperforation is performed. This is done following the anatomy of the midpalatal suture and the transpalatal suture. In some

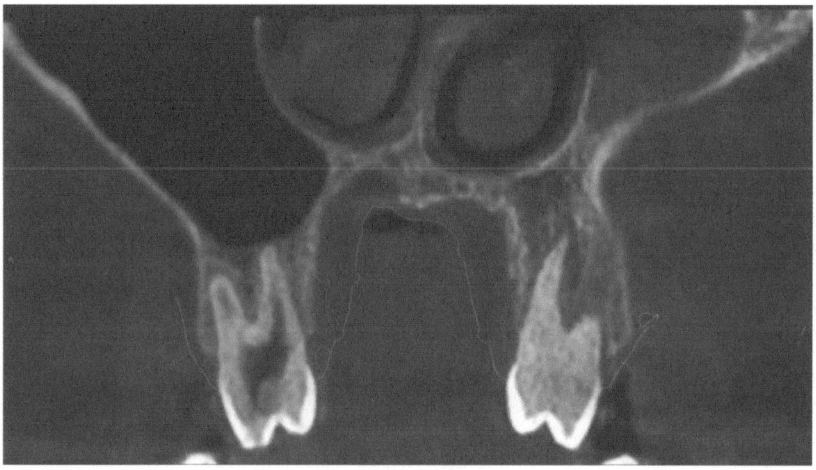

Figure 6.
Nasal septum deviation to the left side of the patient.

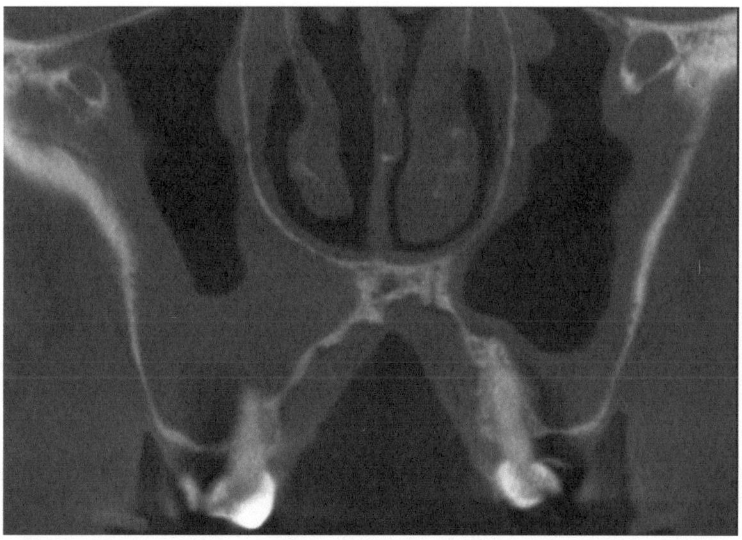

Figure 7.
Alveolar extension of the maxillary sinus and severe transverse deficiency of the maxilla.

patients, the midpalatal suture is inclined and/or sinuous in the coronal direction. We do not use the soft tissue (palatine raphe) as a reference to locate the midpalatal suture, because sometimes they are not coincident (**Figure 11**).

For the simulation of the drilling, we used digital files with a cylindrical format that reproduces the thickness of the widest portion of the drill used. These cylinders are positioned in such a way that they reach bicortical positioning and maintain a uniform distance between them when possible. Each perforation is analyzed in the three-dimensional simulation and checked in each tomography section to ensure that the perforations are bicortical and if there is no collision with important structures such as the nasopalatine duct.

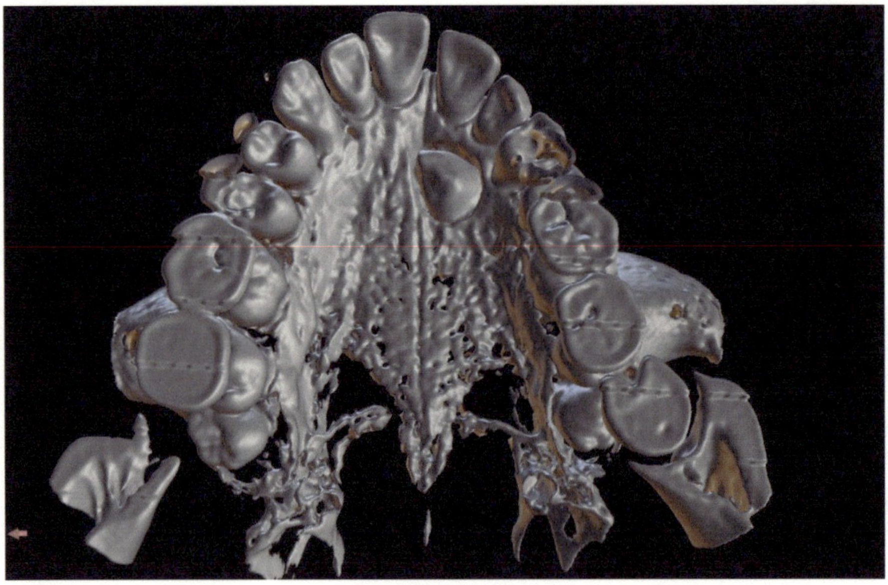

Figure 8.
Impacted tooth in the region near the anterior mini-implant installation placement site.

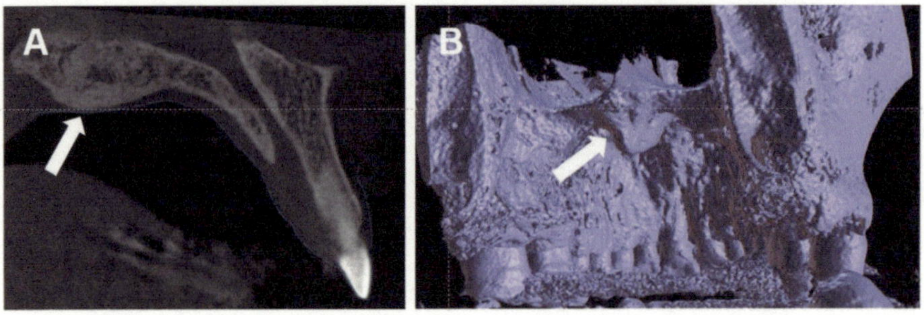

Figure 9.
(A) Sagittal section demonstrating the presence of the palatal torus. (B) Three-dimensional reconstruction of the maxilla illustrating the palatine torus.

When installing drills, we always recommend an inclination that can be performed in the mouth. In this way, we inclined the drills between 10° and 30° with respect to the occlusal plane. The drills are performed precisely following the direction of the suture, either rectilinear or sinuous (**Figure 12**).

It is advisable to maintain a safe distance between the corticoperforation and the region of the MARPE mini-implants as when trying to weaken the suture, we should not weaken the region surrounding the mini-implants, as the tension exerted in this region is high [16] and close perforations can weaken this region, which requires a large bone supply (**Figure 12C**). For this reason, MARPE Guide and Cortex Guide planning should be performed together (**Figure 13**).

After this careful process, it is time to create the guides, which will reproduce both the digital positioning in the prototyped model (MARPE Guide), providing reproducibility to the appliance manufacturing, exactly as done virtually, and the

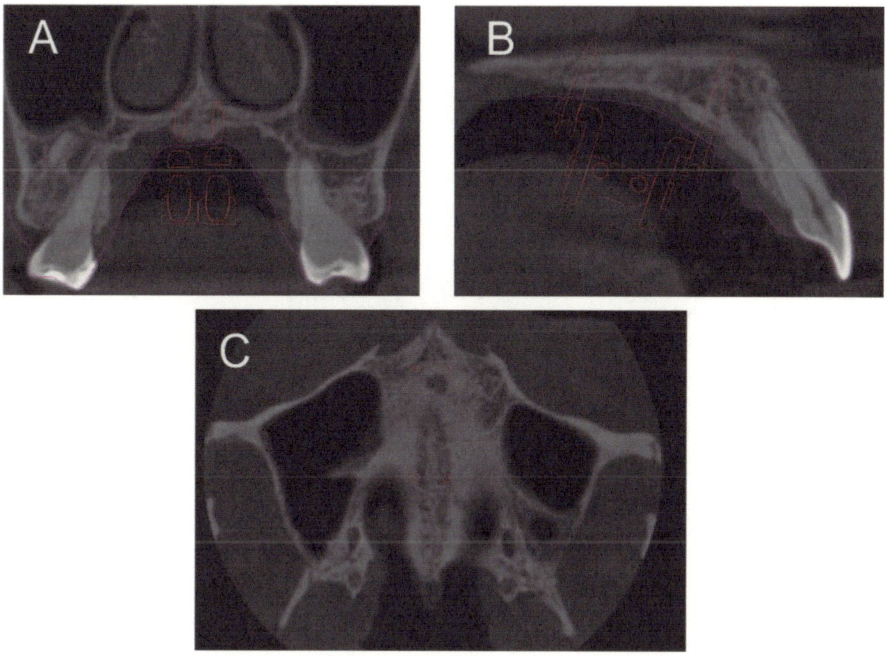

Figure 10.
(A) Coronal section, illustrating the digital placement of MARPE, even in cases of severe atresia and asymmetry. (B) Sagittal section, showing the bicortical position of the mini-implants, respecting a discrete distance from the mucosa to avoid collision during expansion. (C) Placement of the mini-implants, respecting the midpalatal suture, as well as the transpalatal suture and the incisive foramen.

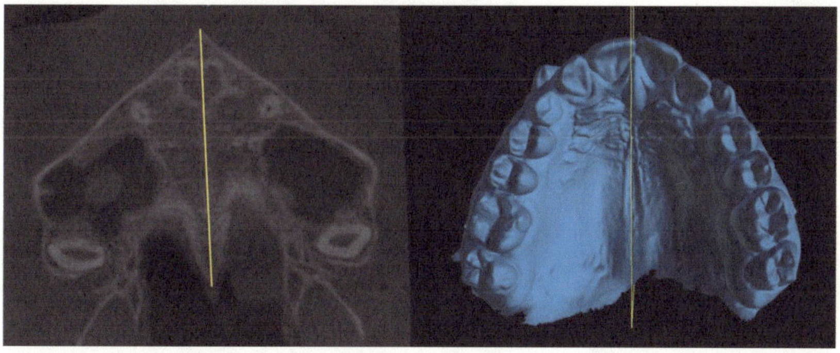

Figure 11.
Palatal raphe and midpalatal suture are not coincident. If the corticoperfortaion is not performed in a guided way. It can lead to an error during the procedure.

corticoperforation guide (Cortex Guide), which reproduces the digital perforation of each point created, with angulation and insertion limits.

2.2 Presentation of a complete planning

Below, we present a complete MARPE Guide and Cortex Guide planning, following all the parameters discussed above (**Figures 14–19**).

Subsequently, the MARPE guide and cortex guide are made as detailed above.

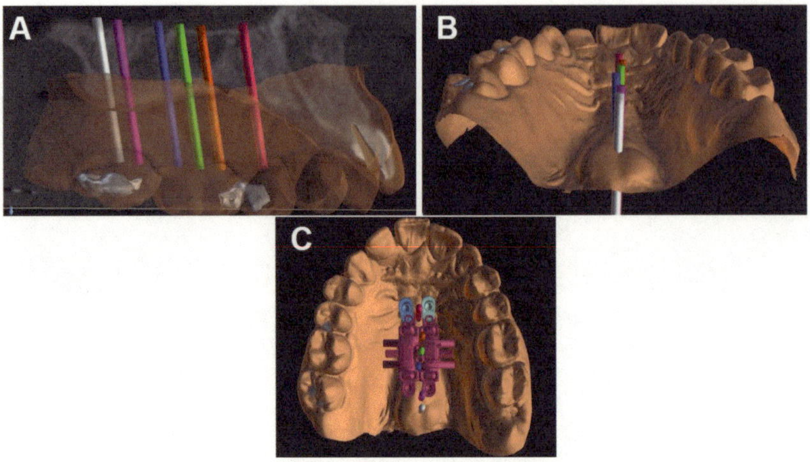

Figure 12.
(A) Perforations performed with bicortical positioning. (B) Note that the positioning respects the suture inclination in both coronal and axial directions. (C) The perforations are performed preserving bone tissue around the MARPE mini-implants.

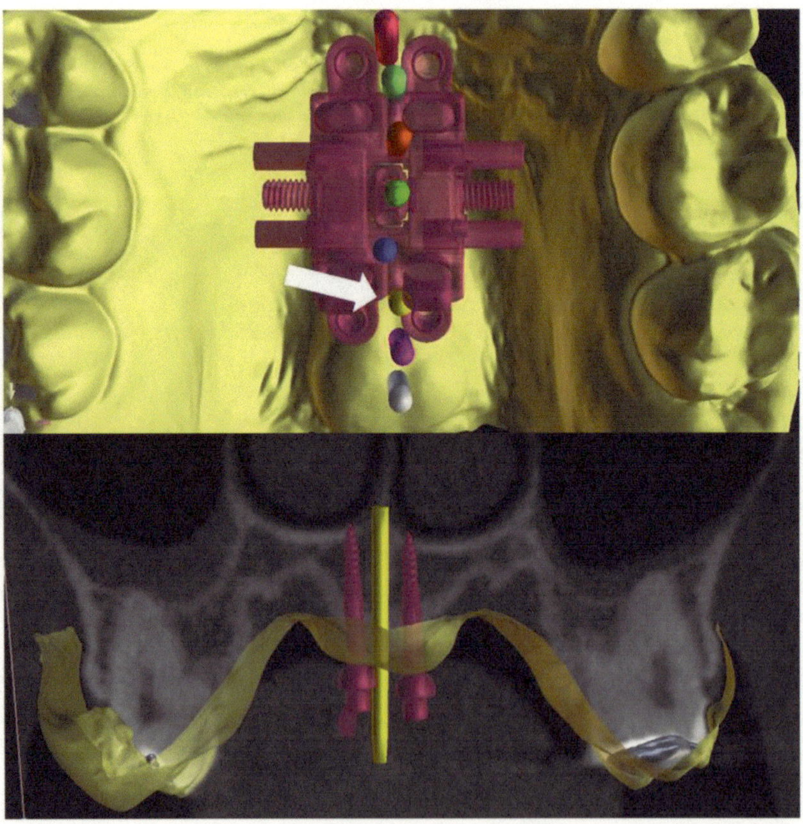

Figure 13.
In the top image we see the simulations of the corticoperforations that would be ideal for this case. However, in the bottom image we note that the perforation in yellow is very close to the posterior mini-implants, which could compromise the technique.

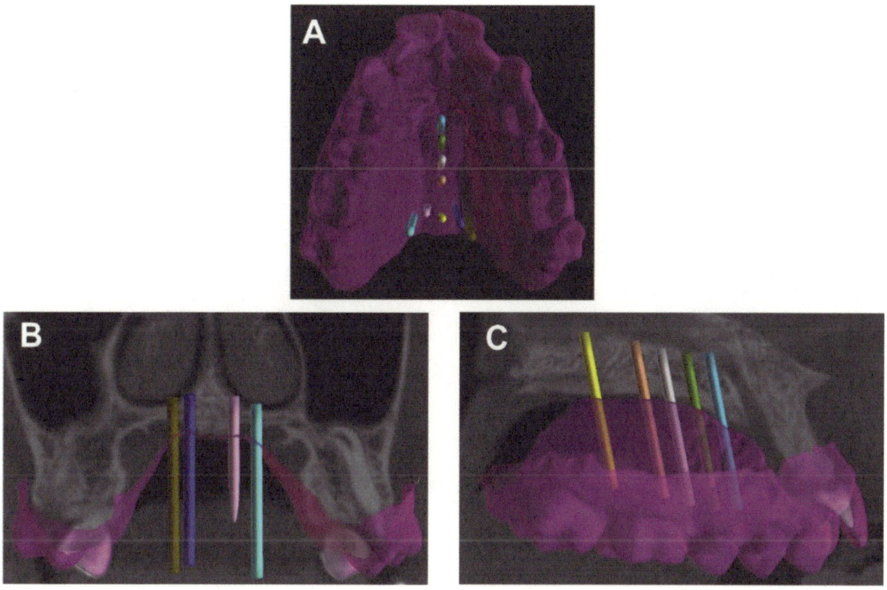

Figure 14.
(A) Virtual corticoperforation drills installed in the midpalatal suture and transpalatal suture. (B) Coronal view (transpalatal suture). (C) Lateral view in sagittal section (midpalatal suture).

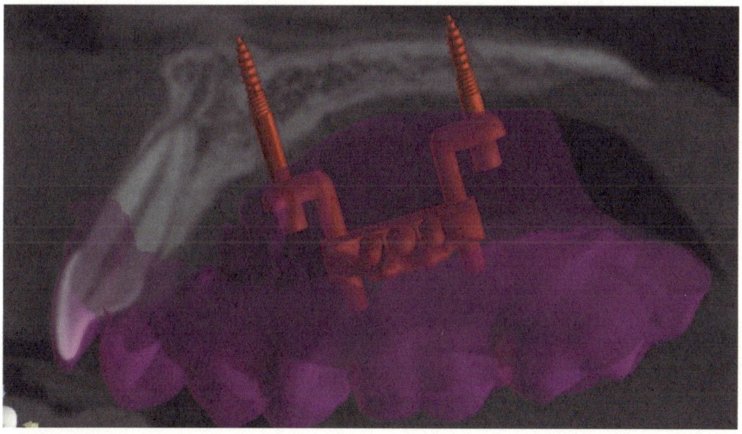

Figure 15.
Sagittal section of the tomography – left side. MARPE installed respecting the bicortical positioning and with the distance of the mini-implant rings from the mucosa.

2.3 MARPE guide

For the virtual placement of MARPE, a concern about injuries caused to the soft tissue due to the contact of the mini-implant rings is resolved with the digital placement (with the MARPE EX and MARPE guide). It has an internal stop that accommodates each mini-implant support ring (**Figure 20**), and its height is established according to the individual's anatomy. It is important to keep the expander screw body as horizontal as possible (**Figure 21**) in the coronal section of the tomography without touching the lateral mucosa.

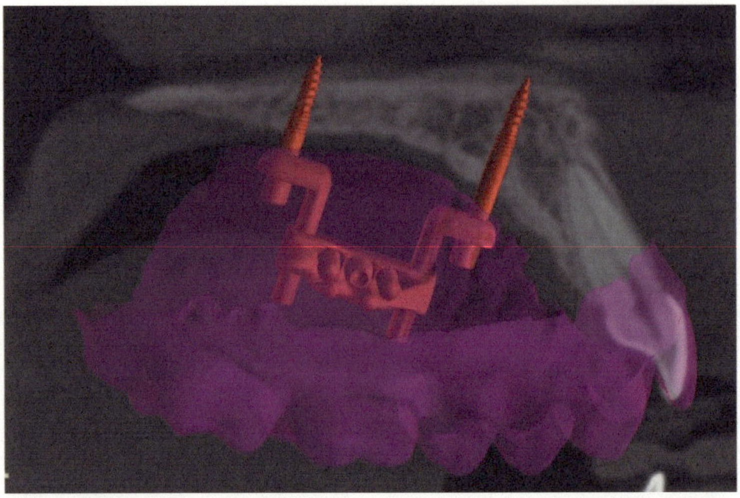

Figure 16.
Sagittal section of the CT scan – left side.

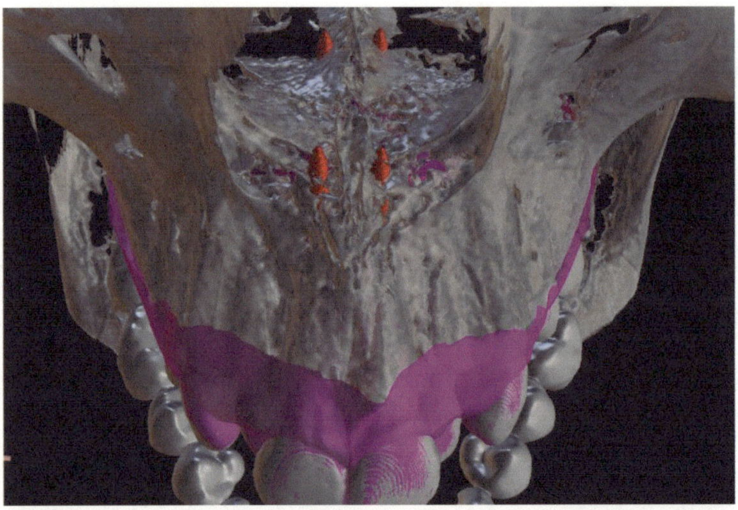

Figure 17.
3D reconstruction of the CT scan illustrating a safe distance of the mini-implants from the transpalatal suture. Note the bicortical positioning of the four mini-implants.

We should be aware of the occlusal plane and nasal floor inclination, which, when altered, can cause asymmetry in the patient. Thus, a stop that holds the expander screw body in position is necessary (**Figure 21**). This guide design is inserted into the patient's STL file, so they are printed at once, which reduces the chances of error by overlapping the guide to the patient's model, in addition to saving printed material.

2.4 Corticoperforation guide

The corticoperforation guide, requires a retentive design (that embraces the posterior teeth), as it will be adapted in the mouth, as a positioner and vertical limiter of each perforation (**Figure 22**) and must remain stable during the process.

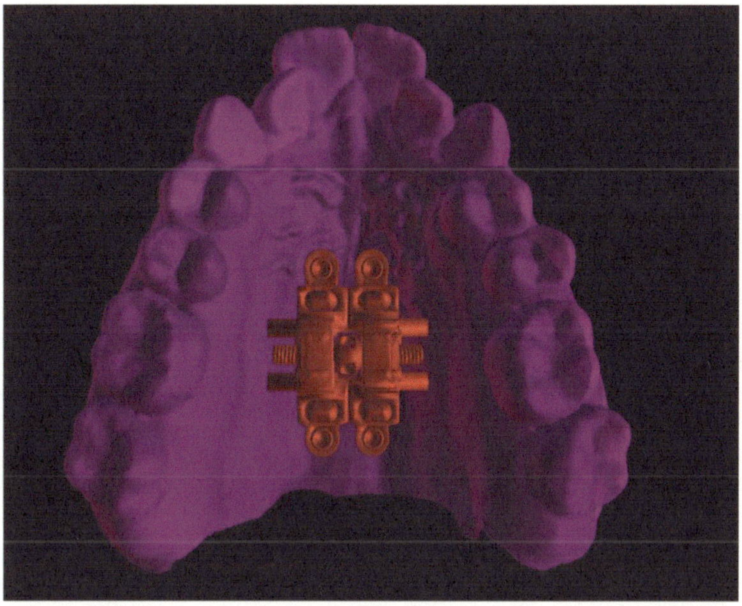

Figure 18.
Occlusal view of the virtually installed MARPE, preserving the lateral tissue and soft palate.

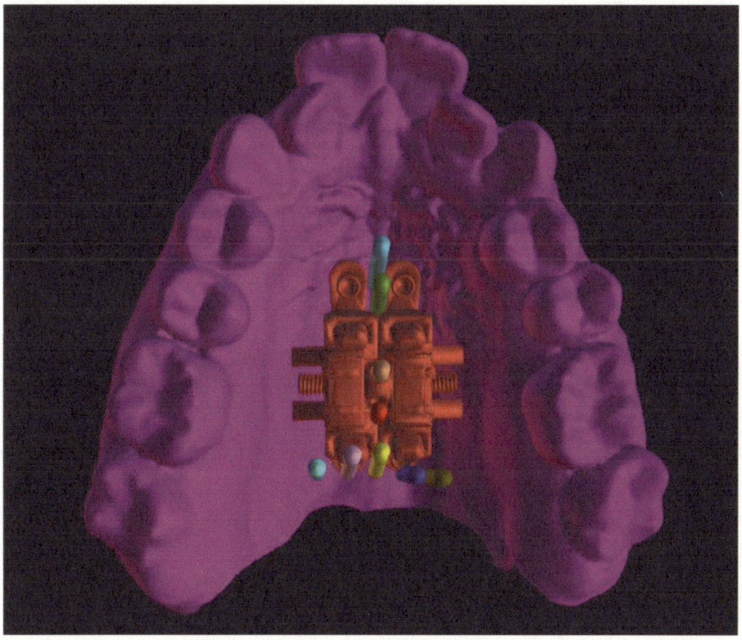

Figure 19.
MARPE guide and cortex guide in the same image to check if there is any collision between the digital plans, such as drilling too close to a mini-implant.

2.5 Laboratory phase – printing the MARPE guide and cortex guide

Finally, it is possible to fabricate MARPE with the reproducibility of each of the precautions taken during the virtual placement. The MARPE EX is made on the guide

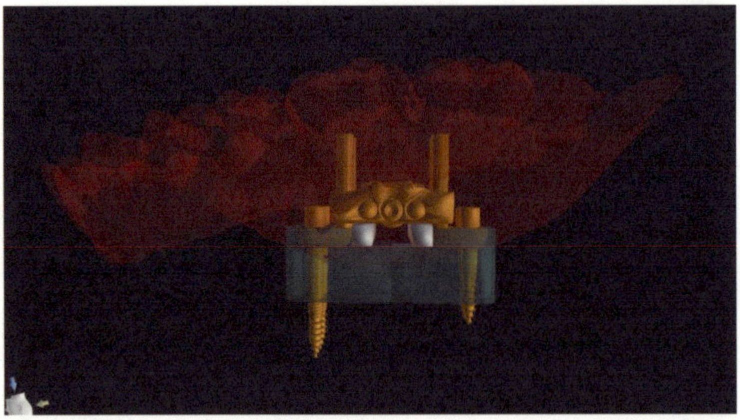

Figure 20.
In green we see the MARPE guide, which accommodates the adjustable mini-implant rings of the MARPE EX, to reproduce the positioning performed during the virtual placement.

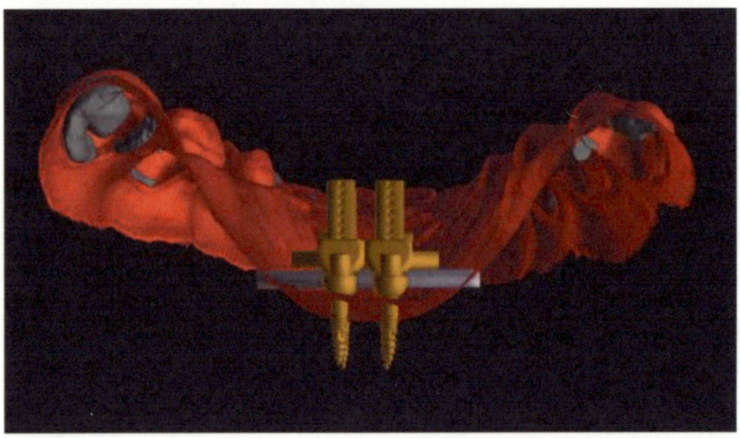

Figure 21.
Digital horizontal support (gray) that are responsible for keeping the MARPE appliance at the planned height during the virtual placement, so that the expander screw does not touch the soft tissue and mainly, remains as horizontal as possible, preventing it from causing any asymmetry in the patient.

template (**Figure 23**), where its mini-implant rings fit exactly inside each small guide, which eliminates transfer errors. It also determines the height and inclination of the expander screw, preventing asymmetries during expansion. Using laser welding, it is possible to weld the MARPE EX to the bands without damaging the prototype model or causing any swelling of the metal of the MARPE EX, owing to the heat of the formerly used silver-based welds.

After this phase, the appliance is polished, and it is ready to reproduce with accuracy the digital planning in the oral cavity. Note that the guide is not used in the oral cavity; it serves as a guide for fabricating the appliance. In the oral cavity the guide for cementation is the bands on the first permanent molars.

To reproduce the corticoperforations in the oral cavity, after designing the guide, it is critical to make an impression of the guide in biocompatible resin (**Figure 24**), and this protocol must be followed even if the guide remains in the oral cavity for some time.

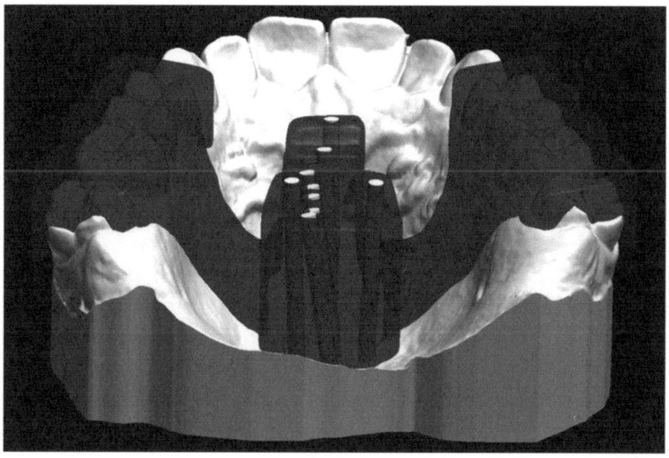

Figure 22.
3D planning of the corticoperforation guide, which reproduces the angulation of each perforation, following the midpalatal suture and transpalatal suture. This guide will also be the limiter for the drill cutter, as soon as it touches the guide, the clinician will know that it has reached the nasal floor cortical.

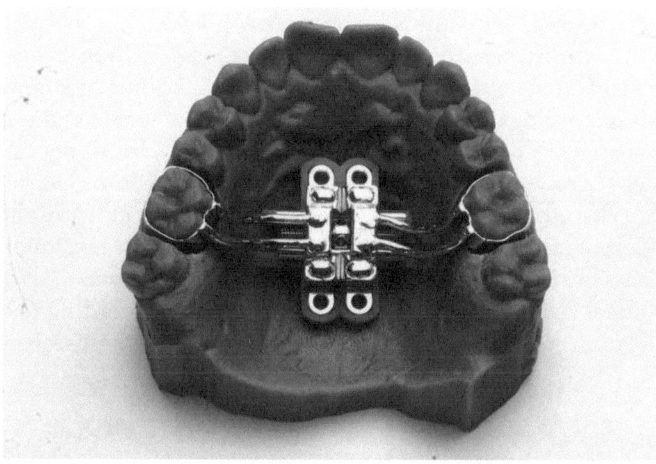

Figure 23.
MARPE device built over the printed MARPE guide template.

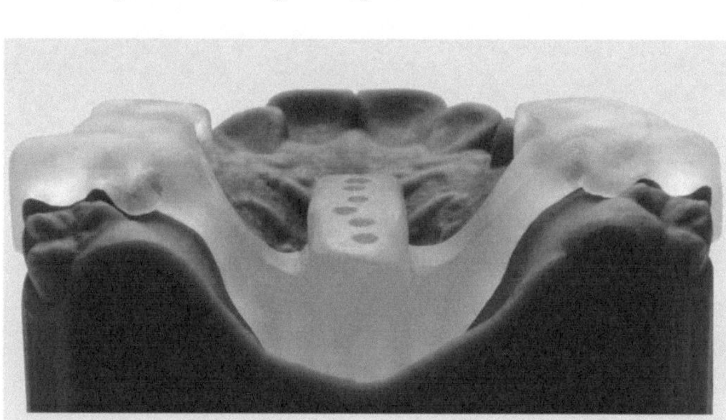

Figure 24.
Cortex guide printed in biocompatible resin.

3. Discussion

For a very short time, the MARPE technique was performed without CT scanning. This type of treatment required three-dimensional (3D) planning since the maxilla contains important structures that must be preserved, both for the patient's safety and success of the technique. The first safety protocols were based on bone and mucosa thickness measurements in the region of first premolars, second premolars, first molars, and second molars [6, 9]. Despite providing important information, these protocols did not show the exact trajectory of MARPE mini-implants. Moreover, the standardization of the patient's head position and evaluation of the tomography sections could not be faithfully reproduced in the oral cavity. This necessitated the creation of digital positioning guides [10–13]. In cases of severe transverse deficiency of the maxilla or asymmetry [23], devices such as the MARPE maxillary skeletal expansion (MARPE MSE) or MARPE SL cannot be indicated because the expander screw does not fit in the palate (**Figure 25**).

Thus, the present study proposes the development of a guide for planning the MARPE technique using MARPE EX [5, 16], to evaluate the capacity of this guide in performing an ideal positioning of the MARPE, prioritizing the adaptation of the mini-implant rings, and respecting the individual anatomy of the patient's palate. The distance between the mini-implants is higher in MARPE EX than that of the other models of MARPE, which, according to a previous study [16], was favorable for better results. Another advantage is that MARPE EX accepts this guide model, where we can place the mini-implant rings away from the palate at customized heights according to the patient's anatomy. This distance from the palate in its closest region is approximately 0.2 mm, both towards the palate (vertical) and towards the lateral mucosa (horizontal) [5]. Therefore, no ring juxtaposed should be left juxtaposed to the tissues.

The EX model was also chosen because it demonstrated less tension in the teeth and mini-implants during RME [16], and it presented more tension, with wide distribution, in the lateral lamina of the pterygoid process [16]. According to Brunetto et al. [18], the lateral lamina of the pterygoid process offers the greatest resistance during

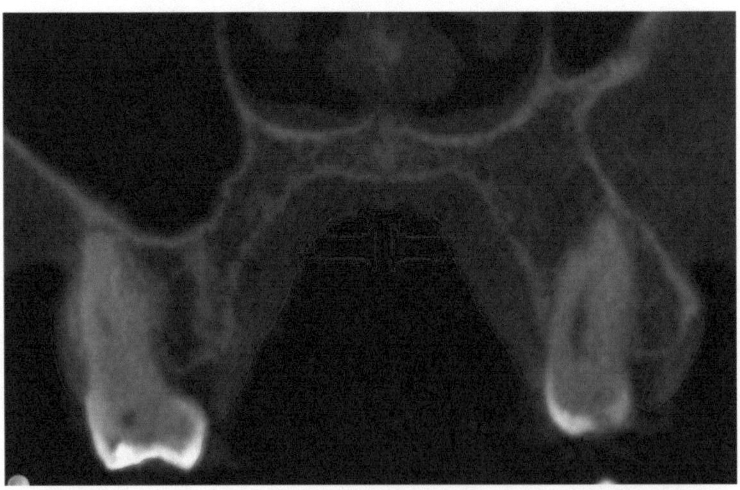

Figure 25.
Model of MARPE without adjustable mini-implant rings. This figure shows that without adjustable mini-implant rings the MARPE does not fit patients with severe transverse disability.

RME. Recent clinical studies have shown that bicortical directly influence treatment with MARPE [8, 24], particularly in patients with advanced maturation stage sutures as the bicortical positioning of mini-implants permits the separation of even the most posterior sutures, such as the lateral lamina from the medial lamina of the pterygoid process [8]. Thus, this demonstrates the importance of a guide that correctly reproduces this bicorticality in the patient, such as the MARPE Guide. It is also important to recognize the importance of the bands, which, in addition to distributing stress, are responsible for transferring the guide model to the oral cavity.

The three initial parameters for placing an MARPE must be discussed. First, it should not touch the midpalatal and transpalatal sutures; second, it should be distant from the incisive foramen; and third, preferably anterior to the transpalatal suture, avoiding collision/perforation of the mini-implants with sutures. We should not touch the incisive foramen to avoid contact with the nerve of the incisive canal, which can result in anterior maxillary paresthesia.

The location of the transpalatal suture does not always coincide with the soft palate; however, if it does, we avoid placing it posteriorly to the transpalatal suture, so that the mini-implants are not inserted in a region of free mucosa, with more chances of inflammation, great difficulty in cleaning, and loss of the mini-implants. However, in some cases of the reduced anteroposterior distance of the maxilla, this becomes unavoidable. The patient's anatomical variation should be considered as it influences the results, such as mini-implants placed in the nasal septum in a patient with palate asymmetry [25] and resulting in a unilateral opening [25]. This highlights the importance of using 3D planning, where insertion in the septum can be easily avoided and bilateral opening can be achieved, eliminating side effects.

While dealing with anatomical variations, it is common to find patients with variations in maxillary sinus extension (**Figure 7**). If the mini-implants are inserted into the sinus cavity, in addition to creating an oral-sinus communication that can generate pain, inflammation, and discomfort, this is a region without trabecular bone, that is, a region that lacks bone volume. Therefore, mini-implants cannot withstand the tension exerted during maxillary expansion [16].

Corticoperforation can be indicated when a torus palatine (**Figure 9**) is detected as it has the potential to decrease the chances of success. Guided corticoperforation, besides allowing perforation of the transpalatal suture, provides accuracy due to the angulation of the guide, which was determined in the virtual simulation, leaving the patient free of perforations outside the suture. Corticoperforations oriented by the palatine raphe may cause asymmetric fractures or even case failure because if performed too close to the mini-implant placement site, they reduce the bone volume required for the tension exerted in the mini-implant region [16]. Another risk of not virtually simulating the corticoperforations and creating a stop guide is to over drill the nasal cavity floor, causing pain to the patient and a bucco-nasal communication, which may lead to sinusitis; in case of inflammation, possibly worsening to bone necrosis or osteomyelitis.

4. Conclusions

The two-dimensional plans do not predict the mini-implant trajectory, and the choice of the mini-implant can be highly subjective and susceptible to errors. The use of the MARPE Guide has already presented interesting results in the literature. By combining the benefits of the MARPE Guide with the MARPE EX and the use of the

Cortex Guide, virtual placement may be performed in a patient with palate asymmetry, bone volume variation, and advanced stage of midpalatal suture classification. This results in tension in the lateral lamina considering the patient's anatomy. Clinical studies are needed to evaluate the results of this new technique in a considerable number of patients.

Conflict of interest

The authors declare no conflict of interest.

Author details

Cristiane Barros André[1*], Bruno de Paula Machado Pasqua[2], José Rino Neto[2] and Fábio Dupart Nascimento[1]

1 Technology Research Center, University of Mogi das Cruzes, Mogi das Cruzes, Brazil

2 School of Orthodontics, University of São Paulo, São Paulo, Brazil

*Address all correspondence to: kika@kikaortodontia.com.br

References

[1] Lee KJ, Park YC, Park JY, Hwang WS. Mini-implants-assisted nonsurgical palatal expansion before orthognathic surgery for a patient with severe mandibular prognathism. Am J Orthod Dentofacial Orthop 2010;(138): 830-839.

[2] Cantarella D, Dominguez-Mompell R, Moschik C, et al. Midfacial changes in the coronal plane induced by micro-implant-supported skeletal expander, studied with cone-beam computed tomography images. Am J Orthod Dentofac Orthop 2018;154(3):337-345.

[3] Celenk-Koca T, Erdinc AE, Hazar S, Harris L, English JD, Akyalcin S. Evaluation of mini-implants-supported rapid maxillary expansion in adolescents: A prospective randomized clinical trial. Angle Orthod 2018;(88):702-709.

[4] Stuart DA, Wiltshire WA. Rapid palatal expansion in the young adult: Time for a paradigm shift? J Can Dent Assoc 2003;(69):374-377.

[5] André CB. MARPE guide: from consolidation to technique evolution. Clin Orthod 2020;19(5):00-00.

[6] André CB. Análise tomográfica para técnica Marpe. Rev Clin Ortod Dental Press 2018;17(4):50-53.

[7] Lee RJ, Moon W, Hong C. Effects of monocortical and bicortical micro-implant anchorage on bone-borne palatal expansion using finite element analysis. Am J Orthod Dentofac Orthop 2017;151(5):887-897.

[8] Li N, Sun W, Li Q, Dong W, Martin D, Guo J. Skeletal effects of monocortical and bicortical mini-implant anchorage on maxillary expansion using cone-beam computed tomography in young adults. Am J Orthod Dentofacial Orthop 2020;157(5):651-661.

[9] Nojima LI, Nojima M, Cunha ACD, Guss NO, Sant'Anna EF. Mini-implant selection protocol applied to MARPE. Dental Press J Orthod 2018;23(5):93-101.

[10] Maino BG, Paoletto E, Lombardo L, Siciliani G. A three-dimensional digital insertion guide for palatal micro-implant placement. J Clin Orthod 2016;50(1): 12-22.

[11] De Gabriele O, Dallatana G, Riva R, Vasudavan S, Wilmes B. The easy driver for placement of palatal micro-implants and a maxillary expander in a single appointment. J Clin Orthod 2017;51(11): 728-737.

[12] André CB. Instalação virtual dos aparelhos: para que serve? Rev Clin Ortod Dental Press 2019;18(5):52-58.

[13] Lombardo L, Occhiuto G, Paoletto E, Maino BG, Sliciliani G. Class II treatment by palatal mini-implants-system appliance: A case report. Angle Orthod 2019;90(2):305-313.

[14] Antonino Lo Giudice, Vincenzo Quinzi, Vincenzo Ronsivalle, Stefano Martina, Orazio Bennici, and Gaetano Isola. Description of a digital work-flow for CBCT-guided construction of micro-implant supported maxillary skeletal expander. Materials 2020(13):1815.

[15] Cantarella D, Savio G, Grigolato L, Zanata P, Berveglieri C, Lo Giudice A, Isola G, Del Fabbro M, Moon W. A new methodology for the digital planning of micro-implant-supported maxillary skeletal expansion. Med. Devices Evid. Res. 2020;13:93-106.

[16] André CB, Rino-Neto J, Iared W, et al. Stress distribution and displacement of three different types of micro-implant assisted rapid maxillary expansion (MARME): A three-dimensional finite element study. Prog Orthod 2021; 22:20.

[17] Suzuki SS, Garcez AS, Reese PO, Suzuki H, Ribeiro MS, Moon W. Effects of corticopuncture (CP) and low-level laser therapy (LLLT) on the rate of tooth movement and root resorption in rats using micro-CT evaluation. Laser Med Sci 2018;33(4):811-821.

[18] Brunetto DP, Sant'Anna EF, Machado AW, Moon W. Non-surgical treatment of transverse deficiency in adults using microimplant-assisted rapid palatal expansion (MARPE). Dental Press J Orthod 2017;22(1):110-125.

[19] Angelieri F, Franchi L, Cevidanes LHS, Toyama-Hino C, Nguyen T, McNamara JA Jr. Zygomaticomaxillary suture maturation: A predictor of maxillary protraction? Part I: Classification method. Orthod Craniofac Res 2017;(20):85-94.

[20] Barbosa NMV, Castro AN, Conti F, Capelozza-Filho L, Almeida-Pedrin RR, Cardoso MA. Reliability and reproducibility of the method of assessment of midpalatal suture maturation: A tomographic study. Angle Orthod 2019;89(1):71-77.

[21] Angelieri F, Franchi L, Cevidanes LHS, Hino CT, Nguyen T, McNamara Jr JA. Zygomaticomaxillary suture maturation: A predictor of maxillary protraction? Part I – A classification method. Orthod Craniofac Res 2017;20(2):85-94.

[22] Cury SEN, Mondelli AL, André CB, Iared W, Guerra JGP, Rovira J, Berni L. Protocolo diferencial para a técnica MARPE em pacientes com variação no volume ósseo do palato. Rev Clín Ortod Dental Press 2019;18(4): 116-129.

[23] Andrade T. MARPE: uma alternativa não cirúrgica para o manejo ortopédico da maxila – parte 2. Rev Clín Ortod Dental Press 2019;17(6):24-41.

[24] Moon HW, Kim, MJ, Ahn, HW, Kim, SJ, Kim, SH, Chung, KR, Nelson, G. Molar inclination and surrounding alveolar bone change relative to the design of bone-borne maxillary expanders: A CBCT study. Angle Orthod 2020;90(1):13-22.

[25] Santos AM, Miranda F, Rocha AD, Cruz AP, Naveda R, Garib D. Mini-implants-assisted rapid palatal expansion in adult patient with severe maxillary constriction: Case report. Clin Orthod 2021;19(6):101-112.

Section 3

Orthodontic Techniques and Trends

Chapter 9

Understanding Orthodontic Bone Screws

Agharsh Chandrasekaran, H.P. Naga Deepti and Harshavardhan Kidiyoor

"Progress is impossible without change, and those who cannot change their minds cannot change anything."

—George Bernard Shaw

Abstract

The field of orthodontia has been witnessing numerous reforms in terms of treatment modalities through the years, under which the concept of absolute anchorage employing mini-implants can be well subsumed. The usage of orthodontic bone screws has witnessed growing popularity and has been deemed to revitalize the management of complex malocclusions. Orthodontic bone screws are larger in diameter (2 mm) in comparison with the average mini-implant and are placed in areas of high bone mineral density like the infrazygomatic crest in the maxilla and the buccal shelf area in the mandible. Owing to a difference in size, they are placed away from the roots and hence, the term extra-radicular implants seem a befitting one. With an expansion of the envelope of discrepancy to skeletal anchorage, the employment of these bone screws in practice will have to be appraised further in terms of biological limits. Orthodontic bone screws have been successfully utilized as an absolute anchorage system in well-chosen cases, pushing the realm of treatment possibilities further ahead in the sands of time. This chapter aims to provide you with a narrative insight into the salient features of orthodontic bone screws starting right from its inception to its contemporary usage in practice.

Keywords: anchorage, orthodontic bone screws, extra-alveolar implants, infrazygomatic crest, buccal shelf

1. Introduction

A universally accepted scientific perspective, the best current explanation of a natural phenomenon, has been termed a paradigm. A paradigm can be thought of as the foundation upon which a scientific structure is erected, similar to laying brick upon brick of new findings and insights. As each newer paradigm replaces an older one, today's "truths" become tomorrow's myths. In orthodontics, at present, we are on the threshold of a paradigm shift that changes the fundamental conceptual underpinnings of orthodontics, and with it, the traditional emphasis on diagnosis and treatment planning.

The goal of any orthodontic treatment is to achieve desired tooth movement with the minimum number of undesirable side effects [1]. Strategies for anchorage control have been a major factor in achieving successful orthodontic treatment since the specialty began. With conventional orthodontics, it is almost impossible to achieve absolute intraoral anchorage. Recently, the use of skeletal anchorage has grown in popularity, especially in challenging situations [2].

The field of orthodontics has had a lot of landmarks in its evolution, but very few can match the clinical impact made by micro-implants and the recently introduced extra-radicular bone screws. Temporary anchorage devices have revolutionized the orthodontic field with their concept of absolute anchorage and have proved to be an adjunct in the hands of a clinician to gain control in handling complex malocclusions and clinical challenges.

It aids in the conversion of borderline surgical cases to cases that can be handled with bone screws in an equally effective way. The purpose of this review chapter is to offer to the reader, an insight into the depths of orthodontic bone screws from cradle to what has been explored till date, while touching upon integral aspects that might prove to be of use in both an academic and a clinical sense [3].

2. History

Creekmore and Eklund (1983) used a small-sized vitallium bone screw to depress the entire anterior maxillary dentition. The screw was inserted just below the anterior nasal spine. Ten days after placement, a light elastic thread was tied from the head of the screw to the archwire. The maxillary central incisors were intruded by about 6 mm. The bone screw did not move during treatment and was not mobile at the time of removal [4].

Shapiro and Kokich (1988) described the possibility of using dental implants for anchorage during orthodontic treatment. Melsen and co-workers (1998) introduced the use of zygomatic ligatures as anchorage in partially edentulous patients. Under local anesthesia, two holes were made in the superior portion of infrazygomatic crest. A double-twisted 0.012″ stainless steel wire was ligated between the two holes and inserted into the oral cavity. After surgery, nickel-titanium coil springs were attached from the zygomatic ligatures to the anterior fixed appliance for intrusion and retraction of maxillary incisors [5].

3. Structure of an orthodontic bone screw

Mindful of the fact that orthodontic bone screws have insertion points in areas with greater quantities of cortical bone, the regular mini-implant has been revamped with the following design features to form a bone screw (**Figure 1**) [2, 3]:

- A length of 10–14 mm that facilitates insertion in areas of high bone density with adequate primary stability. Also, the increased length is owed to its placement steered away from the roots at extra-alveolar sites.

- A diameter of 1.5–2 mm that ensures greater fracture resistance. The resistance to torsional fracture is directly proportional to greater diameter and length and hence, these are crucial design features that have been worked upon.

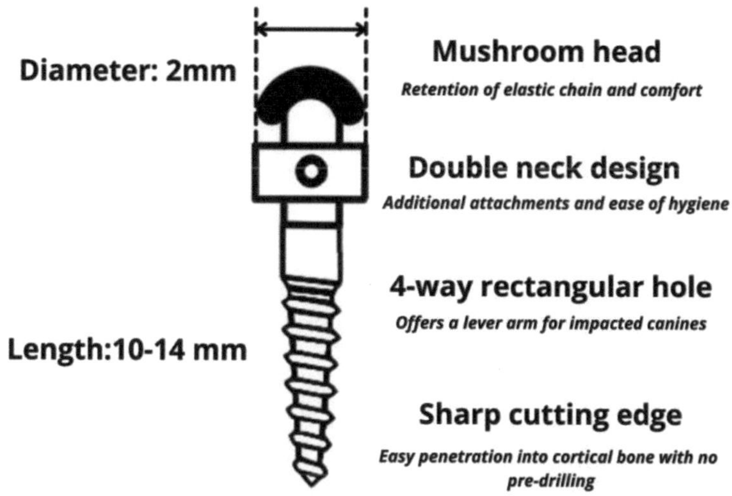

Figure 1.
Diagrammatic representation of orthodontic bone screw.

- Commonly, a mushroom-shaped head is incorporated to allow greater comfort and better ease in the attachment of elastic chains.
- A four-way rectangular hole that offers a lever arm for disimpacting canines.
- A double neck feature that permits better maintenance of oral hygiene and additional attachments.
- A sharp cutting edge that allows for an insertion free of pre-drilling.

4. Material aspects of orthodontic bone screws

Bone screws inserted in extra-alveolar areas are made up of either stainless steel or titanium alloys (Ti-6 AI-4 V). There has been a serious bone of contention over the material of choice. Pure surgical stainless steel has gained more popularity in being the preferred material of choice.

4.1 Why stainless steel?

The reason for stainless steel being the popular material of choice is attributed to the high placement torque that occurs when these screws are placed in areas of high bone density. This demands the requisite of a high fracture resistance, and stainless steel seems to be a befitting choice due to its high modulus of elasticity in comparison with titanium alloy. However, both materials seem to be acceptable materials with a comparable success rate [6].

A popular titanium alternative is the Peclab screw kit that was developed by Almeida [7] that has shown promising results and is inclusive in terms of the armamentarium that is required.

5. Quantity and quality of bone at extra-alveolar sites

The extra-alveolar sites of insertion correspond to D1 site as described by Misch [8], which comprises dense cortical bone of greater than 1250 HU.

According to Park [9], the cortical bone thickness and bone depth are as follows:

Infrazygomatic crest region:

- Cortical bone thickness: 2.2–3.6
- Bone depth: 3.0–6.2

Buccal shelf region:

- Cortical bone thickness: 2.0–4.0
- Bone depth: 12.7–13.9

5.1 Variability of bone thickness at different vertical facial heights

The bone thickness also seemed to vary with different divergence patterns. Infrazygomatic crest region did not show any change with regard to the patient's vertical height. But the bone thickness at the buccal shelf region was found to be higher in short-faced individuals as compared to long-faced individuals [10]. Also, in comparison with the hyperdivergent counterparts, the buccal shelf has greater bone width and lesser bone height in hypodivergent individuals [11].

5.2 Is an initial perforation required in self-drilling screws?

In certain cases, an initial perforation with a clinical probe/spear tip is recommended even with a self-drilling bone screw to minimize the risk of fracture of the screw during placement, since it involves a considerable placement torque [9].

6. Envelope of discrepancy

The envelope of discrepancy is an expression of anteroposterior, vertical, and transverse in terms of the millimetric range of treatment possibilities. It gives us an estimate of tooth movement that can be deemed possible by purely orthodontics alone, orthodontic with dentofacial orthopedics, orthodontics with the employment of skeletal anchorage, and orthodontics with orthognathic surgery. Different colored zones connote the range of possibilities (**Figures 2–4**). The direction of movement in the diagrammatic illustration has been depicted by arrows. The different colors zones are as follows: 1) The pink zone denotes the envelope for orthodontics alone, 2) the yellow zone connotes orthodontics plus orthopedics, 3) the green zone shows skeletal anchorage, and 4) the blue zone any combination of the above with orthognathic surgery. The green zone has been depicted by a "fuzzy" area, as an indication of the paucity of reliable data available at this point to make any claims. The same drawback is why a figure depicting the mandibular transverse envelope does not exist at this juncture [12]. To sum up, the biological limits of the skeletal anchorage system in the management of severe malocclusions albeit proven useful in several case reports needs further research to arrive at a more definitive conclusion in the envelope.

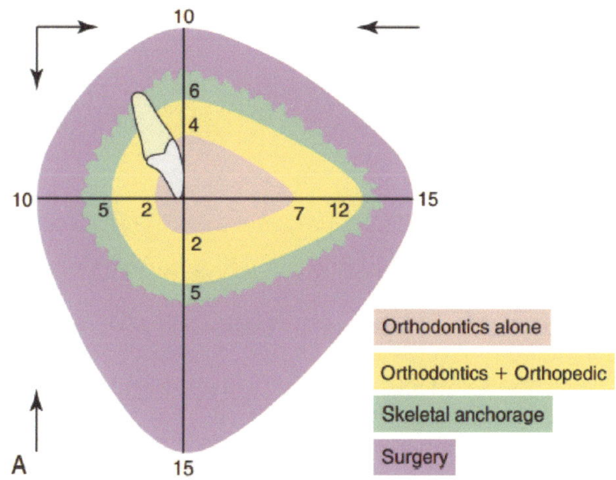

Figure 2.
Revised envelope of discrepency.

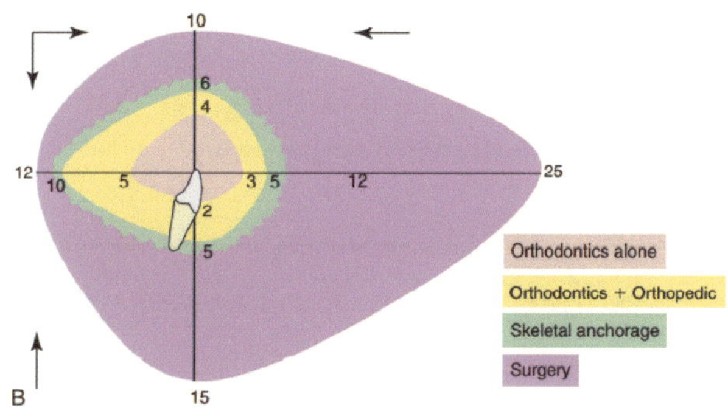

Figure 3.
Revised envelope of discrepency.

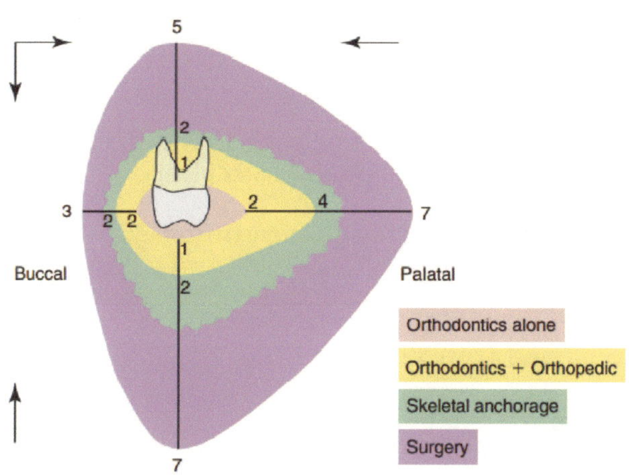

Figure 4.
Revised envelope of discrepency.

7. Indications of orthodontic bone screws

The indications of orthodontic bone screws [13]:

1. Borderline cases,
2. Camouflage treatment,
3. Molar uprighting by crown distalizing or by root mesializing,
4. Anterior open bite treatment with molar intrusion (with or without extractions),
5. Severe transverse discrepancies: severe scissors bite and severe crossbite,
6. Leveling of transverse tipping of occlusal plane,
7. Extraction cases,
8. Distalizing or anchorage after distal movement with other kinds of appliances, such as the pendulum, and
9. Forced eruption of impacted teeth.

8. Contraindications of orthodontic bone screws

8.1 Absolute contraindications

1. Systemic diseases such as diabetes, osteoporosis, osteomyelitis, blood dyscrasias, metabolism disorders,
2. Patient undergoing the radiotherapy in arches,
3. Psychological disorders,
4. Presence of pathological formations in the zone, such as tumors or cysts,
5. Thin cortical bone and insufficient retention,
6. Deficient quality of the bone,
7. Soft tissue lesions, such as lichen planus, leukoplakia,
8. The patient who does not accept bone screw treatment.

8.2 Relative contraindications

1. Tobacco, alcohol, and drugs abuse,
2. Presence of active oral infections,
3. Uncontrolled periodontal disease, and
4. Absence of ability to maintain proper oral hygiene.

9. Concepts of placement of bone screws at different sites

9.1 Infrazygomatic crest (IZC) screws

9.1.1 Anatomy of the infrazygomatic crest (IZC)

The infrazygomatic crest is a crest of bone emanating from the buccal plate of the alveolar process, lateral to the roots of the first and second maxillary molars. It extends superiorly up to 2 cm to the zygomaticomaxillary suture and inferiorly into the areas of first and second maxillary permanent molars. The sites of placement at first or second molar have been much discussed and have been proposed by authors Liou and Lin respectively. Comparisons of both sites have been summarized in **Table 1** [14].

Though both sites have been deemed fit, the IZC 7 site gains an upper hand in terms of having a greater bone thickness over the buccal surface of the second molar. Nevertheless, a CBCT evaluation of the area before placement is an important aspect of treatment planning with these screws.

9.1.2 Insertion technique and angulations

Liou [15] suggested orienting screws about 55–70° inferior to the horizontal plane to achieve maximal buccal bone engagement. During placement, the point of initial insertion is between the first and second molar, 2 mm above the mucogingival junction. The screw is directed first at the right angle to the occlusal plane and after a couple of turns when the initial notch has been made in the bone, the direction of the driver is altered by 55°–70° toward the tooth. This downward change aids in bypassing the roots of the teeth and helps direct the screw to the infra-zygomatic area of the maxilla (**Figure 5**). The bone screw is screwed until only the screw head is visible. The need for pre-drilling, flap raising, or a mucosal vertical slit has been deemed unnecessary.

9.1.3 Magnitude of the employed force

The recommended loading for orthodontic mechanics using miniscrews in the region of the IZC ranges from 220 to 340 g (8–12 oz). The force load can be employed by means of an elastomeric chain or closed coil springs [9].

LIOU-IZC 6	LIN-IZC 7
PLACEMENT: Anterior to the anatomic ridge and buccal to the mesiobuccal root of the maxillary first permanent molar. Small oral cavities are more convenient to place screws at this site. Less predictable as compared to seven sites due to lesser bone thickness over mesiobuccal and distobuccal roots of 6.	PLACEMENT: Distal to the anatomic ridge and buccal to the mesiobuccal root of the maxillary second permanent molar. Large oral cavities and lip reflection are needed for adequate access. More predictable and greater retraction due to greater amount of bone thickness over mesiobuccal and distobuccal roots of 7.

Table 1.
LIOU-LIN concept of IZC site: A comparison.

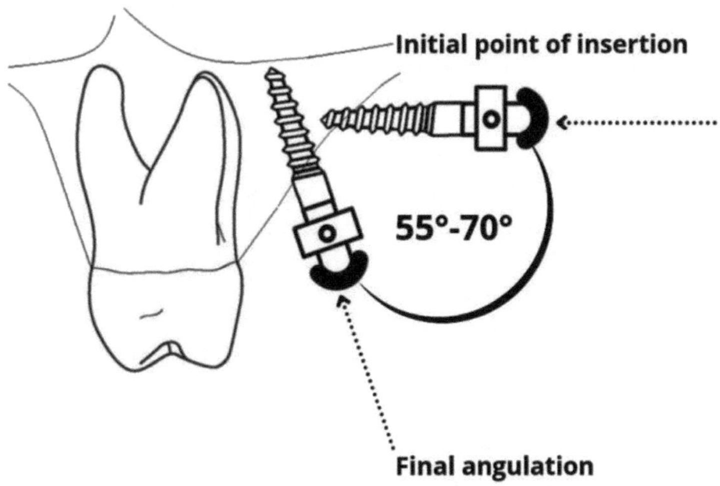

Figure 5.
Insertion of infrazygomatic crest screw.

9.1.4 Anatomical considerations

An important consideration that one cannot overlook during the placement of infrazygomatic crest screws is the soft tissue irritation and this is a frequent occurrence if there is contact or close intimacy between the inferior platform of the screw head and the mucosa.

As a general guideline, 1.5-mm clearance is considered a necessity between the mucosa and the inferior aspect of the screw platform. This is important irrespective of whether the screw is placed in a region of attached gingiva or movable mucosa though the selection of the size of the screw would vary accordingly.

It is vital to assess the anatomy of the IZC site to select an appropriate screw length. The average thickness of the attached gingiva in the maxillary first molar is about 1.0 mm, and the cortical bone thickness is about 1.1–1.3 mm The screw threads must engage cortical bone to insure primary stability. Generalizing the widths, for soft tissue clearance, attached gingiva and cortical bone at 1.5 mm each, reveals that 8–12-mm IZC screws penetrate the medullary bone or sinus from 3.5 to 7.5 mm. Under most clinical conditions, an 8-mm screw is adequate to engage the cortical plate and secure primary stability [14].

9.1.5 Sinus considerations

Cases with the maxillary sinus extending low between the teeth are not ideal candidates for infrazygomatic crest screws. The thickness of the sinus floor is preferred to be over 6 mm to ensure safe insertion. Small uncomplicated penetrations into the sinus heal spontaneously [16]. The penetration into the maxillary sinus with IZC screws was found to be rather high and double cortical engagement with sinus penetration within 1 mm was recommended for adequate primary stability. Penetrations above 3 mm led to thickening of the Scheniderian membrane and sinusitis eventually leading to failure [17].

9.1.6 Guided infrazygomatic crest screws

To ensure greater precision, a number of guides [14] have been made available for easy installation of IZC screws. They are as follows:

- Chen double film radiographic method
- Pin Head soft tissue penetration method
- Double film method with a transparent adhesive patch like comfort brace strips.

9.2 Buccal shelf screws

9.2.1 Anatomy of the buccal shelf

Mandibular buccal shelf area is located in the posterior part of the mandibular body, buccal to the roots of the mandibular, and anterior to the oblique line of the mandibular ramus. The area buccal to the distal root of the mandibular second molar, between 4 and 8 mm from the cementoenamel junction, has been claimed to be the best anatomical location for fixation. However, the region shows significant anatomic variations and also possibly ethnic variations wherein some patients present with a well-defined bony plateau and some with a straight bony profile. This could be better evaluated with a CBCT and clinical examination [9].

9.2.2 Insertion technique and angulations

While placing bone screws in the mandibular buccal shelf, the point of initial insertion is between the first and the second molar, 2 mm below the mucogingival junction. The screw is first directed at the right angle to the occlusal plane at this point and then, the driving direction is altered by 60°–75° toward the tooth. This upward change in direction helps to bypass the teeth roots and directs the screw to the buccal shelf area of the mandible. Pre-drilling or vertical slit in the mucosa may be necessary if the bone density is too thick. However, raising a flap is never required during placement.

9.2.3 Magnitude of the employed force

The recommended loading for orthodontic mechanics using miniscrews in the region of the buccal shelf area ranges from 340 to 450-g. The force load can be employed by means of an elastomeric chain or closed coil springs [9].

9.2.4 Inflection point and limits of mandibular molar distalization

The intersection of the line of occlusion and the internal oblique ridgeline is the inflection point (**Figure 6**). The second molar cannot move on the internal oblique line, and the amount of possible movement depends on the distance of the original position of the second molar to the inflection point. This varies from patient to patient. A comprehensive evaluation of the buccal shelf area and the alveolar housing with the help of a cone-beam computed tomogram seems pivotal to treatment planning [18].

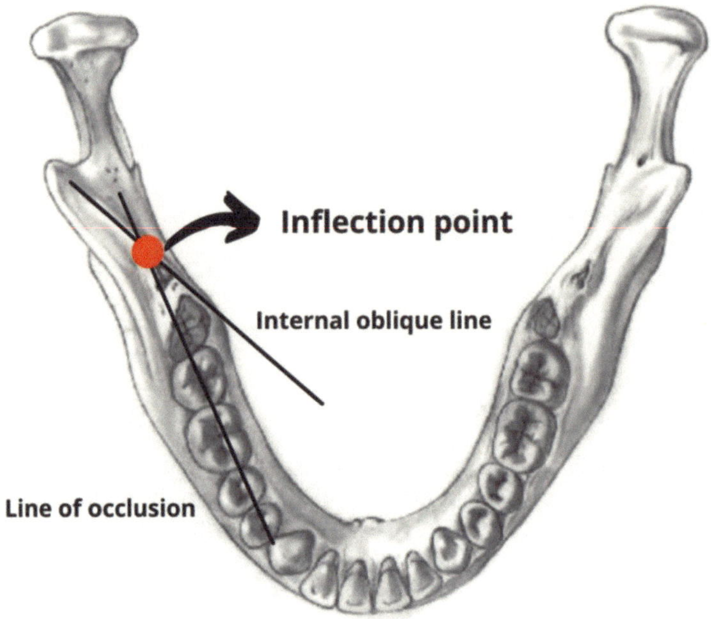

Figure 6.
Limits of mandibular molar distalisation.

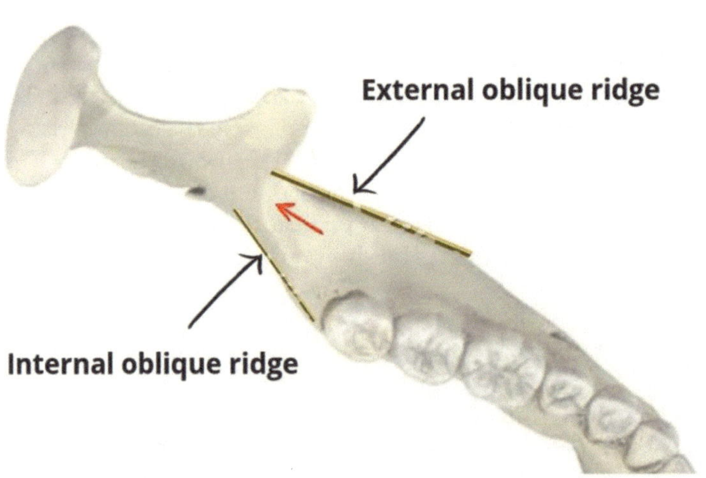

Figure 7.
Ramus Screw insertion.

9.3 Ramus screws

Ramus screws were developed to overcome the difficulties that buccal shelf screws posed during the dis-impaction of horizontally impacted lower molars. From the standpoint of biomechanics, these screws are installed in the anterior ramus of the mandible to offer a traction force that is more superior and posterior in direction.

This coupled with simple yet efficient mechanics to upright the lower molars in tandem with ramus screws has offered a brilliant treatment option in such cases.

9.3.1 Anatomical location point

The insertion site for a ramus screw (red arrows) is between external and internal oblique ridges, about 5–8 mm superior to the occlusal plane (**Figure 7**).

A relatively long (14 mm) ramus screw is selected because of the need to penetrate thick non keratinized mucosa, with an underlying layer of masticatory muscle. For hygiene access, the ramus screws were screwed in until the head of the TAD was ~5 mm above the level of the soft tissue. The average bone engagement for a ramus screw is ~3 mm [19].

10. Biomechanics of orthodontic bone screws

10.1 Generations of biomechanical principles

According to Robert et al. [20]

- First-generation biomechanics: 2D/two-dimensional mechanics based on the third law of Newton and correspond to classical segmented mechanics.

- Second-generation biomechanics/Stress sensor theory: 3D mechanics based on finite elements that determine the exact amount of stress in the periodontium with determinate mechanics. With the aid of determinate mechanics, extra-alveolar bone screws are employed in complex malocclusions in a multivector fashion, which simplifies and eliminates the need of numerous accessory devices that were used in segmented mechanics.

10.2 Employed force magnitude

The force magnitude employed is important in terms of anchorage stability. A force magnitude ranging from 220 to 340 g (8 to 12 oz) for mechanics with mini-implants in the IZC area, and from 340 to 450 g on the ones with mini-implants in the BS area, has been recommended. This is vital to achieve the en masse distalization that bone screws offer popularly in clinical settings. In cases that require partial retraction, force magnitude may be adjusted between 150 and 200 g.

10.3 Biomechanics of buccal shelf screws

Buccal shelf screws are employed for en masse retraction of the entire mandibular dentition since the screws are placed at extra-alveolar sites.

Three critical factors exist for this system to be deemed statically determinate when two screws are inserted into the buccal shelf areas for retraction:

1. Use of rectangular arch (full-size) with torque control during retraction,

2. Relative constant force stemming from superelastic NiTi springs,

3. Force applied directly to the arch.

Biomechanical effects of retraction with anchored buccal shelf screws:

- Molar intrusion and incisor extrusion with a counter-clockwise rotation of the mandibular occlusal plane.
- The axis of rotation was found close to the mandibular canine area.
- The counterclockwise rotation occurs since the line of force is occlusal to the center of resistance and thus causing molar intrusion and incisor extrusion. These movements offer favorable Class III correction presenting with open bite.

10.4 Biomechanics of infrazygomatic crest screws

When two screws are installed in the IZC area for retraction, similar effects were found as in the buccal shelf region. With the retraction force from the coil spring to the screw, retraction occurs along with vertical side effects, that is, molar intrusion and incisor extrusion leading to rotation of the occlusal plane. The axis of rotation in the maxillary arch lies between the premolars and this change is beneficial in Class II cases with the open bite or where bite deepening is required.

10.5 How can the force system be varied to suit the needs of a particular case?

In order to overcome the side effects that are not suited for correction in all cases, the force system can be modified to obtain different kinds of dental movements:

- Height of hooks in the anterior area.
- Height modification in extra-alveolar mini-implants insertion (this often is not a viable option since insertion depends on numerous other factors).

10.6 Height of hooks/power arm

Depending on the force vector and direction required in each case, the height of the hook will help decide the type of tooth movement required along with torque and vertical control.

Short hook: Anterior teeth have a tendency to rotate clockwise when retraction/distalization force is applied by means of a force that passes below the Center of resistance, which leads to torque loss and a vertical extrusion force on the incisors.

Medium hook: The force action line is passing over the anterior teeth's center of resistance, due to the middle positioning. When distalization force is applied to the entire maxilla, with force parallel to the occlusal plane, anterior teeth are likely to keep their initial inclination, minimizing vertical forces.

Long hook: The height of the hook is positioned mesial to the canine allows the force action line to pass above the incisors' center of resistance. The positioning simply produces a counterclockwise anterior moment during retraction and simultaneous extrusion of the incisors. In the clinical scenario, it might be pointed out that this may offer a possibility of injuring the oral mucosa of the patient.

Orthodontic bone screw	Sagittal	Vertical	Transverse
a. IZC screw	1. En masse distalization in Class II malocclsuions 2. Re-treatment cases 3. Segmental retraction of canines 4. Simultaneous retaction and intrusion 5. Mesialization of molars 6. Severe bimaxillary protrusion cases 7. Decompensation for Class III orthognathic cases	1. Vertical maxillary excess correction by posterior rotation and mandibular autorotation. 2. Maxillary molar intrusion in anterior open bite cases.	Expansion of maxillary arch
b. Buccal shelf screw	1. Class III camoflauge cases by enmasse distalization 2. Retraction during extraction space closure 3. Severe bimaxillary protrusion 4. Mesialization of molars 5. Decompensation for Class II orthognathic cases	Molar intrusion in cases requiring mandibular rotation	Expansion of mandibular arch

Table 2.
Clinical applications of extra-alveolar bone screws [2, 3, 4, 9].

10.7 Simultaneous retraction and intrusion

In cases with vertical maxillary excess, in order to facilitate gingival smile correction while also balancing the clockwise rotation effect of the maxillary occlusal plane, it was suggested that two mini-implants were to be installed between central and lateral incisors apart from the IZC screws. This would help counter-effect the anterior extrusion, resulting in the intrusion of the entire maxillary dentition and favoring gingival smile correction (**Table 2**).

11. Conclusion

To encapsulate, orthodontic bone screws have recast the approach to complex malocclusions in a significant way. These have been designed without losing sight of the fact that they are installed in extra-alveolar sites away from the roots and in areas of high amounts of cortical bone to affect tooth movement. While they gain an upper hand in terms of safety to roots and effective tooth movements, it is pivotal that the clinician must focus on the appropriate case selection for the same. One cannot deny their role of marching into the orthodontic field and that too with a roaring success. Considering that there is still a great deal of research that needs to be done about them, they are interesting areas of study to further the understanding and applications of these screws in orthodontic practice.

Author details

Agharsh Chandrasekaran[1*], H.P. Naga Deepti[1] and Harshavardhan Kidiyoor[2]

1 Private Practitioner, Bengaluru, India

2 SDM College of Dental Sciences and Hospital, A Constituent Unit of Shri Dharmasthala Manjunatheshwara University, Dharwad, India

*Address all correspondence to: agharshc@gmail.com

References

[1] Proffit WR. Contemporary Orthodontics. 6th ed. St. Louis: Mosby Yearbook; 1993. p. 307

[2] Jong Lin JL. Text Book of Creative Orthodontics: Blending the Damon System and TADs to Manage Difficult Malocclusions. Yong Chieh: Taipei, Taiwan; 2007

[3] Ghosh A. Infra-zygomatic crest and buccal shelf – Orthodontic bone screws: A leap ahead of micro-implants – Clinical perspectives. The Journal of Indian Orthodontic Society. 2018;**52**:S127-S141

[4] Jae-Hyun Sung. Microimplants in Orthodontics. Department of Orthodontics, School of Dentistry, Kyungpook National University, 2006.

[5] Shapiro PA, Kokich VG. Uses of implants in orthodontics. Dental Clinics of North America. 1988;**32**:539-550

[6] Chang CH, Lin JS, Roberts WE. Failure rates for stainless steel versus titanium alloy infrazygomatic crest bone screws: A single-center, randomized double-blind clinical trial. Angle Orthod. 2019 Jan;**89**(1):40-46.

[7] Almeida MR. Mini-implantes extra-alveolares em Orrtodontia. 1st ed. Maringá: Dental Press; 2018

[8] Misch CE. Density of bone: Effect on treatment plans, surgical approach, and healing, and progressive loading. The International Journal of Oral Implantology. 1990;**6**:23-31

[9] Park JH. Temporary Anchorage Devices in Clinical Orthodontics. 1st ed. Wiley Blackwell; 2020. p. 111

[10] Vargas EOA, Lopes de Lima R, Nojima LI. Mandibular buccal shelf and infrazygomatic crest thicknesses in patients with different vertical facial heights. American Journal of Orthodontics and Dentofacial Orthopedics. 2020;**158**(3):349-356

[11] Gandhi V, Upadhyay M, Tadinada A, Yadav S. Variability associated with mandibular buccal shelf area width and height in subjects with different growth pattern, sex, and growth status. American Journal of Orthodontics and Dentofacial Orthopedics. 2021;**159**(1): 59-70

[12] Graber LW, Vanarsdall RL, Vig KWL, Huang GJ. Orthodontics: Current Principles and Techniques. 6th ed. Amsterdam, Netherlands: Elsevier; 2017

[13] Pablo Echarri, Tae-Weon Kim, Lorenzo Favero, Hee-Jin Kim. Orthodontics & Microimplants: Complete Technique, Step by Step.

[14] Lin J, Roberts WE. Guided Infra-zygomatic screws: Reliable maxillary arch retraction. International Journal Orthodontics Implantology. 2017;**46**:4-16

[15] Liou EJ, Pai BC, Lin JC. Do miniscrews remain stationary under orthodontic forces? American Journal of Orthodontics and Dentofacial Orthopedics. 2004;**126**(1):42-47

[16] Baumgaertel S, Hans MG. Assessment of infrazygomaticbone depth for mini-screw insertion. Clinical Oral Implants Research. 2009;**20**:638-642

[17] Jia X, Chen X, Huang X. Influence of orthodontic mini-implant penetration of the maxillary sinus in the infrazygomatic crest region. American Journal of Orthodontics and Dentofacial Orthopedics. 2018;**153**(5):656-661

[18] Padmanabhan S, Kalia A. An interview with Dr. Junji Sugawara. Journal of Indian Orthodontic Society. 2018;**52**(4_suppl1):62-67

[19] Chang CH, Lin JS, Roberts WE. Forty consecutive ramus bone screws used to correct horizontally impacted mandibular molars. Int J Orthod Implantol. 2016;**41**:60-72

[20] Almeida MR. Biomechanics of extra-alveolar mini-implants. Dental Press Journal of Orthodontics. 2019;**24**(4):93-109

Chapter 10

Effectiveness and Stability of Treatment with Orthodontics Clear Aligners: What Evidence?

Soukaina Sahim and Farid El Quars

Abstract

Clear aligners, as a transparent and removable appliance, offer an alternative to conventional fixed appliance to patients with high demands for esthetics and comfort. Only a few investigations have focused on the efficacy of clear aligner therapy in controlling orthodontic tooth movement. Furthermore, the stability after treatment has not been thoroughly investigated. The purpose of this chapter was to update the knowledge of the available evidence about effectiveness and stability of clear aligners in non-growing subjects. Searches was made in different databases from January 2015 to January 2021. Relevant articles that met the inclusion criteria were selected. The level of evidence of the studies was moderate. The vertical movements of tooth were difficult to accomplish. Mesiodistal tipping showed the most predictability (82.5%) followed by vestibulolingual tipping. Molar distalization was also recorded as the highest accuracy. Derotation was difficult to accomplish with aligners especially of rounded teeth. The effectiveness of aligners in achieving the simulated transverse goals was 45%. The stability of clear aligner therapy was assessed by only two studies. Refinements are likely needed in almost all cases and to ensure treatment stability a retention period using a specific protocol is necessary.

Keywords: clear aligners, effectiveness, efficacy, stability, outcomes

1. Introduction

Orthodontic developments, especially during the last years, have been accompanied by a significant increase in the esthetic demands of the patients [1]. With the significant recent improvements in computer-aided design/computer-aid-ed manufacturing (CAD/CAM) and dental materials, there has been an increase in the demand for plastic systems [2]. Clear aligners provide an esthetic and comfortable treatment experience, facilitate oral hygiene, cause less pain as compared to fixed orthodontic appliances, and reduce the number and duration of appointments [3–5]. The aligner therapy also involves a lower incidence of demineralization, enamel abrasion, periodontal lesions, and mucosal irritations [6].

The concept of clear aligners was introduced by Kesling in 1946 with a tooth positioner fabricated by thermoplastic material molding technology and designed for minor tooth movements during the finishing stages of orthodontic treatment. In 1993, Sheridan and colleagues developed a technique of giving new clear retainers to the patient at each visit, incorporating interproximal reduction to provide the necessary space for tooth movement [3, 7]. With further advancement in orthodontic technology, Align Technology introduce the clear aligner treatment (CAT) rendering Kesling's concept a feasible orthodontic treatment option [8]. A series of removable polyurethane aligners were introduced as an esthetic alternative to fixed labial appliances. Scanned images are converted to physical models by using different stereolithography (STL) techniques to fabricate a series of aligners that sequentially reposition the teeth. Each aligner is programmed to move a tooth or a small group of teeth 0.25–0.33 mm every 14 days [9, 10]. Align Technology provides orthodontists with ClinCheck (Align Technology Inc., Santa Clara, Calif) models, which reflect the treatment outcomes. The aligners incrementally shift the teeth into place based on the outcome the orthodontist expects to achieve [11].

The primary focus of the clear aligner system was initially to solve cases of low and moderate crowding and to close small spaces [1]. However, it has continually evolved through the development of new aligner materials, attachments on teeth, as well as new auxiliaries, such as "Precision Cuts" and "Power Ridges" to address a wider range of malocclusions and to enable additional treatment biomechanics [2, 5, 12].

Despite the available body of literature pertaining to aligner technology, only a few investigations have focused on the efficacy of clear aligner therapy in controlling orthodontic tooth movement. Furthermore, the stability after treatment has not been thoroughly investigated.

The purpose of this chapter was to update the knowledge of the available evidence about effectiveness and stability of clear aligners and to answer the following clinical research question: "Are clear aligners effective in controlling the orthodontic movement in non-growing subjects and what about stability of this treatment modality?"

2. Materials and methods

2.1 Search strategy

A systematic search in the medical literature produced between January 2015 and January 2021 was performed to identify all peer-reviewed articles potentially relevant to the review's question.

The following databases have been used: CENTRAL, MEDLINE, MEDLINE in Process, Embase and Cochrane Library databases.

The search strategy comprised use of the following terms: (invisalign OR clear aligners OR aligners OR transparent aligners) AND (effectiveness OR efficacy) AND (dental changes OR treatment outcome) AND (stability).

Additionally, a manual search was conducted in orthodontic journals of interest, such as The Angle Orthodontist, the American Journal of Orthodontics and the European Journal of Orthodontics. Title and abstract screening was performed to select articles for full text retrieval.

2.2 Eligibility criteria

The following inclusion and exclusion criteria were used:

2.2.1 Inclusion criteria

Study design: meta-analysis, systematic reviews, randomized and non-randomized clinical trials, prospective and retrospective studies were included.

Participants: non growing patients.

Intervention: articles that studied dental movement of cases treated with clear aligners.

Results: the efficacy of clear aligners in performing dental movements and the stability of treatment, superimposing virtual models or radiographs.

2.2.2 Exclusion criteria

We excluded for our study articles older than 6 years, samples with growing patients, articles written in a language other than English, in-vitro studies, author opinions, letters to the editor, isolated cases, series of cases, surgical cases, or reports of patients with syndromes.

2.3 Level of evidence

The grading system described by the Swedish Council on Technology Assessment in Health Care (SBU) [13] was used to assess the methodological quality and the level of evidence of the articles (**Tables 1** and **2**).

Grade A—high value of evidence
All criteria should be met:
Randomized clinical study or a prospective study with a well-defined control group
Defined diagnosis and endpoints
Diagnostic reliability tests and reproducibility tests described
Blinded outcome assessment
Grade B—moderate value of evidence
All criteria should be met:
Cohort study or retrospective case series with defined control or reference group
Defined diagnosis and endpoints
Diagnostic reliability tests and reproducibility tests described
Grade C—low value of evidence
One or more of the conditions below:
Large attrition
Unclear diagnosis and endpoints
Poorly defined patient material

Table 1.
Swedish Council on Technology Assessment in Health Care (SBU) criteria for grading assessed studies.

Level	Evidence	Definition
1	Strong	At least two studies assessed with level "A"
2	Moderate	One study with level "A" and at least two studies with level "B"
3	Limited	At least two studies with level "B"
4	Inconclusive	Fewer than two studies with level "B"

Table 2.
Definitions of evidence level.

3. Results

3.1 Study selection

The selection of articles included in this review is shown in the PRISMA flow chart (**Figure 1**). Study selection procedure was comprised of title-reading, abstract-reading, and full-text-reading stages. After exclusion of not eligible studies, the full report of publications considered eligible for inclusion by the authors was assessed. Eleven studies were included in the qualitative synthesis.

3.2 Study characteristics

Of the eleven included articles, there were five retrospective studies [6, 14–17], two prospective studies [7, 11], two randomized controlled trials (RCT) [18, 19], two systematic reviews [2, 20] and one meta-analysis [20]. Most of the included studies evaluated mild to moderate malocclusions except for one [17] that involved first premolar extraction cases. The majority of studies used the Invisalign® system except two studies that used Nuvola® system [15] and F22 aligners [14].

Data collected from each of the included articles are described in **Tables 3** and **4**. Nine of the covered studies assessed predictability of tooth movements comparing

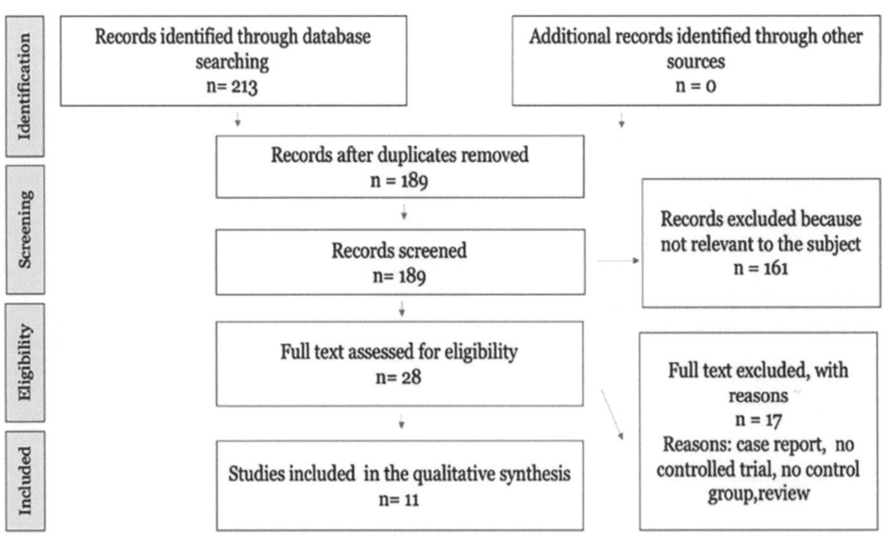

Figure 1.
Flow chart according to the PRISMA statement.

Study	Study design	Participants	Intervention	Results
Buschang et al. 2015 [11]	Prospective clinical trial	27pts	• Post-treatment patient models compared with their ClinCheck models provided by Invisalign • American Board of Orthodontics OGS	• The ClinCheck models overestimated alignment, buccolingual inclinations, occlusal contacts, and occlusal relations
Lombardo et al. 2017 [14]	Retrospective case series	16 pts. F22 aligners	• Pre-treatment, ideal post-treatment and real post-treatment models were analyzed using VAM software • Rotation, mesiodistal tip and vestibulo-lingual tip	• Mesiodistal tipping was the most predictable (82.5%) followed by vestibulolingual tipping • Mesiodistal tip on upper molars and lower premolars was the most predictable • Rotation of the lower canines was extremely unpredictable
Tepedino et al. 2018 [15]	Retrospective case series	39 pts. First phase of treatment made of 12 aligners by Nuvola® aligner system	• Torque of anterior teeth was measured on digital models at T0 (pre-treatment), T1 (post-treatment), and TS (digital setup)	• Clear aligner system was able to produce clinical outcomes comparable to the planning of the digital setup relative to torque movements of the anterior teeth
Charalampakis et al. 2018 [16]	Retrospective case series	20 pts. Class I patients treated with Invisalign and needed refinement	• Superimposition of predicted and achieved models over the initial ones	• Horizontal movements of all incisors seemed to be accurate • The most inaccurate movements were intrusion of the incisors and rotation of the canines
Lopez et al. 2019 [2]	Systematic review	20 studies	• Scientific evidence	• The expression of the programmed movement was not fully accomplished with Invisalign® • Invisalign® was able to alter intercanine, interpremolar, and intermolar width in the presence of crowding • Incisors tended to procline and protrude when crowding was > 6 mm • Molar distalization was recorded as the highest accuracy • Derotation was difficult to accomplish and IPR was recommended, especially in canines

Study	Study design	Participants	Intervention	Results
Dai et al. 2019 [17]	Retrospective case series	30 pts. First premolar extraction treatment with Invisalign	• Superimposition between predicted and achieved tooth positions • Influence of age, attachment and initial crowding	• First molar anchorage control and central incisor retraction were not fully achieved as predicted • Age, attachment, and initial crowding affected the predictability of tooth movement
Zhou et al. 2020 [7]	Prospective clinical trial	20 pts. arch expansion with Invisalign aligners	• Digital models and CBCT records of pretreatment and immediately after the expansion phase	• Aligners could increase the arch width, but expansion was achieved by tipping movement of posterior teeth • The efficiency of bodily buccal expansion for maxillary first molars averaged 36.35%.
Al-Nadawi et al. 2020 [18]	Randomized clinical trial	80 pts. three aligner wear protocols: 7 day, 10 day, and 14 day.	• Digital superimposition of posttreatment scans and final virtual treatment simulations	• Fourteen-day changes were statistically significantly more accurate in some posterior movements • Clinically similar accuracy between the 7-day protocol and 14-day protocol in half the treatment time • 14-day protocol if challenging posterior movements are desired
Riede et al. 2021 [6]	Retrospective case series	30 pts. Aligner treatment (Invisalign®) with the current material (SmartTrack®)	• Pretreatment model, scan-based model, posttreatment clinical model, and CC model reflecting the treatment outcome as simulated were analyzed. • Thirteen transverse parameters • Occlusal contacts	• The effectiveness of achieving the simulated transverse goals was 45% and was generally not found to be better with SmartTrack® than with the previously used Ex30® material • Out of 100 simulated occlusal contacts, 40 will never materialize, and achieving around 60 will adequately ensure a clinically favorable contact pattern

pts, patients; OGS, Objective Grading System; IPR, interproximal reduction; CBCT, Cone beam computed tomography.

Table 3.
Design, participants, type of intervention, and results of studies included in the qualitative analysis.

Study	Study design	Participants	Intervention	Results
Zheng et al. 2017 [20]	Systematic review and meta-analysis	• 4 studies included in qualitative synthesis • 2 studies included in quantitative synthesis (meta-analysis)	Scientific evidence	• Only one study compared the stability of treatment outcome with clear aligners to conventional brackets. • Patients treated with Invisalign relapsed more than those treated with conventional fixed appliances
Graf et al. 2021 [19]	Double-center trial	33pts	• PAR Index measured at baseline (T0), after finishing orthodontic treatment with Invisalign® (T1) and after a mean retention period of 10 months (T2).	• Treatment effects were stable throughout a short-term retention period using a specific retention protocol. • Effectiveness and stability were equally achieved in mild, moderate, and rather severe cases.

pts, patients.

Table 4.
Studies assessing treatment stability of clear aligners.

Study (first author, year)	Evidence level
Buschang, 2015 [11]	C
Lombardo, 2017 [14]	B
Tepedino, 2018 [15]	B
Charalampakis, 2018 [16]	C
Dai, 2019 [17]	C
Zhou, 2020 [7]	B
Al-Nadawi, 2020 [18]	A
Riede, 2021 [6]	C
Graf, 2021 [19]	B

Table 5.
Evidence grade according to Swedish Council on Technology Assessment in Health Care.

post-treatment patient models to the predicted digital planned tooth movement models [2, 6, 7, 11, 14–18]. Two studies assessed the stability of the clear aligner therapy [19, 20].

3.3 Level of evidence of studies

According to the SBU tool (**Tables 1** and **2**), among the selected studies, the methodological quality was low for four studies [6, 11, 16, 17], moderate for four others [7, 14, 15, 19] and high for one study [18] (**Table 5**). Thus, conclusions with a moderate level of evidence could be drawn from the review process.

4. Discussion

In this review, we aimed to provide data on the effectiveness and stability of treatment with clear aligners. The level of evidence was moderate as we identified one study with level «A» and four studies with level «B».

The effectiveness of clear aligners was judged by the predictability of tooth movement which varies with the type of tooth and the type of movement. Lopez et al. [2] found that the expression of the programmed movement was not fully accomplished with Invisalign®.

Concerning **vertical movements**, the study by Lopez et al. [2] revealed that vertical movements are difficult to accomplish with aligners. Extrusion of a single tooth is moderately difficult using clear aligners when compared to fixed-appliance systems, however, some auxiliaries such as buttons, elastics and optimized extrusion attachments can be used to facilitate this movement [5, 21].

Many studies showed that intrusion was the most unpredictable movement especially for the maxillary central and lateral incisors [16, 21]. Invisalign has a bite-block effect, because 2 aligners of 0.38-mm width are interposed between posterior teeth throughout treatment. Unexpected intrusion of the molars would cause the incisors to appear extruded on the posttreatment models after superimposition [16]. In fact, according to Grunheid et al. [22], mandibular incisors tend to be positioned more occlusally than predicted. The bite-block effect may make open bites easier to treat with Invisalign [16].

Concerning **horizontal movements**, mesiodistal tipping showed the most predictability especially of upper molars and lower premolars (82.5%) followed by vestibulolingual tipping [14]. Lingual crown tip (53%) was significantly more accurate than labial crown tip (38%), particularly for maxillary incisors [23]. According to Rossini et al. [8], aligners can easily tip crowns but cannot tip roots because these appliances cause tooth movement by tilting motion rather than bodily movement. In the anterior region, the elasticity of the aligner at the gingival margin results in difficulty in controlling the applied forces [24]. With the use of Power Ridges (Align Technology, Amsterdam, The Netherlands), the aligner can accurately control root torque according to the crown position in the virtual setup [17]. Tepedino et al. [15] also concluded that with Nuvola® aligners, in patients with moderate crowding up to 6 mm, the torque movements for central and lateral incisors and canines of both arches predicted in the digital setup were, in general, clinically achieved. However, molar torque may not be fully achieved, with maxillary second molars often having a clinically relevant magnitude of more facial crown torque than predicted [22].

Molar distalization was recorded as the highest accuracy with no need for attachments. Simon et al. [25] also reported a high accuracy (88%) of the bodily movement of upper molars when a distalization movement of at least 1.5 mm was prescribed.

Several studies agreed that derotation of rounded teeth especially canines was difficult to achieve with aligners [16, 22, 26]. An amount of rotation greater than 15° has been identified as a risk factor for decreased accuracy for rotational prediction [25]. Interproximal contacts of rotated canines might also be considered a significant predictor for the diminished efficacy of tooth movement, especially in the absence of interproximal reduction of the enamel (IPR) [26]. The direction of derotation has been also documented to influence the accuracy of the maxillary canine, with distal movement demonstrating less accuracy than mesial [21]. This is possibly due to the actual contact area between canine and premolar and the potential challenges of providing enamel reduction in this area.

It has been recommended to plan overcorrections, especially if rotations exceed 15°, to use attachments, and to reduce staging to less than 1.5° per aligner [8, 16, 25]. However, although various types or shapes of attachment grips or practices of interproximal enamel reduction have been reported as potential prognostic factors for better efficacy of rotational tooth movement, this does not necessarily translate into an identified substantial effect in practice [26].

Concerning **transverse movements**, the effectiveness of achieving the simulated transverse goals was 45% [6]. Aligners could increase the arch width, but expansion was achieved by tipping movement of posterior teeth rather than bodily expansion. In fact, Invisalign becomes less accurate going from the anterior to the posterior region being more effective in premolar area [27, 28]. Thus, according to the initial torque of the posterior teeth, an appropriate amount of negative torque in the crown could be preset in ClinCheck to improve bodily expansion efficiency. For patients who need a large amount of expansion, clinicians should consider reducing the amount of expansion for each aligner to ensure periodontal health [7].

According to Lopez and al. [2], Invisalign® was also able to alter intercanine, interpremolar, and intermolar width in the presence of crowding. Kravitz et al. [23] recommended to treat cases with severe lower crowding mostly by interproximal reduction (IPR) instead of dentoalveolar expansion. This recommendation comes from the finding that retraction is more accurate than dentoalveolar expansion of the lower anterior teeth. The expansion of the mandibular intercanine width also poses the greatest risk of relapse following treatment [29].

Concerning the effectiveness of the occlusal contacts with clear aligners, the study by Izhar et al. [10] found that the software models do not accurately reflect the patient's final occlusion immediately at the end of active treatment. Kassas et al. [30] also stated that clear aligners were not sufficient for providing ideal occlusal contacts. The deterioration in occlusal contacts was caused by the thickness of aligners, which interferes with the settling of the occlusal plane.

As far as the malocclusion type is concerned, the study by Graf et al. [19] showed that Invisalign® treatments are able to significantly reduce malocclusions in adult patients. The study found that all types of sagittal malocclusion (class I, class II, and class III) were 'greatly improved' with a rate of 77.44%. Graf and al. [19] also concluded that conventional attachments and the combination with optimized attachments equally led to treatment effectiveness regarding the total PAR score reduction with equally achieved effectiveness in mild, moderate, and rather severe cases. However, for Class II malocclusion, Patterson et al. [31] reported that there was no significant Class II correction or overjet reduction with elastics for an average of 7-month duration in the adult population. Additional refinements may be necessary to address problems created during treatment mainly posterior open bite.

One study of our review by Dai et al. [17] assessed the effectiveness of Invisalign in first premolar extraction treatment. According to this study, first molar anchorage control and central incisor retraction were not fully achieved as predicted. Only medium anchorage control was achieved as the first molars actually moved mesially. The G6-optimized attachment showed similar control in first molar angulation and mesiodistal translation as did 3- and 5-mm horizontal rectangular attachments. On the other hand, setting a distal tipping of 6.6 mm on the first molars might help clinically maintain the tooth angulation, leading to bodily tooth movement. According to the same study [17], the incisors inclined lingually under the retraction force.

Accordingly, the use of power ridges or attachments as well as overcorrection by setting greater buccal crown inclination during the virtual setup should be considered to achieve optimal incisor torque control.

Current evidence does not support the clinical use of aligners as a treatment modality that is equally effective to the gold standard of braces [32]. However, clear aligners have advantage in segmented movement of teeth and shortened treatment duration, but are not as effective as braces in producing adequate occlusal contacts, controlling teeth torque, and retention [5, 33].

Many variables influence the accuracy of dental movements, but very few studies have analyzed these parameters in treatments with clear aligners. According to Tepedino et al. [15], several factors determine successful tooth movement such as the attachment's shape and position, the aligner's material and thickness, the amount of activation present in each aligner, and the techniques used for the production of the aligners. Treatment outcomes depend also on the patient's characteristics, bone density and morphology, crown and root morphology of the teeth, as well as on factors related to the clinician. Orthodontists have to incorporate their expert knowledge in determining proper sequencing of tooth movements, tooth attachment design and placement, and prescribing overcorrection when needed for difficult tooth movements to increase efficiency and achieve better treatment outcomes [22, 34]. Patient compliance is also mandatory to achieve good results by wearing the aligners 22 hours a day or more [28].

One study from this review with a high level of evidence [18] evaluated the impact of wear protocol on the accuracy of clear aligners. It has concluded that fourteen-day changes were statistically significantly more accurate in some posterior movements mainly maxillary intrusion, distal-crown tip and buccal-crown torque, and in mandibular intrusion and extrusion.

As in all types of orthodontic treatment, stability is one of the most important issues to discuss regarding clear aligners. According to the systematic review by Zheng et al. [20], only one study compared the post-retention dental changes between patients treated with Invisalign and those treated with conventional fixed appliances. They found that the change in the total alignment score in the Invisalign group was significantly larger than that for the Braces group. There were significantly larger changes in maxillary anterior alignment in the Invisalign group than in the conventional bracket group. Tamer et al. [5] also reported that maxillary anterior leveling relapsed in the Invisalign group. On average, the posttreatment models lost twice as many points for alignment than the respective ClinCheck models. In other words, a full finishing phase of treatment may be needed to achieve the results indicated in the ClinCheck model [11].

The type and degree of tooth movement, the duration of active treatment and the retention protocol are among major influencing factors of posttreatment stability and relapse. The study by Graf et al. [19] is the first one to assess the stability of clear aligners outcome throughout a retention period of 10 months. The retention protocol involved a mandibular multistrand fixed retainer (0.0155 inch; stainless steel, 24 K gold plated) bonded on each lingual surface from canine to canine and a removable modified Hawley retainer for the upper arch (with mandatory Adams clasps on first molars). The study showed that the treatment outcome can be stable throughout this retention protocol. It has also concluded that treating patients with respect to their physiological boundaries and maintaining their original arch form would be key to treatment stability. Overexpansion of the dental arch, especially in the lower arch and in adult patients, is a potential risk for stable results.

5. Conclusion

There is current evidence with a moderate level of certainty regarding the effectiveness of clear aligner therapy for certain tooth movements. Clear aligners can safely straighten dental arches in terms of leveling and derotating the teeth, except for canines and premolars. The crown tipping can be easily performed. However, important limitations include arch expansion through bodily tooth movements, extraction space closure, corrections of occlusal contacts, and larger antero-posterior and vertical discrepancies. The use of additional attachments might be more effective for various types of movement, such as bodily expansion of the maxillary posterior teeth, canine and premolar rotational movements, incisors torque control and extrusion of maxillary incisors. Overcorrections might also improve the effectiveness of orthodontic movement. However, overcorrections are not as simple for all movements and need to be made on a case-by-case basis depending on the goal of treatment.

Studies on effectiveness of clear aligners had methodological heterogeneity as they assessed predictability of different types of tooth movements for different teeth by using different materials like Invisalign, F22 aligner and Nuvola system. Retention and stability studies regarding aligners also remain limited in the literature. Therefore, further well-designed and reported researches are required on this subject.

Acknowledgements

Special thanks to the department of Orthodontics of the Faculty of the dentistry of the University Hassan II of Casablanca. We would also like to acknowledge the support of Professor Farid Bourzgui for the realization of this work and for sharing and discussing the initial idea of the project.

Conflict of interest

The authors declare no conflict of interest.

Author details

Soukaina Sahim* and Farid El Quars
Department of Orthodontics, Faculty of Dentistry, University Hassan II, Casablanca, Morocco

*Address all correspondence to: souki-2s@hotmail.fr

References

[1] Papadimitriou A, Mousoulea S, Gkantidis N, Kloukos D. Clinical effectiveness of Invisalign® orthodontic treatment: A systematic review. Prog Orthod. 2018 Sep 28;19(1):37. DOI:10.1186/s40510-018-0235-z. PMID: 30264270; PMCID: PMC6160377.

[2] Galan-Lopez L, Barcia-Gonzalez J, Plasencia E. A systematic review of the accuracy and efficiency of dental movements with Invisalign®. Korean J Orthod. 2019 May;49(3):140-149. DOI:10.4041/kjod.2019.49.3.140. Epub 2019 May 21. PMID: 31149604; PMCID: PMC6533182.

[3] Kau CH, Feinberg KB, Christou T. Effectiveness of clear aligners in treating patients with anterior open bite: A retrospective analysis. J Clin Orthod. 2017 Aug;51(8):454-460. PMID: 29112503.

[4] Lione R, Paoloni V, Bartolommei L, Gazzani F, Meuli S, Pavoni C, Cozza P. Maxillary arch development with Invisalign system. Angle Orthod. 2021 Jul 1;91(4):433-440. DOI:10.2319/080520-687.1. PMID: 33570617; PMCID: PMC8259755.

[5] Tamer İ, Öztaş E, Marşan G. Orthodontic treatment with clear aligners and the scientific reality behind their marketing: A literature review. Turk J Orthod. 2019 Dec 1;32(4):241-246. DOI:10.5152/TurkJOrthod.2019.18083. PMID: 32110470; PMCID: PMC7018497.

[6] Riede U, Wai S, Neururer S, Reistenhofer B, Riede G, Besser K, Crismani A. Maxillary expansion or contraction and occlusal contact adjustment: effectiveness of current aligner treatment. Clin Oral Investig. 2021 Jul;25(7):4671-4679. DOI:10.1007/s00784-021-03780-4. Epub 2021 Jan 20. PMID: 33474622; PMCID: PMC8310473.

[7] Zhou N, Guo J. Efficiency of upper arch expansion with the Invisalign system. Angle Orthod. 2020 Jan;90(1):23-30. DOI:10.2319/022719-151.1. Epub 2019 Aug 1. PMID: 31368778; PMCID: PMC8087062.

[8] Rossini G, Parrini S, Castroflorio T, Deregibus A, Debernardi CL. Efficacy of clear aligners in controlling orthodontic tooth movement: A systematic review. Angle Orthod. 2015 Sep;85(5):881-889. DOI:10.2319/061614-436.1. Epub 2014 Nov 20. PMID: 25412265.

[9] Caputo M, Di Luzio C, Bellisario A, Squillace F, Favale M. Evaluation of the effectiveness of clear aligners therapy in orthodontic tooth movement. WebmedCentral ORTHODONTICS 2017;8(11): WMC005359

[10] Izhar A, Singh G, Goyal V, Singh R, Gupta N, Pahuja P. Comparative assessment of clinical and predicted treatment outcomes of clear aligner treatment: An in vivo study. Turk J Orthod. 2019 Dec 1;32(4):229-235. DOI:10.5152/TurkJOrthod.2019.19019. PMID: 32110468; PMCID: PMC7018496.

[11] Buschang PH, Ross M, Shaw SG, Crosby D, Campbell PM. Predicted and actual end-of-treatment occlusion produced with aligner therapy. Angle Orthod. 2015 Sep;85(5):723-727. DOI:10.2319/043014-311.1. Epub 2014 Nov 5. PMID: 25372019.

[12] Putrino A, Barbato E, Galluccio G. Clear aligners: Between evolution and efficiency—A scoping review. Int J Environ Res Public Health. 2021 Mar

11;18(6):2870. DOI:10.3390/ijerph18062870. PMID: 33799682; PMCID: PMC7998651.

[13] Alexanderson K, Norlund A. Swedish Council on Technology Assessment in Health Care (SBU). Chapter 2. Methods used for the systematic literature search and for the review of relevance, quality, and evidence of studies. Scand J Public Health Suppl. 2004; 63:31-35. DOI:10.1080/14034950410021826. PMID: 15513651.

[14] Lombardo L, Arreghini A, Ramina F, Huanca Ghislanzoni LT, Siciliani G. Predictability of orthodontic movement with orthodontic aligners: A retrospective study. Prog Orthod. 2017 Nov 13;18(1):35. DOI:10.1186/s40510-017-0190-0. PMID: 29130127; PMCID: PMC5682257.

[15] Tepedino M, Paoloni V, Cozza P, Chimenti C. Movement of anterior teeth using clear aligners: A three-dimensional, retrospective evaluation. Prog Orthod. 2018 Apr 2;19(1):9. DOI:10.1186/s40510-018-0207-3. PMID: 29607469; PMCID: PMC5879033.

[16] Charalampakis O, Iliadi A, Ueno H, Oliver DR, Kim KB. Accuracy of clear aligners: A retrospective study of patients who needed refinement. Am J Orthod Dentofacial Orthop. 2018 Jul;154(1): 47-54. DOI:10.1016/j.ajodo.2017.11.028. PMID: 29957318.

[17] Dai FF, Xu TM, Shu G. Comparison of achieved and predicted tooth movement of maxillary first molars and central incisors: First premolar extraction treatment with Invisalign. Angle Orthod. 2019 Sep;89(5):679-687. DOI:10.2319/090418-646.1. Epub 2019 Mar 28. PMID: 30920875; PMCID: PMC8111827.

[18] Al-Nadawi M, Kravitz ND, Hansa I, Makki L, Ferguson DJ, Vaid NR. Effect of clear aligner wear protocol on the efficacy of tooth movement. Angle Orthod. 2021 Mar 1;91(2):157-163. DOI:10.2319/071520-630.1. PMID: 33296455; PMCID: PMC8028485.

[19] Graf I, Puppe C, Schwarze J, Höfer K, Christ H, Braumann B. Evaluation of effectiveness and stability of aligner treatments using the Peer Assessment Rating Index. J Orofac Orthop. 2021 Jan;82(1):23-31. English. DOI:10.1007/s00056-020-00249-z. Epub 2020 Sep 22. PMID: 32960313.

[20] Zheng M, Liu R, Ni Z, Yu Z. Efficiency, effectiveness and treatment stability of clear aligners: A systematic review and meta-analysis. Orthod Craniofac Res. 2017 Aug;20(3):127-133. DOI:10.1111/ocr.12177. Epub 2017 May 26. PMID: 28547915.

[21] Haouili N, Kravitz ND, Vaid NR, Ferguson DJ, Makki L. Has Invisalign improved? A prospective follow-up study on the efficacy of tooth movement with Invisalign. Am J Orthod Dentofacial Orthop. 2020 Sep;158(3):420-425. DOI:10.1016/j.ajodo.2019.12.015. Epub 2020 Jun 30. PMID: 32620479.

[22] Grünheid T, Loh C, Larson BE. How accurate is Invisalign in nonextraction cases? Are predicted tooth positions achieved? Angle Orthod. 2017 Nov;87(6):809-815. DOI:10.2319/022717-147.1. Epub 2017 Jul 7. PMID: 28686090; PMCID: PMC8317555.

[23] Kravitz ND, Kusnoto B, BeGole E, Obrez A, Agran B. How well does Invisalign work? A prospective clinical study evaluating the efficacy of tooth movement with Invisalign. Am J Orthod Dentofacial Orthop. 2009 Jan;135(1):27-35. DOI:10.1016/j.ajodo.2007.05.018. PMID: 19121497.

[24] Zhang XJ, He L, Guo HM, Tian J, Bai YX, Li S. Integrated three-dimensional digital assessment of accuracy of anterior tooth movement using clear aligners. Korean J Orthod. 2015 Nov;45(6):275-81. DOI:10.4041/kjod.2015.45.6.275. Epub 2015 Nov 20. PMID: 26629473; PMCID: PMC4664903.

[25] Simon M, Keilig L, Schwarze J, Jung BA, Bourauel C. Treatment outcome and efficacy of an aligner technique—Regarding incisor torque, premolar derotation and molar distalization. BMC Oral Health. 2014 Jun 11; 14:68. DOI:10.1186/1472-6831-14-68. PMID: 24923279; PMCID: PMC4068978.

[26] Koletsi D, Iliadi A, Eliades T. Predictability of rotational tooth movement with orthodontic aligners comparing software-based and achieved data: A systematic review and meta-analysis of observational studies. J Orthod. 2021 Jun 27:14653125211027266. DOI:10.1177/14653125211027266. Epub ahead of print. PMID: 34176358.

[27] Morales-Burruezo I, Gandía-Franco JL, Cobo J, Vela-Hernández A, Bellot-Arcís C. Arch expansion with the Invisalign system: Efficacy and predictability. PLoS One. 2020 Dec 10;15(12): e0242979. DOI:10.1371/journal.pone.0242979. PMID: 33301484; PMCID: PMC7728268.

[28] Houle JP, Piedade L, Todescan R Jr, Pinheiro FH. The predictability of transverse changes with Invisalign. Angle Orthod. 2017 Jan;87(1):19-24. DOI:10.2319/122115-875.1. Epub 2016 Jun 15. PMID: 27304231.

[29] Phan X, Ling PH. Clinical limitations of Invisalign. J Can Dent Assoc. 2007 Apr;73(3):263-266. PMID: 17439714.

[30] Kassas W, Al-Jewair T, Preston CB, Tabbaa S. Assessment of Invisalign treatment outcomes using the ABO Model Grading System. Journal of the World Federation of Orthodontists. 2013 Jun 1;2(2): e61–e64. DOI:10.1016/j.ejwf.2013.03.003

[31] Patterson BD, Foley PF, Ueno H, Mason SA, Schneider PP, Kim KB. Class II malocclusion correction with Invisalign: Is it possible? Am J Orthod Dentofacial Orthop. 2021 Jan;159(1):e41-e48. DOI:10.1016/j.ajodo.2020.08.016. Epub 2020 Nov 19. PMID: 33223374.

[32] Papageorgiou SN, Koletsi D, Iliadi A, Peltomaki T, Eliades T. Treatment outcome with orthodontic aligners and fixed appliances: A systematic review with meta-analyses. Eur J Orthod. 2020 Jun 23;42(3):331-343. DOI:10.1093/ejo/cjz094. PMID: 31758191.

[33] Ke Y, Zhu Y, Zhu M. A comparison of treatment effectiveness between clear aligner and fixed appliance therapies. BMC Oral Health. 2019 Jan 23;19(1):24. DOI:10.1186/s12903-018-0695-z. PMID: 30674307; PMCID: PMC6343314.

[34] Boyd RL. Esthetic orthodontic treatment using the invisalign appliance for moderate to complex malocclusions. J Dent Educ. 2008 Aug;72(8):948-967. PMID: 18676803.

Chapter 11

The Value of Self-Ligating Brackets in Orthodontics: About the Damon Protocol

Suvetha Siva, Shreya Kishore, Suganya Dhanapal, Janani Ravi and Chandhini Suresh

Abstract

In orthodontics there has been a change in the treatment plan of crowding cases from extraction protocol. This was mainly due to the introduction of self-ligating bracket and temperature activated wires. Even though there are certain exceptions, the self-ligating bracket have evolved in orthodontics because of its advantages such as low friction, shorter treatment duration and increased efficacy. Damon's self-ligating system has been in existence since 1930 but it has been well developed in the past 30 years with the introduction of newer systems. Damon's self-ligating brackets have been designed to overcome the drawbacks of conventional bracket system and are often considered as the pinnacle of bracket technology. The main advantage of Damon's system was low friction and shorter treatment duration. But the efficiency of the appliance is influenced by several factors such as Biomechanics, frequency of dental visits and patient comfort. The chapter will highlight the efficiency of the appliance, the various possible outcomes and its influence on the ease of orthodontic therapy.

Keywords: self-ligating bracket, Damon's system, Damon brackets, passive self-ligating bracket, Damon philosophy

1. Introduction

Orthodontics and orthodontists have always worked towards delivering better care for patients. This has led to the invention of various bracket systems along with the changes in the protocol of management of extraction cases.

The Self Ligating Brackets (SLB) has come into orthodontic practice since 1930's with the invention of Boydband bracket. These bracket systems along with the thermally activated NiTi wires have reduced the treatment duration, chair-side time, and improved the treatment efficacy and patient co-operation. This led to the invention of Damon's system by Dr. Dwight Damon in the year 1996. It is called as "System" rather than "Brackets" because it utilizes the benefits of both the brackets and copper NiTi wires, thus delivering a "low force- low friction" mechanics for the management of dental malocclusion [1].

There has been lot of evidence in literature which states that "atraumatic" remodeling of periodontal tissues was rarely achieved using conventional orthodontic bracket system. This is mainly because the tooth was always moved in group. In Damon's system, the tooth is allowed to move individually, yet stay in the group. The bracket system allows for easy sliding of the tooth along the path of least or no resistance thus leading to faster leveling and alignment and reduced treatment duration [2]. The aim of this chapter is to describe the bracket prescription, efficiency of the appliance, the possible outcomes and its influence on orthodontic therapy.

2. Why choose Damon?

Damon philosophy uses the concept of passive self-ligation technique which claims to have the lowest frictional resistance of any ligation system. Reduction in friction helps the force to transmit directly from the arch wires to the teeth and its supporting structures without any force dissipation by the ligature system [3].

Comparing the other prescriptions, Damon system has lots of benefits:

- Limitations in the use of intraoral expansion appliances such as quad-helix or jack-screw as the optimal forces from the arch wires completely allows the connective tissue and alveolar bone to follow tooth movement with uninterrupted vascular supply to the tooth and its surrounding system thereby providing the necessary expansion [3–5].

- In a study stated that Damon System produced a significant transversal increase in the posterior region of the arches with differences in teeth buccolingual inclinations at post-treatment [6].

- Faster alignment of teeth as passive self-ligation produces lower resistance thus allowing a wire to slide.

- Reduced amount of pain experienced by patients, and higher treatment efficiency as this friction-free system produces less forces on the teeth [4, 5].

- Reduction in the need for extraction as the force applied is minimal that the pressure from lips can control unwanted tipping of incisors during alignment stage [5].

- Decreased demand for the use of anchorage devices comparing the conventional appliances as there is reduced friction between the ligation for better tooth control [7].

- Reduction in the overall duration of orthodontic treatment up to 7 months and also reduced number of appointments have been found in few researches [8, 9].

- Control of tooth position because there is an edgewise slot of adequate width and depth [3].

- Decreased discomfort experienced by the patients with the Damon prescription as the forces applied to the teeth are kept minimal throughout the treatment [4].

- More efficient chair-side due to reduced ligation time [10].
- Promotes periodontal health with better infection control [11].

3. Classification of Damon's system

In orthodontics achieving ideal inclination of anterior using the edgewise system is challenging. In an attempt to overcome this drawback, Damon's system has different torque prescription. This includes:

3.1 High torque brackets

These brackets can be used in cases where the incisors or cuspids are severely retroclined or palatally placed. Examples are:

- Class I extraction cases with proclined of anterior.
- Class II division 1 malocclusion.
- Class II division 2 malocclusion with retroclined incisors.
- Palatally placed incisors or cuspids.

3.2 Standard torque brackets

These brackets can be used in cases where the inclination of anterior is satisfactory and when there will not be any obvious change in the inclination during the course of the treatment.

3.3 Low torque brackets

- Examples of the cases include:
- Anterior open bite cases with severe proclination of anteriors.
- Moderate and severe crowding.
- Treatment mechanics which may result in proclination of anteriors.
- Incisors with palatally positioned roots.
- In class II fixed functional cases or class II elastics cases where control of lower incisor proclination is necessary.
- Lingually placed lower incisors [3].

4. Tip and torque

The tip and torque values of Damon's system are as in **Tables 1** and 2.

Upper arch						
U1	**U2**	**U3**	**U4**	**U5**	**U6**	**U7**
+5°	+9°	+6°	+2°	+2°		
Lower arch						
L1	L2	L3	L4	L5	L6	L7
+2°	+2°	+5°	+2°	+2°		

Table 1.
Tip values in Damon's system.

	Upper arch						
	U1	**U2**	**U3**	**U4**	**U5**	**U6**	**U7**
High torque	+17°	+10°	+7°				
Standard torque	+12°	+8°	0°	−7°	−7°	−18°	−27°
Low torque	+7°	+3°					
	Lower arch						
	L1	L2	L3	L4	L5	L6	L7
High torque			+7°				
Standard torque	−1°	−1°	0°	−12°	−17°	−28°	−10°
Low torque	−6°	−6°					

Table 2.
Torque values in Damon's system.

5. Advantages and disadvantages

5.1 Advantages

- Clinically proven
- Enhances facial esthetics
- More comfortable than traditional braces
- Reduced friction and faster tooth movement
- Shorter treatment duration
- Lesser visits

5.2 Disadvantages

- Expensive than traditional braces
- "Metal Mouth" look

6. Arch wire sequencing

The phases of tooth movement are generally.

- Initial leveling and aligning – where initial round wires made of multistranded steel or NiTi are used, starting from the smaller dimensions then proceeded with the larger dimensions.
- Retraction and space closure – where rigid rectangular wires are used for major mechanics like torque expression and space closure.
- Finishing and detailing – round steel wires are usually used.

There are two sequences which are generally followed in pre-adjusted edgewise prescription.

6.1 Universal arch wire sequencing

An older concept of a sequence which initially uses round steel wires from sizes.014, .016, .018 and .020 followed by rectangular steel wires from dimensions.018 × .025, .019 × .025 and.021 × .025 in.022 slots.

Multi-stranded wires of dimensions .015 and .0175 were used for initial aligning before .014 round Steel wire came into practice and finishing and detailing was done with.014 steel wires.

Later with the introduction of MBT prescription, arch wire sequencing started with initial .016 CuNiTi wire followed by .019 × .025 CuNiTi and then .019 × .025 Steel wire was used for major biomechanics and detailing was done with .014 round steel wire [12, 13].

A clinical research by Mandall, in which three wire sequences were randomly allocated to patients to compare are as follows:

Group A - 0.016 NiTi, 0.018 × 0.025nNiTi, and .019 × 0.025 Steel wires.

Group B- 0.016 Niti, 0.016 SS and finally 0.020-inch Steel wires.

Group C - 0.016 × 0.022 CuNiTi wire, followed by 0.019 × 0.025 CuNiTi, and ending with 0.019 × 0.025 Steel wire,

And found that all sequences were equally effective. However, the CuNiTi may be preferred by the clinicians as it reduces the number of appointments [14].

In another study by Ong, the three different archwire sequences were applied are as follows:

- 0.014 Niti, 0.017×0.017 HANT, 0.016×0.022 Steel
- 0.014 Sentalloy, 0.016×0.022 Bio force, 0.016×0.022 Steel
- 0.014 CuNiTi, 0.014×0.025 CuNiTi, 0.016×0.022 Steel,

And found that there were no differences among the archwire sequences in terms of aligning or discomfort [15].

6.2 Damon arch wire sequencing

Phase 1: Light Round Wires

This phase of treatment uses 0.013, 0.014, or 0.016 CuNiTi arch wires. The aim of this first phase of treatment is to achieve tooth alignment including rotation correction except second molars, level the arches and initiate arch development with light forces to permit the soft tissues to desired arch shape. This phase of treatment normally extends from 10 to 20 weeks and the intervals between appointments are about 10 weeks.

Phase 2: High Rectangular Wires

Phase 2 uses two arch wires: 0.014 × 0.025 CuNiTi followed by 0.018 × 0.025 CuNiTi wires. In case of well aligned arches only 0.016 × 0.025 CuNiTi are used in this phase. If intrusion of anteriors is planned, 0.017× 0.025 or 0.019× 0.025 CuNiTi arch wires with preformed curves or reverse curves of Spee or additional torque can be applied anteriorly in this stage.

The main purposes of this phase are:

- Continue arch development
- achieve complete alignment of all teeth including second molars,
- consolidate anterior spaces and maintain tooth contact,
- Initiate torque control and bite opening,

The duration of this phase ranges from 20 to 30 weeks. The first archwire is placed from 8 to 10 weeks and the second is from 4 to 6 weeks.

Phase 3: Major Mechanics

Preposted stainless steel arch wires of size 0.019 × .025 are used. Presence of cross bite at this stage when persisted can be corrected with the use of 0.016 × 0.025 preposted stainless steel arch wire with the use of cross elastics where buccal and lingual tipping can be achieved at this stage.

The main purposes of this phase are:

- Finish torque control,
- Consolidate posterior space and
- Maintain the arch form which developed during the initial two phases,
- Completely correct the tooth position in all the three relationships.

This phase of treatment extends from 8 to 10 weeks with an interval about 10-weeks between appointments.

Phase 4: Finishing and Detailing

The stainless steel arch wires continued in this phase with elastics for achieving proper interdigitation. But for individual teeth position 0.019× 0.025 ß-titanium arch wires may also be used [2, 3, 16].

In a study by Handem, used the arch sequence with initial round wires 0.014 or 0.016, followed by rectangular 0.016 × 0.025, 0.018 × 0.025, and 0.019 × 0.025 CuNiTi arch wires subsequently, rectangular 0.017 × 0.025 or 0.019 × 0.025 Steel arch wires [17].

DOI: http://dx.doi.org/10.5772/intechopen.100536

7. Bracket placement in Damon system

Various clinicians have put forth bracket placement methodologies of the Damon bracket system to achieve the desired smile arc protection, functional occlusion and enhancing the facial esthetics.

Standard bracket placement by Dwight Damon [18]:

According to him, the arch wire slot should be at the distances mentioned below from the incisal edge.

Maxillary

U-1 4.75 mm.

U-2 4.50 mm.

U-3 5.00 mm.

U-4 4.50 mm.

U-5 4.25 mm.

Mandibular

L-1 4.75 mm.

L-2 4.50 mm.

L-3 5.00 mm.

L-4 4.50 mm.

L-5 4.25 mm.

7.1 Placement tips

- The upper brackets open occlusally and the lower brackets open gingivally.

- The mesiodistal width of the pad and the mesiodistal edges of the teeth should be given importance.

- Panorex view prior to bracket placement allows to identify root position.

- The internal slot and the horizontal components should be parallel to the occlusal plane. This is of greater importance in the lower anteriors.

- The scribe line of the bracket and crown long axis should be focused while placing the bracket.

Dr. Dwight Damon advises placement of the bracket within the green zone (in between the green lines). The Damon prescription has variable torque prescriptions to foster the need for different clinical cases. A clinician can place the upper and lower mid-bracket slot within the green lines without dramatically impacting torque.

Dr. Thomas. R. Pitts Protocol [19]:

Dr. Thomas. R. Pitts worked with a philosophy of "beginning with the end in mind". He believed that developing acumen in precise bracket placement is the single most important protocol to achieve an esthetically pleasing smile and functional occlusion.

Basic principles of the Pitts placement protocol:

Detailed bonding plan before the day of bonding and to select brackets of appropriate torque based on the demand of the case.

Ensure tray setup entails all items for an efficient bonding.

Use two assistants to assist in bonding.

Recontour teeth for esthetics and bracket fit.

Follow an exacting placement protocol to achieve an ideal smile arc in the anteriors and leveling buccal cusps and marginal ridges in the posteriors.

Dr. Pitts bonds the maxillary anteriors to achieve a consonant smile arc at the end of the treatment, the mandibular anteriors for overjet and overbite and the remaining teeth for a good occlusion. He first bonds the mandibular teeth, from the second molar to canine on one side, and repeats the same on the opposite side, followed by lateral to lateral. This is followed to achieve symmetry on either side. The same sequence is repeated in the upper arch. He believed in keying off the maxillary canine to ensure that the canine-lateral and canine- premolar contacts are esthetic and functional.

In the posteriors, to achieve leveled marginal ridges and contact points, the teeth are bonded using the contact points as reference. This is done up to the canine and then the incisors are bonded based on the slot of the maxillary canine to give a sweep in the smile arc which gives a pleasing appearance **Figures 1** and **2**.

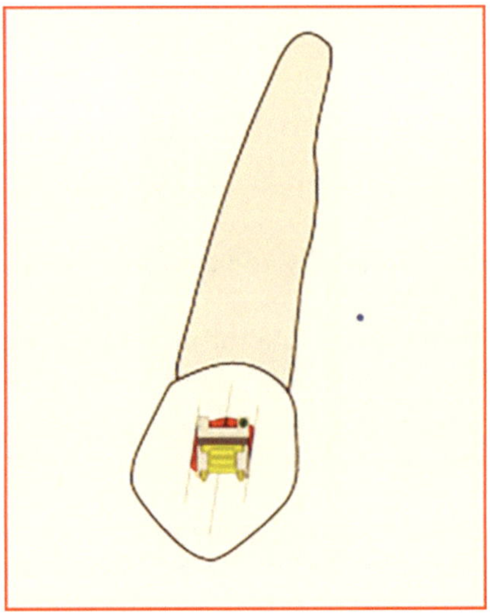

Figure 1.
Standard bracket placement of damon bracket.

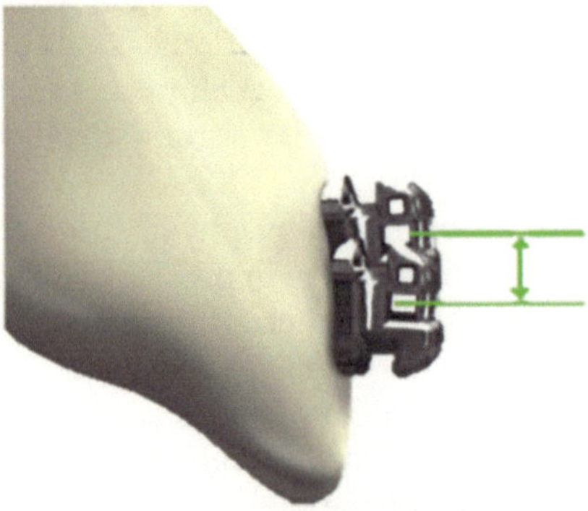

Figure 2.
Picture depicting the "green zone" for bracket placement in the Damon system.

Dr. Pitt's occluso gingival positioning of brackets is slightly more gingival to the conventional placement on both arches. He believed positioning the brackets more incisally will prevent us from achieving the ideal smile arc and hinders torque control (**Figure 3**). Dr. Pitts along with Dr. Mike Steffan developed a method to making the bracket positioning easier by drawing lines on the stone models from contact points for the canine, premolars and molars to prevent mistakes in bracket positioning in the transition of contact points from posteriors to anteriors (**Figure 4**).

7.2 Maxillary anteriors

The position of the maxillary canine is given the prime importance for the sweep in the smile arc. Based on the positioning of this bracket, other anterior brackets were placed. In this method, the incisal edge of the canine bracket wing needs to be placed on a line drawn from mesial to distal contact at the height of contour interproximally. This line was called the mesiodistal (M-D) contact line. The level of the slot of this bracket was used as a reference for maxillary central and lateral incisor positioning. The maxillary lateral incisor bracket is placed 0.5 mm gingival to the canine bracket and central incisor bracket 0.25 mm gingival to this to achieve the ideal smile arc (**Figure 5**) Further to avoid the bracket positioning error, the author advises the use of a two inch large front surface mirror to avoid any error in bracket positioning (**Figure 6**).

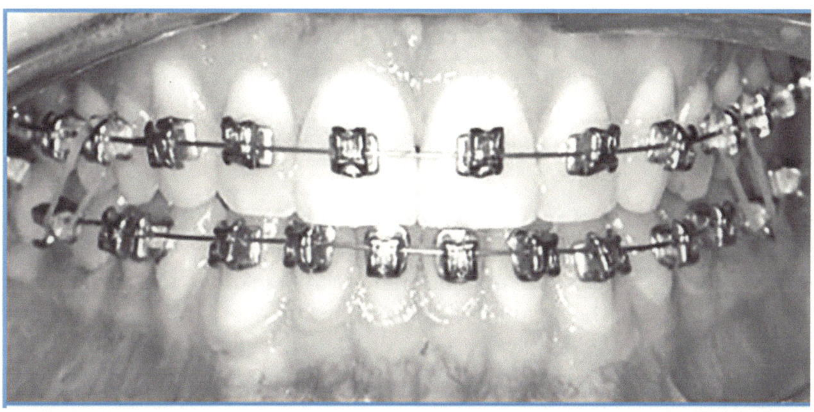

Figure 3.
Gingival bracket placement for smile arc protection by Dr. Thomas Pitts.

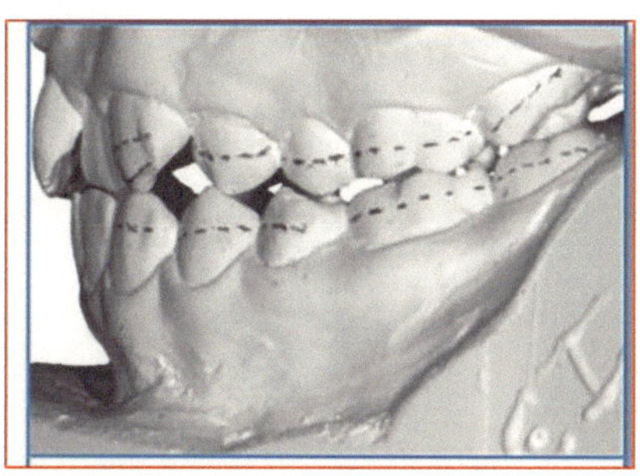

Figure 4.
Marking the contact points reference for establishing occlusogingival positioning of brackets.

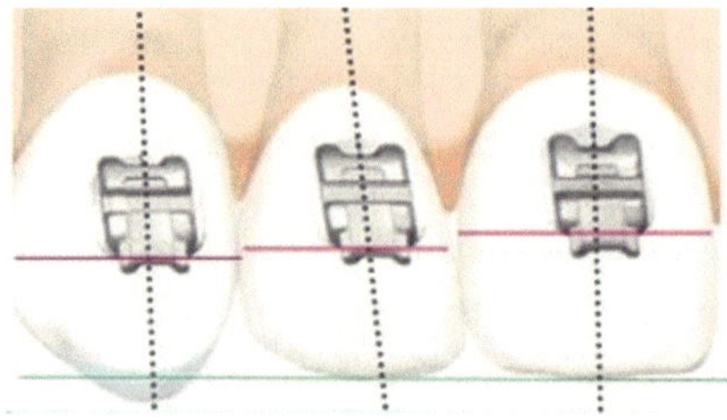

Figure 5.
Bracket positioning in the maxillary incisors and canines.

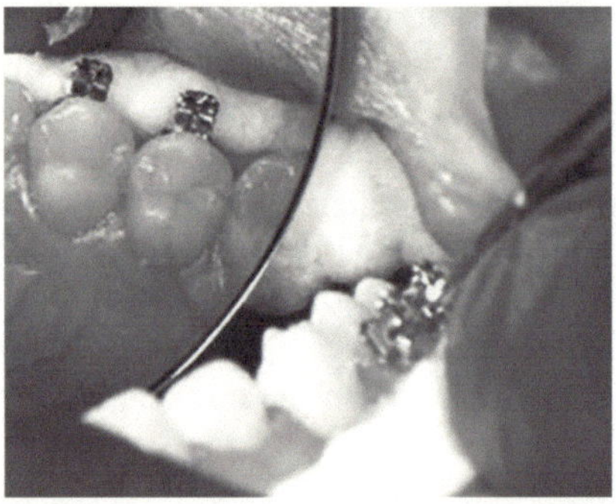

Figure 6.
Use of a large front surface mirror to prevent errors in bracket positioning.

7.3 Maxillary premolars

The maxillary premolars are positioned by aligning the scribe line with the crown long axis at the height of contour paralleling the central groove and the M-D buccal line angle. Following correct bracket placement, the bracket on the first premolar would seem too distal to the height of contour and the second premolar at times would appear mesial to the height of contour when viewed from the buccal aspect. The occlusal edge of the brackets should touch the M-D contact line (**Figure 7**).

7.4 Maxillary molars

The mesiodistal positioning of the buccal tube is done by centering the buccal tube pad over the buccal groove of the teeth and the occluso gingival positioning is done

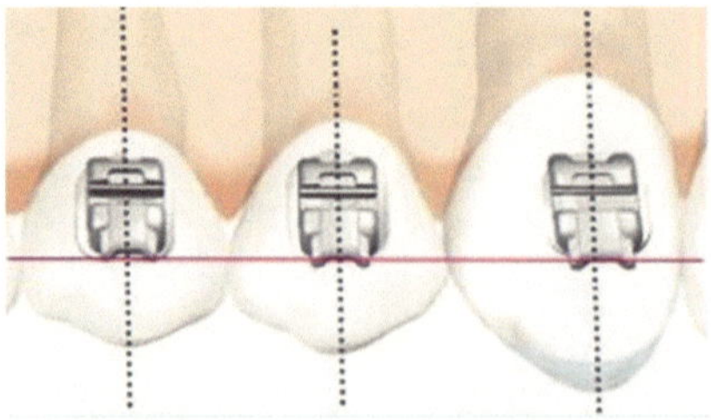

Figure 7.
Bracket positioning in the maxillary premolars.

by placing the occlusal edge of the pad on the M-D contact line of the first molar. The second molars follows the same rule for mesiodistal positioning but placed 1.5 mm more occlusally to the first molar tube (**Figure 8**).

7.5 Mandibular incisors

The mandibular incisors are placed such that the scribe line is aligned with the long axis of the tooth. The bracket position is viewed from the incisal aspect. For deep bite, the position of the top of the slot is 3.5 mm from the incisal edge to reverse the curve of spee and for open bite; the position of the top of the slot is 5 mm from the incisal edge to open the curve of spee (**Figure 9**).

7.6 Mandibular canines

The mesiodistal positioning is done by aligning the scribe line to the long axis of the crown at the height of contour. The position is verified by viewing from the incisal

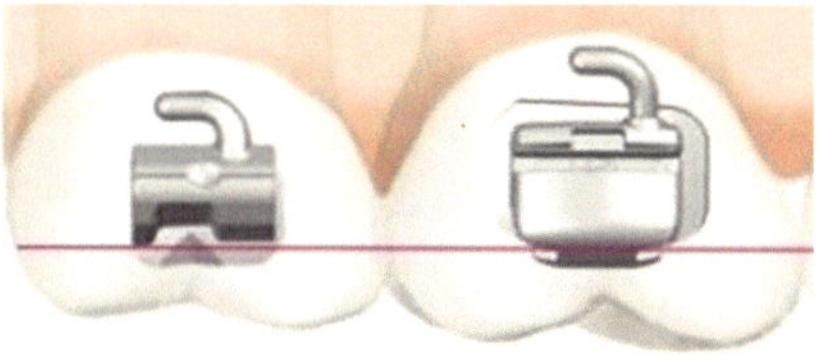

Figure 8.
Bracket positioning in the maxillary molars.

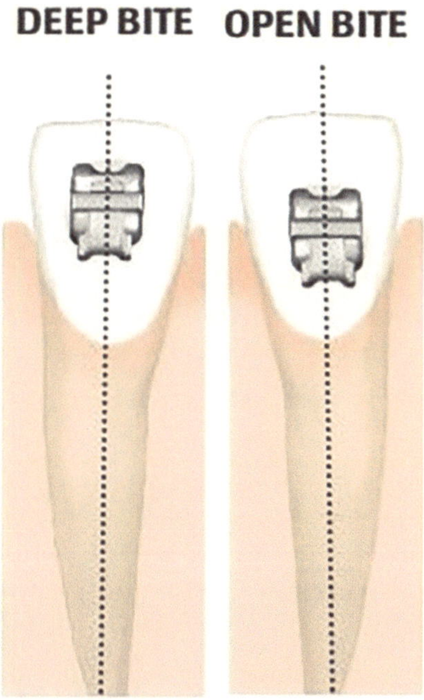

Figure 9.
Bracket positioning in the mandibular anteriors.

aspect. The occluso gingival positioning is placing the incisal edge of the bracket wing at the M-D contact line (**Figure 10**).

7.7 Mandibular premolars

The mesiodistal positioning is done by aligning the scribe line to the crown long axis and viewed from the occlusal aspect. The occluso gingival positioning is based on positioning the occlusal edge of the bracket wing 0.5 mm gingival to the M-D contact line (**Figure 11**).

7.8 Mandibular molars

The mandibular molars are placed in the same way as the maxillary molars in terms of mesiodistal positioning by orienting the center of the buccal tip of the buccal tube with that of the buccal groove of the tooth. Unlike the maxillary molars, both the mandibular molars are placed at the same height, which is 0.5 mm gingival to the M-D contact line (**Figure 12**).

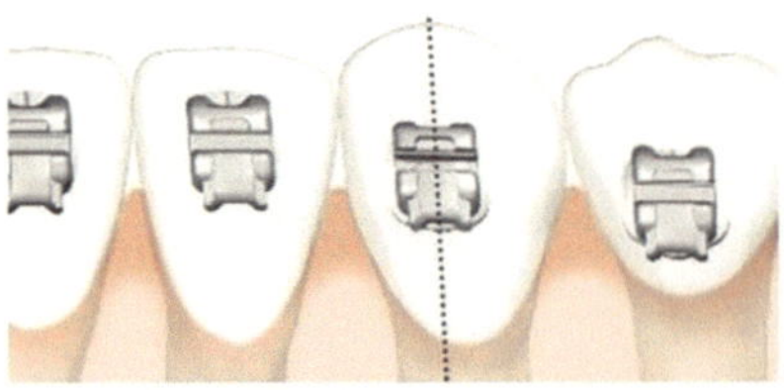

Figure 10.
Bracket positioning in the mandibular canine.

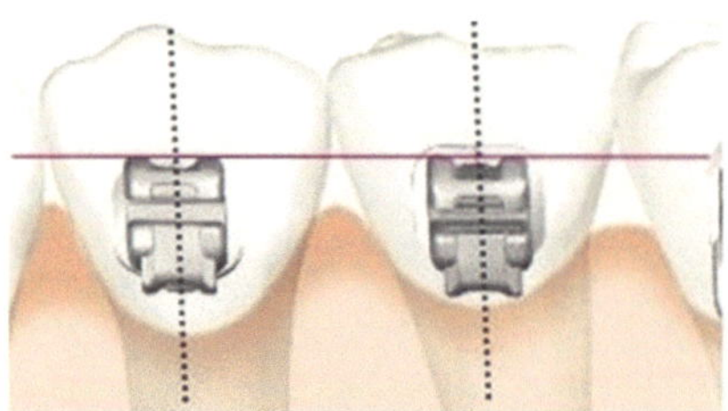

Figure 11.
Bracket positioning in the mandibular premolars.

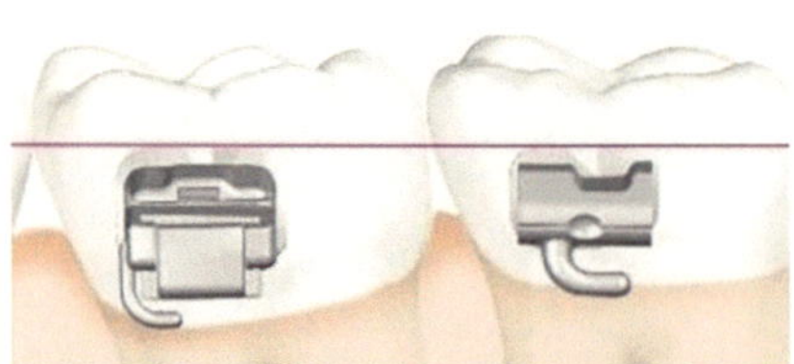

Figure 12.
Bracket positioning in the mandibular molars.

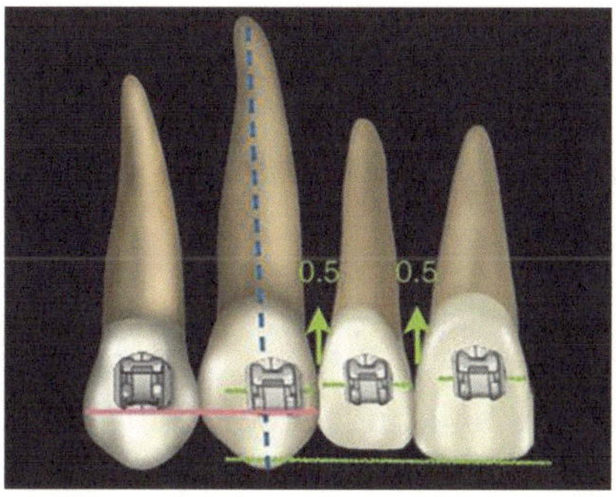

Figure 13.
Figure showing placement of brackets in the maxillary anteriors.

Another technique that was proposed was the bracket placement in Beethoven's Orthodontic center. The bracket placement was similar to that given by Dr. Pitts except some modifications that were made in the maxillary canines. According to him, the maxillary canine bracket is placed by aligning it 1 mm mesially away from the long axis of the crown. The slot of the canine was used as a reference for placing the incisor brackets. The slots of the central and lateral incisor brackets are raised 0.5 mm consecutively (**Figure 13**).

8. Ideal cases for Damon

Dr. Damon has said that force applied to the bracket should be as light as possible to stimulate tooth movement. His philosophy was to employ the concept of biological adaptation and facially driven treatment plan that focuses on facial esthetics as a critical foundation for diagnosis.

The treatment objective in Damon cases is to

- Gain maxillary and mandibular arch length.
- Establish upper and lower incisor position to give lip support.
- Establish maxillary and mandibular posterior arch width to support mid-face.
- Establish ideal maxillary lip-to-tooth relationship.
- Design treatment mechanics to eliminate need for higher force rapid palatal expansion.
- With low-force mechanics to work with the orofacial muscle complex, bone, and tissue to establish a physiologic tooth position

Damon system can be used in the following cases

- Class I- Non Extraction- Young patient with severe crowding and a flat profile
- Class I- Non Extraction- Adult patient with severe crowding and a flat profile

- Class I- Non Extraction- Young patient- Open bite with posterior crossbite and very narrow deep palate.
- Class I- Non Extraction- Adult patient- Open bite with posterior crossbite and very narrow deep palate.
- Class I- Extraction- Bimaxillary protrusion and crowding.
- Class II division I subdivision with functional shift- Non Extraction
- Class II division I- Severe crowding and deep bite
- Class II division II- Severe crowding and deep bite
- Class III- Severe crowding.

Using the light forces from the Copper NiTi wires and friction less passive self-ligating brackets along with Superelastic NiTi open coil springs wherever required we can achieve a desired treatment outcome with the Damon system.

In case of Class II patients with retrognathic mandibles we can go for Phase 1 therapy with functional appliances or fixed functional appliances.

9. Recent advances

The Damon self-ligating appliances have certain characteristics such as ease in ligation, wire engagement without undesirable force relaxation of elastomeric modules, which helps in maintaining a constant active status of engaged wires. This makes the Damon appliance more suitable than conventional appliances. This is in agreement with the findings by various other orthodontists, Berger [20], Harradine [9], Turnbull and Birnie [4].

Ormco, Damon Company keeps evolving over the years, coming out with different and more compatible bracket systems. Starting from Damon 3©, to Damon 3mx©, to Damon Q©, to Damon Q2© followed by the latest development, the Damon Ultima™© system. In clear ceramic braces from Damon clear© they have recently developed the Damon Clear 2© system.

9.1 Damon Clear2 ©

They are completely esthetic passive self-ligating brackets made of polycrystalline alumina (PCA) material, which is resistant to staining from coffee, mustard, red wine and other agents. It eliminates the need for the use of elastomers (modules) which generally stain and collect bacteria during the course of the treatment.

Damon Clear 2© brackets have a sturdy base with a fortified slide, window channel and tie wings for extra strength and durability. The four solid walls enable effective torque expression and rotation control for a good and meticulous finishing (**Figures 14** and **15**).

The base design of the Damon Clear 2© brackets is a patented laser etched pad that provides optimal bond strength for greater reliability (**Figure 16**). The contours

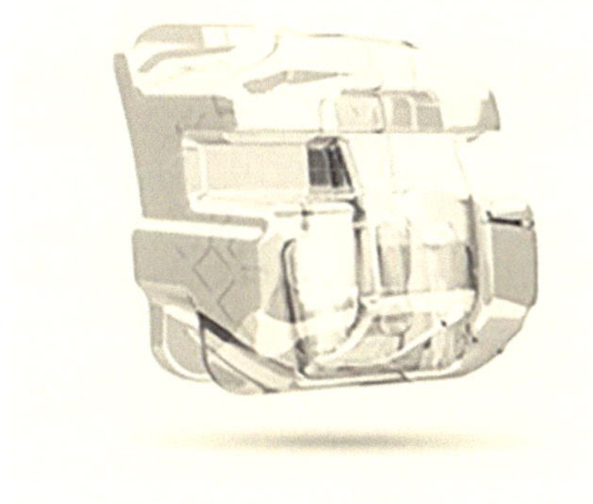

Figure 14.
Damon clear 2© bracket.

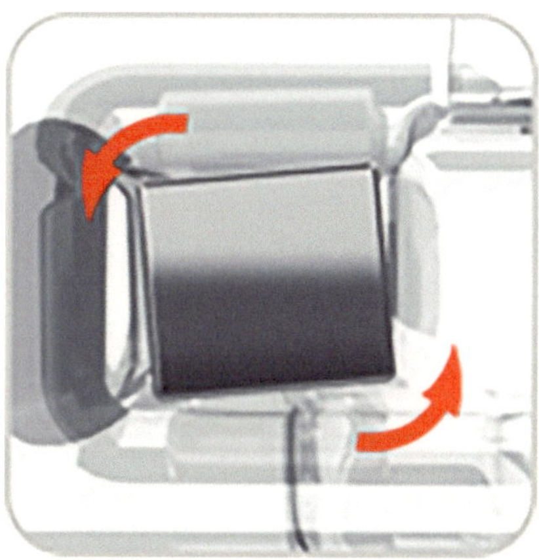

Figure 15.
Enhanced strength for effective torque expression.

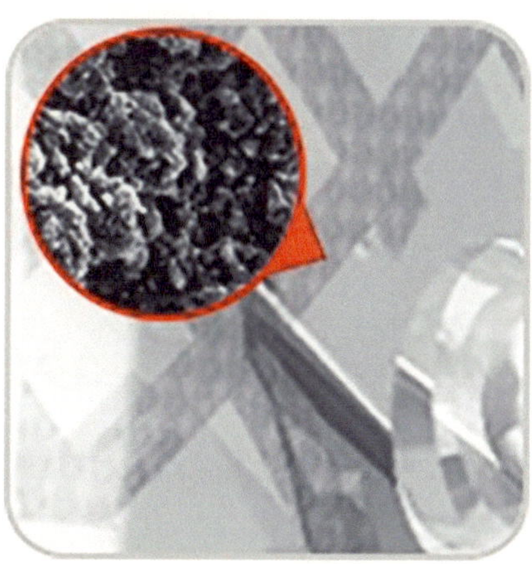

Figure 16.
Laser etched base for enhanced stability.

of the brackets are smooth and rounded, which ensures patient comfort. The is an option to switch to brackets that have discrete contoured hooks for elastics and other auxiliaries (**Figure 17**).

Generally ceramic brackets are thought of as messy, while debonding as they tend to crack and splutter while using a debonding plier to remove the bracket. Whilst, for Damon Clear 2©, Ormco has a patented debonding instrument, the Damon Clear Debonding Instrument ©, which results in fast and comfortable debonding experience for patients (**Figure 18**). There is also no requirement for removing flash after the debonding procedure.

Removable positioning gauge with scaler notch is present in each of the clear brackets for easy and efficient placement of the bracket (**Figure 19**). There are color-coded positioning gauges on brackets (13–23) present that denote torque values.

For a higher efficient and quality treatment, proper wire sequencing must be employed. The initial arch wires being the Damon Optimal-Force Copper Ni-Ti® to low-friction TMA and stainless-steel arch wires. Each wire must have sufficient time to express itself before progression to the next wire. For anterior torque expression,

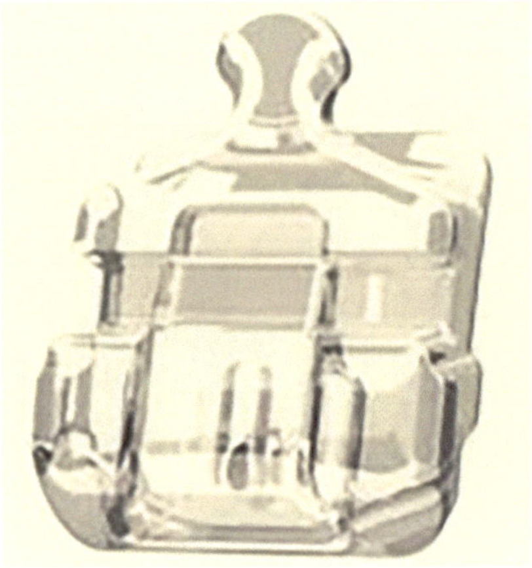

Figure 17.
Discrete contoured hooks for auxiliaries.

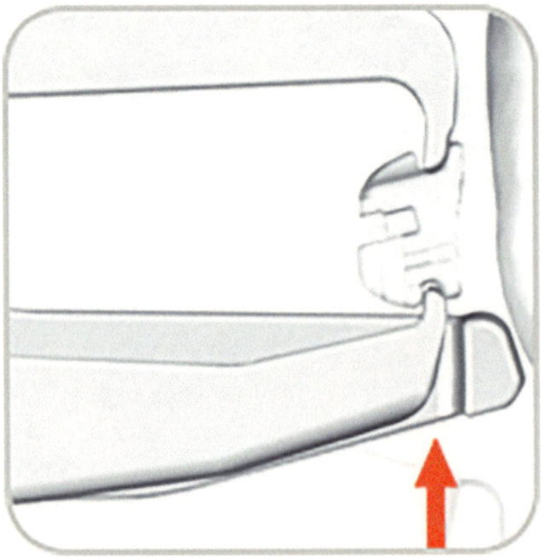

Figure 18.
Debonding of the bracket with Damon clear Debonding instrument ©.

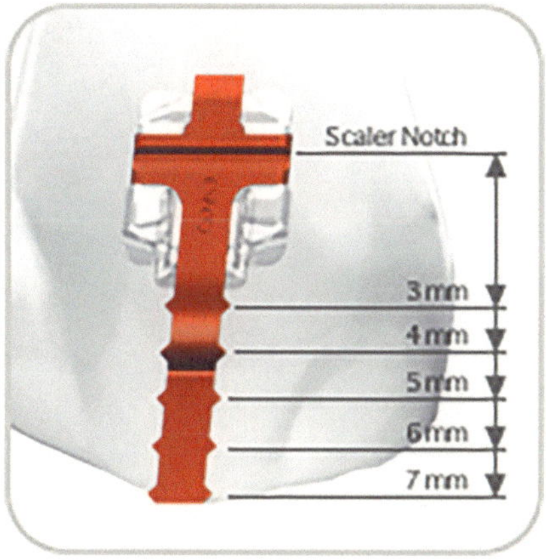

Figure 19.
Removable position gauge with scalar notch.

either pre-torqued nickel titanium arch wires or TMA arch wires are to be used. For rotational bends, TMA arch wires or titanium niobium arch wires are to be used. However, care should be taken in employing finishing bends in stainless steel wires, since such bends may result in fractures.

9.2 Damon Ultima ©

Damon Ultima ™ © was designed and introduced for a faster and a more precise finishing. Traditional passive self-ligating brackets and wires have significant play which generally results in poor control, manual adjustments and extended treatment time. The Damon Ultima ™© system is the first system that is completely reengineered to virtually eliminate play, for a precise control of rotation, angulation and torque [3].

The enhanced features in Damon Ultima ™© are as follows:

- Completely re-engineered tie-wing is said to improve the ability to engage and ligate elastomeric chains (**Figure 20**).

- Smoother tie wings were designed for a better patient comfort and minimal occlusal interference (**Figure 21**).

- The base of the bracket with 80 gauge mesh designed for reliable and increased bond strength throughout treatment and for a predictable debonding experience (**Figure 22**).

- Easy to open and close the slot door design with low reciprocal forces and tactile feedback. The bracket door and wire are designed to reduce door closure interference (**Figure 23**).

- Rhomboid shaped pad with enhanced scribe line help in guiding bracket placement (**Figure 24**).

- Presence of vertical slot for convenient placement of drop-in hooks (**Figure 25**).

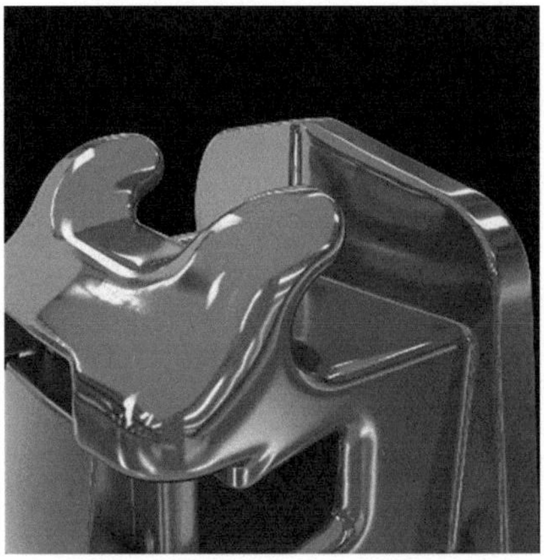

Figure 20.
Reengineered tie wing in Damon Ultima ™©.

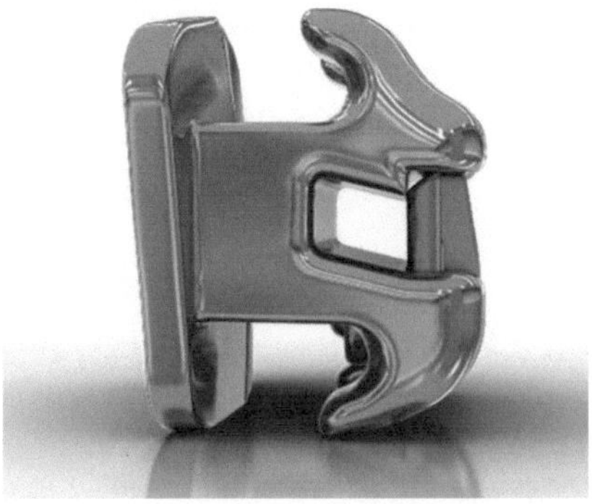

Figure 21.
Smoother tie wings for patient comfort.

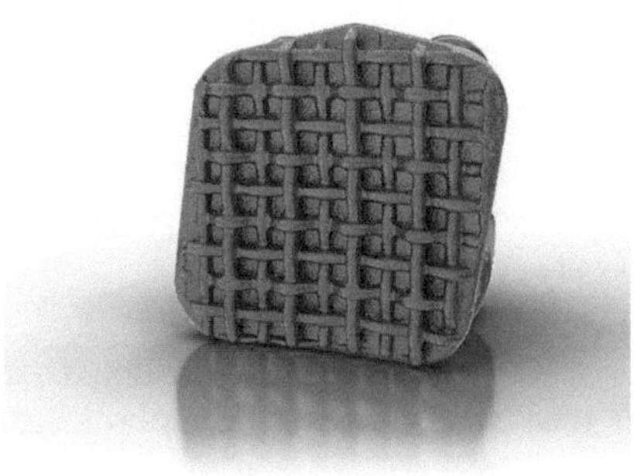

Figure 22.
Base of the bracket of Damon Ultima ™©.

The retrocline and procline bracket options were introduced for enhanced torque control. Brackets were designed from the centre point of the clot to the line-up with the FA point to express desired torque and provide easier and more precise placement (**Figure 26**).

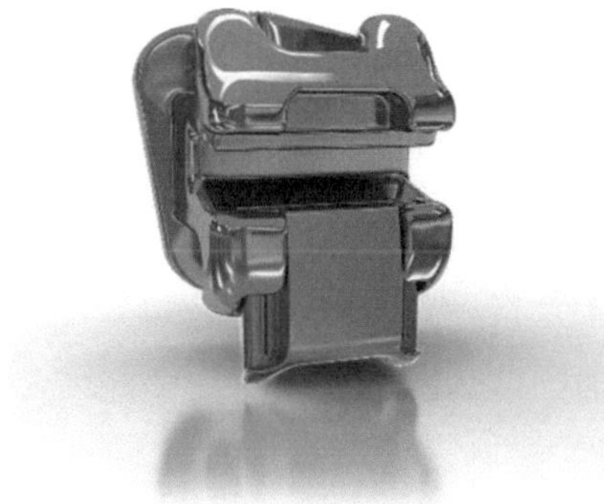

Figure 23.
The enhanced bracket door design.

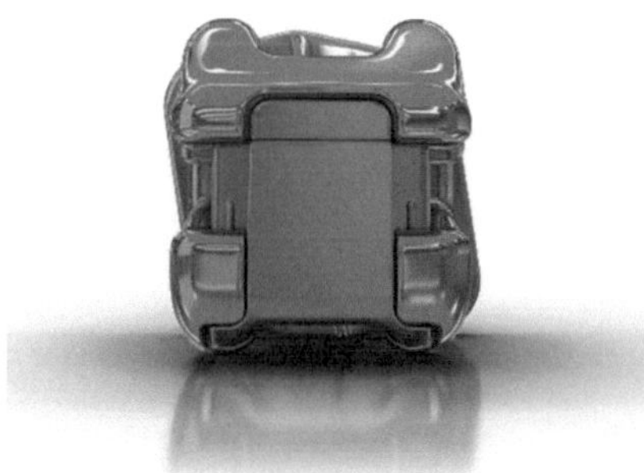

Figure 24.
Rhomboid shaped pad in Damon Ultima ™©.

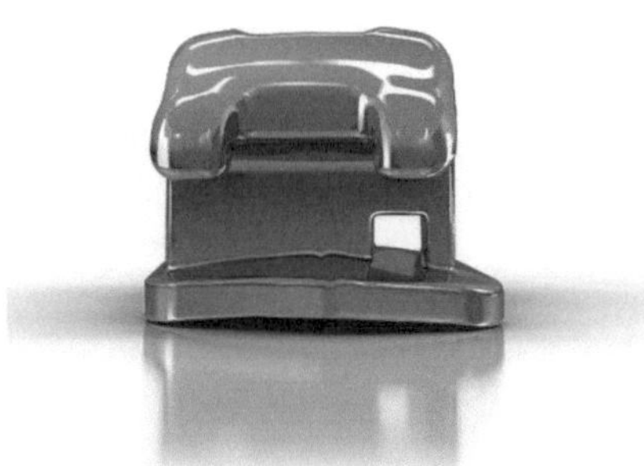

Figure 25.
Vertical slot for placement of drop-in hooks.

Additionally, extra arch wire options were included, for torque control when needed. Sizes available are: 0.019*0.0275, 0.0020*0.0275, and 0.021*0.0275 in Copper NiTi, TMA and SS (**Figure 27**).

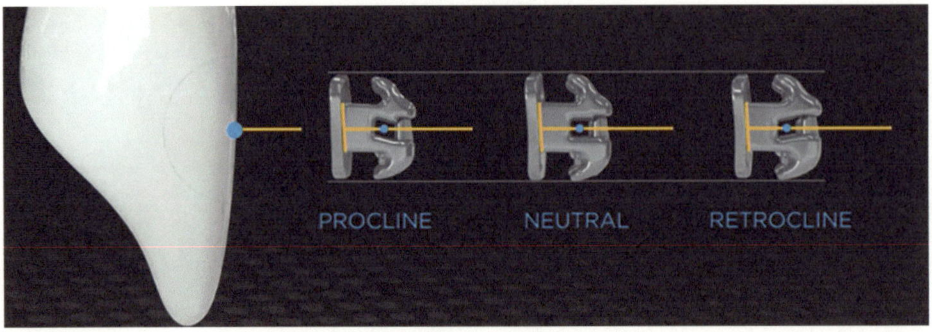

Figure 26.
Adversity of procline and retrocline brackets in the Damon Ultima ™© system, that can be used to incorporate torque whenever needed.

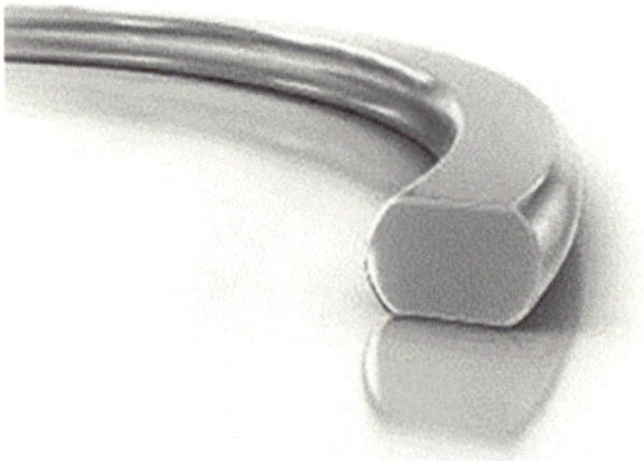

Figure 27.
Reengineered arch wire for better torque control.

10. Conclusion

Passive self-ligation offers the most direct transmission of force from the arch wire to the tooth with very low friction, a very secure ligation along with excellent control of tooth position. Every contemporary modality of orthodontic treatment achieves tooth alignment; however passive self-ligation achieves the results effectively and efficiently. With the evolution of various systems like Damon Clear2 and Damon Ultima ©, the orthodontic tooth movement is achieved at its best.

Conflict of interest

Dr. Suvetha Siva- No conflict of interest with the product (ORMCO).
Dr. Shreya Kishore- No conflict of interest with the product (ORMCO).
Dr. Suganya Dhanapal- No conflict of interest with the product (ORMCO).
Dr. Janani Ravi- No conflict of interest with the product (ORMCO).
Dr. Chandhini Suresh- No conflict of interest with the product (ORMCO).

Author details

Suvetha Siva[1*], Shreya Kishore[1], Suganya Dhanapal[2], Janani Ravi[1] and Chandhini Suresh[1]

1 SRM Dental College, Ramapuram, Chennai, India

2 Sri Ramakrishna Dental College, Coimbatore, India

*Address all correspondence to: suvetha150992@gmail.com

References

[1] Ramachandra. C. S. Damon system protocol for management of class I, class II & class III malocclusions [Modular based learning].

[2] Damon DH. The rationale, evolution and clinical application of the self-ligating bracket. Clin Orthod Res. 1998 Aug;**1**(1):52-61

[3] Birnie D. The Damon Passive Self-Ligating Appliance System. Semin Orthod. 2008 Mar 1;**14**(1):19-35

[4] Turnbull NR, Birnie DJ. Treatment efficiency of conventional vs self-ligating brackets: effects of archwire size and material. Am J Orthod Dentofacial Orthop. 2007 Mar;**131**(3):395-399

[5] Gianoni-Capenakas S, Flores-Mir C, Vich ML, Pacheco-Pereira C. Oropharyngeal 3-dimensional changes after maxillary expansion with 2 different orthodontic approaches. Am J Orthod Dentofacial Orthop. 2021 Mar;**159**(3):352-359

[6] Lineberger MB, Franchi L, Cevidanes LHS, Huanca Ghislanzoni LT, McNamara JA Jr. Three-dimensional digital cast analysis of the effects produced by a passive self-ligating system. Eur J Orthod. 2016 Dec;**38**(6): 609-614

[7] Srinivas S. Comparison of canine retraction with self-ligated and conventional ligated brackets-a clinical study. India: Thesis in fulfillment of postgraduate degree, Tamilnadu Medical University, Chennai; 2003

[8] Eberting JJ, Straja SR, Tuncay OC. Treatment time, outcome, and patient satisfaction comparisons of Damon and conventional brackets. Clin Orthod Res. 2001 Nov;**4**(4):228-234

[9] Harradine NW. Self-ligating brackets and treatment efficiency. Clin Orthod Res. 2001 Nov;**4**(4):220-227

[10] Maijer R, Smith DC. Time savings with self-ligating brackets. J Clin Orthod. 1990 Jan;**24**(1):29-31

[11] Carels C, Willems G. The Future of Orthodontics. Leuven University Press; 1998. 281 p.

[12] McLaughlin RP, Bennett JC, Trevisi HJ. Systemized Orthodontic Treatment Mechanics. Mosby; 2001. 324 p.

[13] Fleming PS, DiBiase AT, Sarri G, Lee RT. Comparison of mandibular arch changes during alignment and leveling with 2 preadjusted edgewise appliances. Am J Orthod Dentofacial Orthop. 2009 Sep;**136**(3):340-347

[14] Mandall N, Lowe C, Worthington H, Sandler J, Derwent S, Abdi-Oskouei M, et al. Which orthodontic archwire sequence? A randomized clinical trial [Internet]. Vol. 28, The European Journal of Orthodontics. 2006. p. 561-6. Available from: http://dx.doi.org/10.1093/ejo/cjl030

[15] Ong E, Ho C, Miles P. Alignment efficiency and discomfort of three orthodontic archwire sequences: a randomized clinical trial. J Orthod. 2011 Mar;**38**(1):32-39

[16] Rahmani A, Oz U. The Effect of Copper Aided Nickel--Titanium Arch-Wire Sequences on Upper Jaw Expansion: A Comparison with Conventional

Nickel--Titanium Wire Systems in Medical Decision Support Systems in Medical Internet of Things. Journal of Medical Imaging and Health Informatics. 2020;**10**(1):238-243

[17] Handem RH, Janson G, Matias M, de Freitas KMS, de Lima DV, Garib DG, et al. External root resorption with the self-ligating Damon system—a retrospective study. Prog Orthod. 2016 Jul 1;**17**(1):20

[18] de Freitas KMS, Vaz de Lima D. Comparison of changes in dental arch dimensions in cases treated with conventional appliances and self-ligating Damon system. Open Dent J [Internet]. 2018; Available from: https://opendentistryjournal.com/VOLUME/12/PAGE/1137/

[19] Pitts T. Begin with the end in mind: Bracket placement and early elastics protocols for smile arc protection. Clin Impressions. 2009;**17**(1):1-11

[20] Berger J. Self-ligation in the year 2000. J Clin Orthod. 2000;**34**(2):74-81

Chapter 12

Pain Perception in Patients Treated with Ligating/Self-Ligating Brackets versus Patients Treated with Aligners

Farid Bourzgui, Rania Fastani, Salwa Khairat, Samir Diouny, Mohamed El Had, Zineb Serhier and Mohamed Bennani Othmani

Abstract

This study compared the perception of pain experienced by patients undergoing orthodontic treatment with conventional, self-ligating brackets and aligners, and investigated the impact that pain had on their daily lives. 346 consecutive patients were included in the study: 115 patients treated with conventional brackets, 112 Patients treated with self-ligating brackets, and 119 patients treated with aligners. The quantitative aspect of pain was assessed using the Visual Analogue Scale, while the qualitative aspect of pain was evaluated using the Moroccan Short Form of McGILL Pain questionnaire. In all three groups experienced pain after activation tended to decrease in the following week. This pain was greater in patients with conventional braces and less in patients with aligners. Using the M-SF-MPQ to describe the qualitative aspect of the pain revealed that the "cramping مزير," "aching تيألم" aspect was most accentuated in the 3 groups. Medication intake was correlated with the intensity of pain experienced in all 3 systems. As for the impact of pain on daily activities, patients in groups of conventional and self-ligating braces showed more pain than those in the aligners group. Overall, aligners were less painful than conventional and self-ligating appliances. Patients did not suffer from an alteration in their quality of life due to orthodontic treatment.

Keywords: orthodontics, corrective, clear aligner appliances, facial pain, pain measurement, Morocco

1. Introduction

Pain is defined as "an unpleasant sensory and emotional experience associated with actual or potential tissue damage, or described in terms of such damage." (IASP) [1]; it: "is a mutually recognizable somatic experience that reflects a person's apprehension of threat to their bodily or existential integrity" [2].

Orthodontic tooth movement requires the application of force to the tooth, which usually results in a painful sensation [3]. It is important to note that there are individual differences in pain sensitivity related to the subjective aspect of pain perception [4].

Recently, orthodontic practices have evolved considerably. In addition to conventional or self-ligating appliances, aligners represent an esthetic and comfortable alternative option for orthodontic treatment. Even though these methods have revolutionized orthodontics practices, practitioners are still confronted with the painful aspect of the treatment. Some patients perceive orthodontic pain as discomfort or inconvenience; others continue to be in so much pain that it can cause them to discontinue treatment [5]. This feeling of discomfort could impact the quality of life of patients and their cooperation. Also, for some patients, factors such as comfort and pain during orthodontic treatment are as important as esthetic considerations. In most cases, the quality of information given to patients about the likely discomfort during orthodontic treatment is somewhat satisfactory, though many patients complain that they are not well informed before the onset of treatment [5].

Previous studies have investigated orthodontics pain and its components for each system there is a dearth of studies that have compared the character and type of pain experienced in qualitative and descriptive terms between the different options used in orthodontics, i.e., conventional appliances, self-ligating appliances, and aligners.

Against this background, the aim of this study was two-fold: First, to compare the perception of pain experienced by patients treated with conventional brackets, self-ligating brackets, and those treated with aligners. Second, to investigate the impact that pain had on their daily lives.

2. The perception of pain experienced by patients treated with conventional braces, self-ligating braces, and those treated with aligners

2.1 Patients and methods

A cross-sectional stud was performed to compare the perception of pain between patients treated with self-ligating fixed appliances and those treated with aligners treated at both the Department of Orthodontics at Casablanca Ibn Rochd University Hospital, and at a private orthodontic office. The study lasted 4 months (November 2019–February 2020). All the patients underwent orthodontic treatment for a period exceeding 2 months, the chief complaint was purely aesthetic and all patients were in class I dento-maxillary disharmony. In relation to our inclusion criteria, we have chosen patients in the process of treatment, avoiding patients at the beginning of treatment where adaptation is not yet established, as well as patients at the end of treatment, as they may be accustomed to their orthodontic appliances.

Exclusion criteria included patients under 8 years of age, those at the beginning of treatment or less than 2 months or at the end of treatment, and those with no medical contraindications or the presence of systemic diseases that influence pain perception (including nervous system disorders).

The study group consisted of 346 consecutive patients: 115 treated with conventional brackets. 112 were treated with self-ligating brackets and 119 were treated with aligners.

The data collection tool was a self-made questionnaire consisting of the socio-economic characteristics of patients, the type of appliance worn, and temporal characteristics of pain during the week of activation, qualitative factors influencing pain after activation, actors influencing pain during the week of activation, the impact of pain on the patient's daily, professional and school life, the patient's attitude to pain, the most distressing element during the treatment stages. The patients were informed about the purpose of the study, and verbal consent was obtained.

The quantitative aspect of the pain was assessed using the Visual Analogue Scale (VAS). The scale used is a graduated ruler whose extremities represent the absence of pain 0 and the maximum imaginable pain 10. The VAS scale was presented to the patients by the operator after explaining the instructions for use, in two stages: After the activation appointment and during the week that followed.

To evaluate the qualitative aspect of pain, we used the M-SF-MPQ "the Moroccan Short Form of McGill Pain questionnaire" [6], previously translated from English and culturally adapted and validated in Moroccan Arabic.

Data were analyzed using SPSS statistical 16.0 software. The comparison of pain perception between the different types of systems was done using the Chi-square test, or Fischer's exact test when the theoretical numbers were low. The comparison of pain intensity according to the VAS score was carried out using the Kruskal Wallis test.

2.2 Results

Table 1 contains the age distribution of our sample. The dominant age range for each type of appliance was: 16–25 years, 58 patients (50.4%) for conventional brackets, 8–15 years, 62 patients (55.4%) for self-ligating brackets, and more than 25 years 71 patients (59.7%) for Aligners. The statistical association between age group and type of appliance was significant ($p<0.001$). Of 346 patients, 137 (39.6%) were male and 209 were female (60.4%). We noted that the female gender was the most dominant in the three groups, respectively: 63 patients (54.8% with the conventional brace, 60 patients (53.6%) with self-ligating braces, and 86 patients (72.3%) with aligners: The statistical association between gender and the type of appliance was significant ($p<0.001$) (**Table 2**).

The socio-economic level in the sample was high in 63%, medium in 24.6%, and low in 12.4%. The association between socioeconomic level and the type of appliance used was statistically significant ($p<0.001$) (**Table 3**).

With respect to the duration of treatment, for 87 patients (25.1%) the beginning of treatment ranged between 2 and 8 months ago, and 259 patients (74.9%) started treatment more than 8 months ago. The comparison between the duration of treatment and the type of appliance used was statistically significant ($p<0.001$).

	Conventional brackets		Self-ligating		Aligner		The whole	
Age group (years)	**N**	**%**	**N**	**%**	**N**	**%**	**N**	**%**
8–15	45	39.1	62	55.4	17	14.3	124	35.8
16–25	58	50.4	39	34.8	31	26.1	128	37
>25	12	10.4	11	9.8	71	59.7	94	27.2
				P<0.001				

Table 1.
Distribution of the sample by age group according to the type of appliance used.

	Conventional brackets		Self-ligating		Aligner		The whole	
Gender	**N**	**%**	**N**	**%**	**N**	**%**	**N**	**%**
Male	52	45.2	52	46.4	33	27.7	137	39.6
Female	63	54.8	60	53.6	86	72.3	209	60.4
				P<0.001				

Table 2.
Distribution of the sample by gender according to the type of appliance used.

Socio-economic status	Conventional brackets		Self-ligating		Aligner		The whole	
	N	**%**	**N**	**%**	**N**	**%**	**N**	**%**
High	35	30.4	94	83.9	89	74.8	218	63
Medium	43	37.4	16	14.3	26	21.8	85	24.6
Low	37	32.2	2	1.8	4	3.4	43	12.4
				P<0.001				

Table 3.
Distribution of the sample by the socio-economic status according to the type of appliance used.

The vulnerability to pain showed that 295 patients (85.3%) were able to tolerate pain, while 51 patients (14.7%) could not tolerate pain. The statistical correlation between pain vulnerability and the type of appliance used was significant, ($p<0.001$) (**Table 4**).

As for pain conditioning, 262 patients (75.7%) already knew someone who had undergone orthodontic treatment, 176 (66.18%) of which reported that this person had experienced pain. Only 84 patients 24.3%. did not know a person, who had received orthodontic treatment. The statistical correlation between the knowledge of a person who underwent orthodontic treatment and the type of appliance used was significant ($p<0.001$).

303 patients reported pain after orthodontic activation, representing 87.6% of the total sample. The statistical association between the presence of pain after activation and the type of appliance was significant ($p<0.001$) (**Table 5**). The intensity of this pain after activation had an average of 6 for conventional and self-ligating braces and 3 for aligners. Despite this intensity, 297 patients (85.8%) reported a reduction in pain the week following the activation. 106 patients (92.2%) with conventional braces, 101 patients (90.2%) with self-ligating braces, and 90 patients (75.6%) with aligners reported a decrease in pain the week following activation. The statistical association

Vulnerability to pain	Conventional brackets		Self-ligating		Aligner		The whole	
	N	**%**	**N**	**%**	**N**	**%**	**N**	**%**
Cannot tolerate	17	14.8	15	13.4	19	16	51	14.7
Can tolerate	98	85.2	97	86.6	100	84	295	85.3
				P<0.001				

Table 4.
Distribution of the sample according to vulnerability to pain by type of appliance.

Pain	Conventional brackets		Self-ligating		Aligner		The whole	
	N	%	N	%	N	%	N	%
No	3	2.6	11	9.8	29	24.4	43	12.4
Yes	112	97.4	101	90.2	90	75.6	303	87.6
				P<0.001				

Table 5.
Distribution of the sample according to the presence of pain after activation.

between pain reduction in the week following the activation appointment and the type of appliance was significant ($p<0.001$). During the second week, we found a median of 2, a minimum value of 0, and a maximum of 8 for conventional braces, a median of 0 and a maximum value of 8 for self-ligating, and a median of 0 and a maximum value of 7 for aligners.

The qualitative aspects of pain for the three types of orthodontic appliances are outlined in **Table 6**. The association of the different qualitative aspects of pain according to the type of appliance was statistically significant ($p<0.001$).

Table 7 presents the distribution of the sample according to the most painful aspect during orthodontic treatment according to the type of appliance used. The statistical correlation between the most distressing aspect during orthodontic treatment and the type of appliance was significant ($p<0.001$). Patients' reactions to pain after activation, at 24 hours, after 3 days, and at one week are reported in **Table 8**.

2.3 Discussion

The aim of this study was to compare the pain perception of patients treated during orthodontic alignment with three different orthodontic appliance types. The results showed that the aligner system was less painful than the vestibular fixed appliances. There were minor differences in the reported pain intensity between conventional and self-ligating systems. Analgesics were mostly used by patients who reported severe pain. Despite the pain experienced by different patients, there was no impact on their quality of life, except for eating and chewing, where the aligners group showed promising results.

Several studies have analyzed the pain levels experienced with different types of brackets. In most of these studies, it was estimated that appliance-related pain was higher for the first 24 hours–3 days of appliance activation, then decreased to low levels within 5–6 days [4]. Scheurer et, al. [7] reported a trend of high pain within 2 days of appliance activation and a trend of pain relief after 5 days. This trend was confirmed in this study. The pain was higher after activation and significantly decreased within 3 days, then to zero within 7 days. Tecco et al. [3] suggested that regardless of the type of fixed appliance used (conventional or self-ligating), the highest intensity of pain was reported in the first two to three days after the initial activation of the appliance. Fleming et al. [8] confirmed that the subjective experience of pain at 4 hours, 24 hours, 3 days, and 7 days after placement of a fixed orthodontic appliance was independent of bracket type. Johal et al. [4] found a slight reduction in pain scores as the orthodontic therapy went on, although these differences were not statistically significant. Nevertheless, this suggests that orthodontic pain may decrease in intensity during treatment, or may reflect some degree of adaptation to discomfort.

Aspect of pain	Conventional brackets		Self-ligating		Aligner		The whole	
	N	%	N	%	N	%	N	%
THROBBING كيزدح								
No	49	42.6	71	63.4	92	77.3	212	61.3
Yes	66	57.4	41	36.6	27	22.7	134	38.7
SHOOTING كضرب بحال اضو								
No	62	53.9	87	77,7	105	88,2	254	73,4
Yes	53	46.1	25	22.3	14	11.8	92	26.6
STABBING بحال الطعنة ديال الخنجر								
No	93	80.9	89	79.5	107	89.9	289	83.5
Yes	22	19.1	23	20.5	12	10.1	57	16.5
SHARP ماضي								
No	60	52.2	77	68.8	98	82.4	235	67.9
Yes	55	47.8	35	31.2	21	17.6	111	32.1
CRAMPING مزير								
No	7	6.1	12	10.7	13	10.9	32	9.2
Yes	108	93.9	100	89.3	106	89.1	314	90.8
GNAWING كياكل								
No	85	73.9	97	86.6	103	86.6	285	82.4
Yes	30	26.1	15	13.4	16	13.4	61	17.6
HOT BURNING تحرق بزاف								
No	60	52.2	85	75.9	110	92.4	255	73.7
Yes	55	47.8	27	24.1	9	7.6	91	26.3
ACHING تيالم								
No	28	24.3	27	24.1	63	52.9	118	34.1
Yes	87	75.7	85	75.9	56	47.1	228	65.9
HEAVY تقيل								
No	78	67.8	76	67.9	88	73.9	242	69.9
Yes	37	32.2	36	32.1	31	26.1	104	30.1
TENDER خفيف								
No	72	62.6	61	54.5	68	57.1	201	58.1
Yes	43	37.4	51	45.5	51	42.9	145	41.9
SPLITTING تقطع								
No	78	67.8	77	68.8	94	79	249	72
Yes	37	32.2	35	31.2	25	21	97	28
TIRING-EXHAUSTING تهلك								
No	77	67	85	75.9	109	91.6	271	78.3
Yes	38	33	27	24.1	10	8.4	75	21.7

SICKENING كمرض								
No	83	72.2	75	67	90	75.6	248	71.7
Yes	32	27.8	37	33	29	24.4	98	28.3
FEARFUL كخلع								
No	101	87.8	95	84.8	117	98.3	313	90.5
Yes	14	12.2	17	15.2	2	1.7	33	9.5
PUNISHING-CRUEL تعدب بزاف								
No	64	55.7	74	66.1	107	89.9	245	70.8
Yes	51	44.3	38	33.9	12	10.1	101	29.2
			P < 0.001					

Table 6.
Distribution of the sample according to the qualitative aspect of pain.

	Conventional brackets		**Self-ligating**		**Aligner**		**The whole**	
Painful aspects	**N**	**%**	**N**	**%**	**N**	**%**	**N**	**%**
Pain								
No	51	44.30	54	48.20	99	83.20	204	59.00
Yes	64	55.70	58	51.80	20	16.80	142	41.00
Aesthetics								
No	94	81.70	85	75.90	93	78.20	272	78.60
Yes	21	18.30	27	24.10	26	21.80	74	21.40
Brushing								
No	87	75.70	81	72.30	95	79.80	263	76.00
Yes	28	24.30	31	27.70	24	20.20	83	24.00
Discomfort								
No	48	41.70	60	53.60	72	60.50	180	52.00
Yes	67	58.30	52	46.40	47	39.50	166	48.00
The volume of the appliance								
No	88	76.50	94	83.90	109	91.60	291	84.10
Yes	27	23.50	18	16.10	10	8.40	55	15.90
Bad taste								
No	103	89.60	101	90.20	111	93.30	315	91.00
Yes	12	10.40	11	9.80	8	6.70	31	9.00
Not being able to eat								
No	48	41.70	71	63.40	76	63.90	195	56.40
Yes	67	58.30	41	36.60	43	36.10	151	43.60
				P<0.001				

Table 7.
Distribution of the sample according to the most painful aspect during orthodontic treatment according to the type of appliance.

	Conventional brackets		Self-ligating		Aligner		The whole	
Patient's attitude	**N**	**%**	**N**	**%**	**N**	**%**	**N**	**%**
After activation								
Abstention	78	67.80	84	75.00	108	90.80	270	78.00
Self-medication	31	27.00	28	25.00	7	5.90	66	19.10
Consult your orthodontist	5	4.30	0	0.00	3	2.50	8	2.30
Consult another practitioner	1	0.90	0	0.00	1	0.80	2	0.60
					P=0			
After 24 hours								
Abstention	105	91.30	106	94.60	116	97.50	327	94.50
Self-medication	8	7.00	6	5.40	2	1.70	16	4.60
Consult your orthodontist	2	1.70	0	0.00	1	0.80	3	0.90
Consult another practitioner	0	0.00	0	0.00	0	0.00	0	0.00
					P=0.136			
After 3 days								
Abstention	113	98.30	112	100.00	117	98.30	342	98.80
Self-medication	1	0.90	0	0.00	1	0.80	2	0.60
Consult your orthodontist	1	0.90	0	0.00	1	0.80	2	0.60
Consult another practitioner	0	0.00	0	0.00	0	0.00	0	0.00
					P=1			
After 7 days								
Abstention	114	99.10	112	100.00	119	100.00	345	99.70
Self-medication	0	0.00	0	0.00	0	0.00	0	0.00
Consult your orthodontist	1	0.90	0	0.00	0	0.00	1	0.30
Consult another practitioner	0	0.00	0	0.00	0	0.00	0	0.00
					P=0.656			

Table 8.
Patients' reaction to pain according to the type of appliance used.

White et al. [9] showed that discomfort after the first and second monthly adjustments was also consistently lower for the aligner than for conventional treatment. For both groups, the levels of discomfort reported at subsequent adjustments reached lower levels than after the initial placement, or when the aligner was first worn.

Patients treated with self-ligating brackets reported significantly less pain than those treated with conventional brackets. These results were consistent with a study conducted by Pringle et al. [10] who reported that the self-ligating appliance (Damon

3, Ormco) resulted in lower pain intensity, on average, compared to the conventional appliance (Tru Straight, Ormco Europe, Amersfoort, The Netherlands). However, Fleming et al. [8] found that significant discomfort was experienced during the insertion and removal of the archwire with the self-ligating device (SmartClip) compared to the conventional system (Victory). Other studies pointed out that there was no statistically significant difference in perceived discomfort levels between the two types of system, namely Damon3 and Synthesis [11] and SmartClipTM and Victory [12].

After activation, patients in the conventional brackets group reported more pain than those in the aligner group. This is in agreement with the results reported in White et al. [9] who maintained that conventional appliances produced significantly more discomfort than aligners. Fujiyama et al [13] noted that patients experienced less pain with Invisalign treatment than with conventional appliances during treatment. Shalish et al. [14] indicated that the results were opposite to those found previously. A greater proportion of patients treated with Invisalign aligners reported more severe pain than did vestibularly treated patients.

In this study, the pain experienced after wearing aligners was lower than that experienced by patients with self-ligating appliances. This finding was consistent with a study by Almasoud [15] who reported that during the first week of orthodontic treatment, patients treated with Invisalign experienced less pain than those treated with a passive self-ligating system. Similarly, in a systematic review, Cardoso et al.; [16] concluded that patients treated with Invisalign seemed to experience lower levels of pain than those treated with fixed appliances during the first days of treatment, and no difference was reported in the next 3 months. In fact, patients treated with aligners reported lower pain levels for a longer period of time, as the fixed appliance was activated once a month and the aligners were changed every 15 days.

The M-SF-MPQ is a very reliable tool for measuring pain in its two sensory and affective components [7]. The use of this criterion makes it possible to establish a comparative profile of the quality of the pain experienced by each group. It was noted that in all 3 systems, the sensory description "cramping مزير " was most reported by all patients in all 3 groups. Comparisons revealed that sensory and affective descriptors were used more in patients in the conventional group, than in the self-ligating or aligner group. Overall, patients in the conventional group identified 6 sensory descriptors, and those in the following descending order: 'cramping مزير', 'aching تيألم', 'throbbing كيزدح', 'sharp ماضي', 'hot burning تحرق بزاف' and 'shooting كضرب بحال اضو'. In contrast, patients in the self-ligating and aligner system identified 3 sensory descriptors: 'cramping مزير' followed by 'aching تيألم' and 'tender خفيف'. However, the proportion of subjects in each group who selected the descriptors was consistently lower in the aligner group than in the self-ligating group. For effective components, the self-ligating and aligner systems did not really raise this aspect of pain, while for the conventional system the most used description was "punishing-cruel تعدب بزاف". Tecco et al. [3] reported that the other two pain descriptors "shooting" and "dull" were used to a lesser extent. Whereas in Bergius et al.'s study [17], the terms "shooting" and "dull" were never used to describe the pain of their patients.

This study showed that tooth brushing could cause pain in patients with fixed appliances. Although the pain was generally minimal, it was experienced by a greater proportion of the sample in the conventional group than in the self-ligating group. However, patients in the aligner group reported almost no discomfort when brushing. The results of the Rakhshan et al. study [17] indicated that tooth brushing mainly induced mild pain. This result was consistent with other studies which suggested that orthodontic pain may have a negative effect on oral hygiene [18, 19].

Pain intensity scores and their impact on daily work/school activities had a minimal effect that peaked at a 24-hour period. In the following days, the number of patients reporting such an effect decreased. Scheurer et al. [7] found that the insertion of fixed appliances seemed to have only a minor effect on the patients' daily life. This is consistent with our results. Shalish et al. [14] noted that the levels of disturbance in oral symptoms and general activities with Invisalign were similar to those of patients with fixed appliances. In contrast, Miller et al. [20] found that the fixed appliance group reported more negative impact than the Invisalign group.

A correlation between pain intensity scores and analgesic use was also observed. In general, analgesics were mostly used by patients who reported more severe pain. In this study, a large proportion of patients did not use medication, as reported in Firestone [21] and Bergius's studies [22]. During orthodontic treatment, analgesic consumption differs according to the period of treatment. Wu et al [23] noted that analgesics were used more frequently during the initial phases of treatment, when pain intensity was highest, supporting the hypothesis that the pain experienced later in orthodontic treatment was relatively low. In our study, after activation, 27% of the patients treated with conventional appliances, 25% of the patients treated with a self-ligating system, and 5.9% treated with aligners used medication after activation. A small percentage of patients used analgesics at 24 hours and 3 days. These patients mainly took paracetamol and a few used non-steroidal anti-inflammatory drugs (ibuprofene) to relieve pain. Most patients used self-medication. Scheurer et al. [7] stated that perceived pain and analgesic consumption would decrease if the patient were effectively informed of the discomfort in advance.

At the end of this chapter, we are aware that our study was a descriptive study with significant selection bias with respect to the confounding factors of need for orthodontic treatment, stage of treatment, age, and undetectable susceptibility to pain and even to orthodontic treatment. A cohort study with three groups benefiting from the three therapeutic choices, taking into account age, gender, type of malocclusion, and facial typology, is the following step to move to observational studies for more epidemiological inference.

3. Conclusion

Orthodontic treatment creates pain at different stages, which seems to be particularly intense at the beginning of treatment and tends to diminish during the course of treatment. Its intensity and duration may be influenced by the type of appliance worn. The results of this study showed that the aligner system was less painful than fixed brackets. There were only minor differences in the reported pain intensity between the conventional and self-ligating appliances. This pain was characterized in all 3 systems by the descriptors "cramping مزير" and "Aaching تيألم".

The daily quality of life of patients treated with aligners was, therefore, better than that of patients treated with fixed appliances. The consumption of analgesics, correlated with the intensity of the pain experienced. Depending on the patient's pain threshold and psychological profile, clinicians should consider prescribing analgesics to alleviate patients' unpleasant experiences.

These observations can be used in clinical situations by informing patients in advance of a specific complaint associated with a particular type of device and will give practitioners and patients additional information that can be used when choosing the type of device. This can help reduce negative experiences of therapy and increase patients' confidence in their orthodontist. Pain is not inevitable, it can be prevented and treated as well as possible.

Conflict of interest

Ethical clearance was obtained from the Ethics Committee of the Faculty of Dentistry, University of Hassan II University, and all participants and their respective teachers were informed about the aims of the study. Access to schools was granted by the Casablanca Regional Academy of Education and training. The parental consent and authorization of all students were also obtained. All authors stated that no conflict could influence their participation in this study.

Acronyms and abbreviations

IASP	International Association for the Study of Pain
VAS	Visual Analogue Scale
M-SF-MPQ	The Moroccan Short Form of McGIll Pain questionnaire.

Author details

Farid Bourzgui[1*], Rania Fastani[2], Salwa Khairat[3], Samir Diouny[4], Mohamed El Had[5], Zineb Serhier[6] and Mohamed Bennani Othmani[6]

1 Department of Orthodontics, Dental School, University Hassan II, Casablanca, Morocco

2 Private Practice Rés. les collines, Casablanca, Morocco

3 Private Practice, Casablanca, Morocco

4 Neurolinguistics and Psychology of Language Hassan II University, Clinical Neuroscience and Mental Health Lab, Casablanca, Morocco

5 Orthodontist Private Practice, Casablanca, Morocco

6 Faculty of Medicine and Pharmacy, Laboratory of Medical Informatics, University Hassan II, Casablanca, Morocco

*Address all correspondence to: farid.bourzgui@etu.univh2c.ma

References

[1] Merskey H, Albe Fessard D, Bonica JJ, Carmon A, Dubner R, Kerr FWL, et al. Pain terms: A list with definitions and notes on usage. Recommended by the IASP subcommittee on taxonomy. Pain. 1979;**6**:249-252

[2] Cohen M, Quintner J, van Rysewyk S. Reconsidering the international association for the study of pain definition of pain. Pain Reports. 2018;**3**(2):e634

[3] Tecco S, D'Attilio M, Tetè S, Festa F. Prevalence and type of pain during conventional and self-ligating orthodontic treatment. European Journal of Orthodontics. 2009;**31**(4):380-384

[4] Johal A, Fleming PS, Al Jawad FA. A prospective longitudinal controlled assessment of pain experience and oral health-related quality of life in adolescents undergoing fixed appliance treatment. Orthodontics & Craniofacial Research. 2014;**17**(3):178-186

[5] Ngan P, Kess B, Wilson S. Perception of discomfort by patients undergoing orthodontic treatment. American Journal of Orthodontics and Dentofacial Orthopedics. 1989;**96**(1):47-53

[6] Bourzgui F, Diouny S, Rguigue O, Aghutan H, Serhier Z, Othmani MB. Cross-cultural adaptation and validation of the Moroccan Short Form McGill Pain Questionnaire (SF-MPQ). International Journal of Medical Reviews and Case Reports. 2020;**4**(11):81-86. DOI: 10.5455/IJMRCR.McGill-Pain-Questionnaire

[7] Scheurer PA, Firestone AR, Bürgin WB. Perception of pain as a result of orthodontic treatment with fixed appliances. European Journal of Orthodontics. 1996;**18**(4):349-357

[8] Fleming PS, Dibiase AT, Sarri G, Lee RT. Pain experience during initial alignment with a self-ligating and a conventional fixed orthodontic appliance system. A randomized controlled clinical trial. The Angle Orthodontist. 2009;**79**(1):46-50

[9] White DW, Julien KC, Jacob H, Campbell PM, Buschang PH. Discomfort associated with Invisalign and traditional brackets: A randomized, prospective trial. The Angle Orthodontist. 2017;**87**(6):801-808

[10] Pringle AM, Petrie A, Cunningham SJ, McKnight M. Prospective randomized clinical trial to compare pain levels associated with 2 orthodontic fixed bracket systems. American Journal of Orthodontics and Dentofacial Orthopedics. 2009; **136**(2):160-167

[11] Scott P, Sherriff M, Dibiase AT, Cobourne MT. Perception of discomfort during initial orthodontic tooth alignment using a self-ligating or conventional bracket system: A randomized clinical trial. European Journal of Orthodontics. 2008;**30**(3): 227-232

[12] Rahman S, Spencer RJ, Littlewood SJ, O'Dywer L, Barber SK, Russell JS. A multicenter randomized controlled trial to compare a self-ligating bracket with a conventional bracket in a UK population: Part 2: Pain perception. The Angle Orthodontist. 2016;**86**(1):149-156

[13] Fujiyama K, Honjo T, Suzuki M, Matsuoka S, Deguchi T. Analysis of pain level in cases treated with Invisalign aligner: Comparison with fixed edgewise appliance therapy. Progress in Orthodontics. 2014;**15**(1):64

[14] Shalish M, Cooper-Kazaz R, Ivgi I, Canetti L, Tsur B, Bachar E, et al. Adult patients' adjustability to orthodontic appliances. Part I: A comparison between Labial, Lingual, and Invisalign™. European Journal of Orthodontics. 2012;**34**(6):724-730

[15] Almasoud NN. Pain perception among patients treated with passive self-ligating fixed appliances and Invisalign® aligners during the first week of orthodontic treatment. Korean Journal of Orthodontics. 2018;**48**(5): 326-332. DOI: 10.4041/kjod.2018. 48.5.326

[16] Wiedel AP, Bondemark L. A randomized controlled trial of self-perceived pain, discomfort, and impairment of jaw function in children undergoing orthodontic treatment with fixed or removable appliances. The Angle Orthodontist. 2016;**86**(2):324-330

[17] Rakhshan H, Rakhshan V. Pain and discomfort perceived during the initial stage of active fixed orthodontic treatment. Saudi Dent Journal. 2015;**27**(2):81-87. DOI: 10.1016/j. sdentj.2014.11.002

[18] Krukemeyer AM, Arruda AO, Inglehart MR. Pain and orthodontic treatment. The Angle Orthodontist. 2009;**79**(6):1175-1181. DOI: 10.2319/ 121308-632R.1

[19] Sergl HG, Klages U, Zentner A. Pain and discomfort during orthodontic treatment: Causative factors and effects on compliance. American Journal of Orthodontics and Dentofacial Orthopedics. 1998;**114**(6):684-691. DOI: 10.1016/s0889-5406(98)70201-x

[20] Miller KB, McGorray SP, Womack R, Quintero JC, Perelmuter M, Gibson J, et al. A comparison of treatment impacts between invisalign aligner and fixed appliance therapy during the first week of treatment. American Journal of Orthodontics and Dentofacial Orthopedics. 2007;**131**(3): 302.e1-302.e9. DOI: 10.1016/j.ajodo. 2006.05.031

[21] Firestone AR, Scheurer PA, Bürgin WB. Patients' anticipation of pain and pain-related side effects, and their perception of pain as a result of orthodontic treatment with fixed appliances. European Journal of Orthodontics. 1999;**21**(4):387-396

[22] Bergius M, Berggren U, Kiliaridis S. Experience of pain during an orthodontic procedure. European Journal of Oral Sciences. 2002;**110**(2):92-98. DOI: 10.1034/j.1600-0722.2002.11193. x

[23] Wu AK, McGrath C, Wong RW, Wiechmann D, Rabie AB. A comparison of pain experienced by patients treated with labial and lingual orthodontic appliances. European Journal of Orthodontics. 2010;**32**(4):403-407. DOI: 10.1093/ejo/cjp117

Chapter 13

Effects of Various Dentofacial Orthopedic and Orthognathic Treatment Modalities on Pharyngeal Airway

Tejashri Pradhan and Aarti Sethia

Abstract

The function of respiration is highly relevant to orthodontic diagnosis and treatment planning. Significant relationships between pharyngeal, craniofacial as well as dentofacial structures have been reported in several studies. Many authors have emphasized that mouth breathing is concomitantly associated with constricted airway causing obstructive sleep apnoea. Associated symptoms can be cured with correction of either skeletal or dental problems or both. Therefore it would be very intriguing to understand and interpret the airway during diagnosis and treatment planning for a clear view of changes in the airway dimensions during the course of orthodontic treatment using various treatment modalities. Therefore a complete understanding of the concept of airway should be considered as an important one. This chapter gives us an insight to the intricate detailing on how the various orthodontic and dentofacial orthopedic treatment signifies the changes in the dimensions of pharyngeal airway.

Keywords: pharyngeal airway, skeletal changes, dental changes, functional appliances, Orthognatic surgeries, expansion

1. Introduction

Orthodontia being one of its kind specialty has always aimed at correcting the dento-facial esthetics which involves achievement of: ideal jaw relationship, normal oral function, proximal and occlusal contact of teeth. But the core aspect of function and performance has been taken up by the function of respiration or breathing which in fact is the top most important function for humans. The synchrony of ideal health and facial development is based on accurate posture of tongue and nasal breathing. Therefore the recent protocols be it Preventive, interceptive or corrective orthodontics, factoring the dire need of pharyngeal airway space improvement in addition to improvement in smile and facial appearance [1].

Today Orthodontists play a very crucial and integral role in the interdisciplinary team management of airway and sleep related disorders. Commencement of Sleep

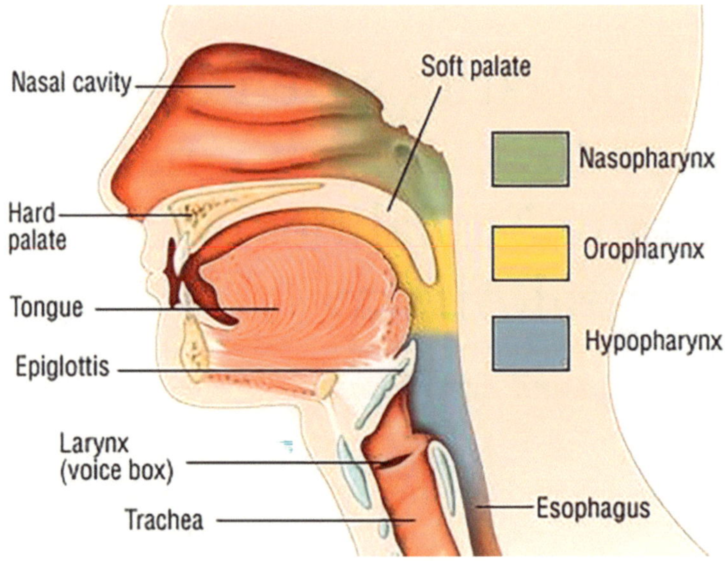

Figure 1.
Anatomy of the pharyngeal airway space.

Medicine as a speciality has brought about a very clear understanding of transformative or developmental biology, medicine; the jaw size and its spatial orientation has surfaced as the important factor of optimizing upper airway physiology. Airway passage, type of breathing and craniofacial formation are so interconnected during growth and development that form follows the function and function follows the form [2]. So the specialty of orthodontics,is well balanced to treat ideally form and function both in children and adults so that the function is optimized for life. The conventional treatment in orthodontics has always priortised primarily on teeth esthetics. This method, seldom addresses symptoms and as a result the airway is ignored. Therefore it is necessary to focus more at physiologic adaptations and its muscle to resolve sleep disordered breathing [3].

The nasal airway analysis requires adequate anatomical dimensions for the overall pharyngeal airway space [4]. Oral breathing in relation to nasal obstruction is a well known entity among orthodontic patients [5]. Obstruction of nasopharyngeal pathway is associated with various craniofacial features, such as backward and upward growth of condyle, backward and downward rotation of mandible, divergent gonial angle, anterior open bite and spacing w.r.t mandibular anteriors [6]. The eradication of respiratory obstruction and aquiring adequate functional nasal breathing with precise patterns of swallowing boosts the stability and functional balance of orthodontic treatment (**Figure 1**) [7, 8].

2. Anatomy of airway

The airway, or respiratory tract, describes its organs that allow airflow during ventilation. They pass through the nares and buccal opening till the blind end of the alveolar sacs. This respiratory tract is subdivided into different regions and various organs and tissues to perform specific functions. The airway passage is subdivided into the upper and lower airway, each of which has numerous compartments.

The pharynx is the mucosal lined portion of the airway that is situated between the base of the skull and the esophagus. It is subdivided as follows:

- Nasopharynx [rhino-pharynx], is the muscular tubular structure from the nares, including the posterior nasal cavity, that divides from the oropharynx by the palate and lining the skull base superiorly.

- Oro-pharynx is the region that joins the nasopharynx and hypopharynx. It is the region situated between the palate and the hyoid bone, which anteriorly gets divided from the oral cavity by the tonsillar arch.

- Hypopharynx is the region which connects the oropharynx to the esophagus and the larynx, the region of pharynx below the hyoid bone.

Boundary between nasopharynx and oropharynx is known as soft palate, similarly the boundary between the oropharynx and laryngopharynx is the epiglottis. The soft palate is dangled at the posterior corner of the hard palate, and its top and bottom are comprises of the mucosal tissues. The centre portion of the soft palate includes muscles, aponeurosis, blood vessels, nerves, lymph and mucosal tissues. During the process of deglutition and injestion, the soft palate develops postero-superiorly and separates the nasopharynx and oropharynx. The mandible is interconnected to the hyoid bone, tongue, and soft palate by the strong musculature. Therefore, the location of the mandible can affect the size of the pharyngeal airway space.

3. Pharyngeal airway space (PAS)

Pharyngeal airway space is divided into three compartments: (**Figure 2**).

Upper pharyngeal width (UPW): Its is the smallest distance between the posterior border of the soft palate to the nearest point on the posterior pharyngeal wall.

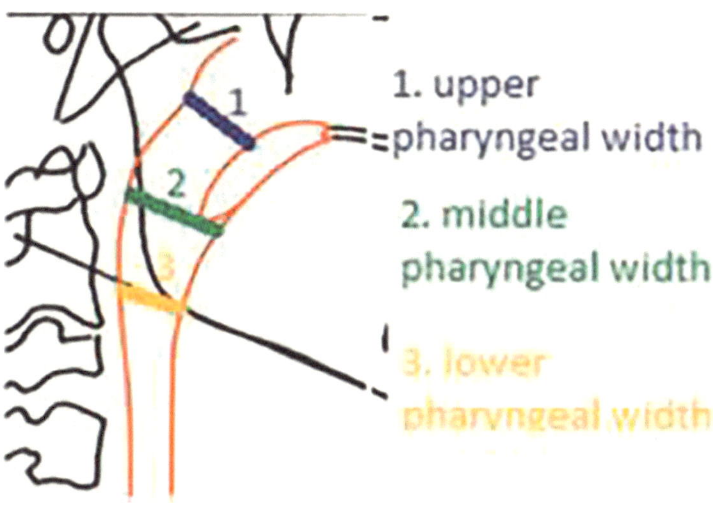

Figure 2.
Various compartments of the pharyngeal airway space [9].

Middle pharyngeal width (MPW): It is the smallest distance between the posterior borders of the tongue to the nearest point on the posterior pharyngeal wall, through the tip of the soft palate.

Lower pharyngeal width (LPW): It is the smallest distance from the intersection of posterior border of tongue and inferior border of the mandible to the closest point on the posterior pharyngeal wall.

Normal upper pharyngeal airway space is 15–20 mm while middle and lower pharyngeal airway (LPA) space is 11–14 mm [9].

Literature supports the hypothesis that mandibular deficiency is analogous to a narrower PAS. It is generally observed that a retrognathic mandible and reduced space between the cranial column and the corpus of the mandible often leads to a posteriorly placed tongue and soft palate, which inturn increases the chances of impaired respiratory function and possibly causing nocturnal breathing problems. Alterations in PAS have been described with various sleeping disorders such as obstructive sleep apnea. Advancement and setback surgeries are standard procedures for the correction of mandibular position whether its retrognathism and prognathism, respectively. Operation for the mandibular deformity changes hard and soft tissue components, including the PAS [10].

4. Diagnosis

Malocclusion can be perceived in several ways which more likely includes patients with enlarged adenoids, obstructive sleep apnoea (OSA), snoring and clefts. The relation between respiratory pattern and form of malocclusion is still disputed. Patients with craniofacial disorders including a short cranial base, reduction in the cranial base angle, bimaxillary retrusion, and retrognathic mandibles show common finding of narrow airways [11].

5. Various methods for assessment

The methods described to assess the airway include: nasal endoscopy, rhinomanometry, acoustic rhinomanometry, cephalometry, computed tomography (CT), magnetic resonance imaging (MRI) and cone-beam computed tomography (CBCT).

6. Two dimensional versus three dimensional imaging

Lateral cephalograms can provide us with useful, credible and replicable airway measurements while minimizing patient costs and radiation exposure. Studies have shown that while cephalometric measurements provide two-dimensional data, cephalometry is a reliable method for airway assessment and adenoid size estimation [12]. Another comparative study to assess the linear measurements with lateral cephalograms and CBCT was carried out and the conclusions drawn: that airway linear measurements are reliable, with both lateral cephalograms and CBCT reconstruction, as there is a positive correlation with the respective area measurements on axial slices [13].

7. Changes in pharyngeal airway space using functional appliance therapy

In 1934, Pierre Robin proposed that use of an intraoral appliance helps in bringing the lower jaw forward in newborns with mandibular deficiency. This helps in preventing the posterior relocation of the tongue during sleep and the occurrence of oropharyngeal collapse [14]. This concept is now often used in adult obstructive sleep apnea (OSA) patients to avoid an upper airway collapse during sleep with the help of various myofunctional appliances [15]. Moreover, the idea to relocate the mandible anteriorly is applied in dentofacial orthopedics by the use of various myofunctional appliances which helps in stimulating mandibular growth in skeletal Class II growing patients with mandibular deficiency [16]. Several authors have hypothesized that the functional orthopedic treatment of growing patients with short mandibles may lead to increased oropharyngeal airway dimensions, and some have suggested a possible reduction in the risk of future respiratory problems (**Figures 3** and **4**) [17–20].

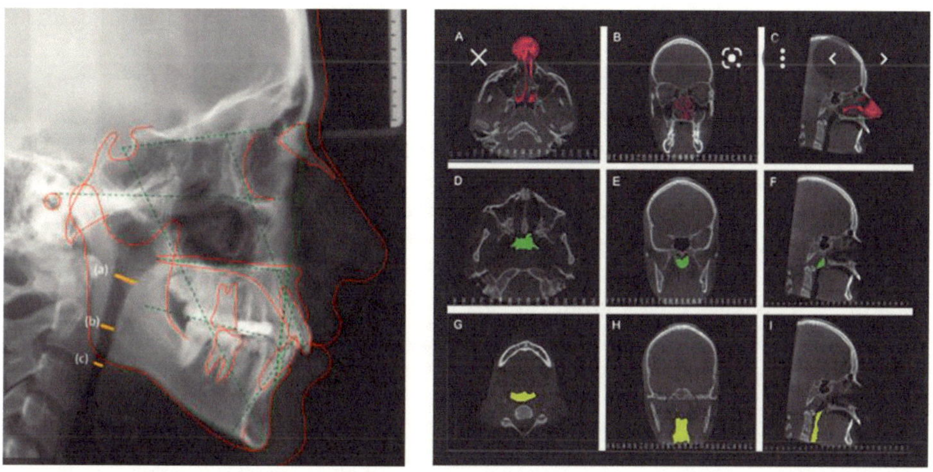

Figure 3.
Two dimensional lateral cephalometric evaluation versus three dimensional CBCT evaluation.

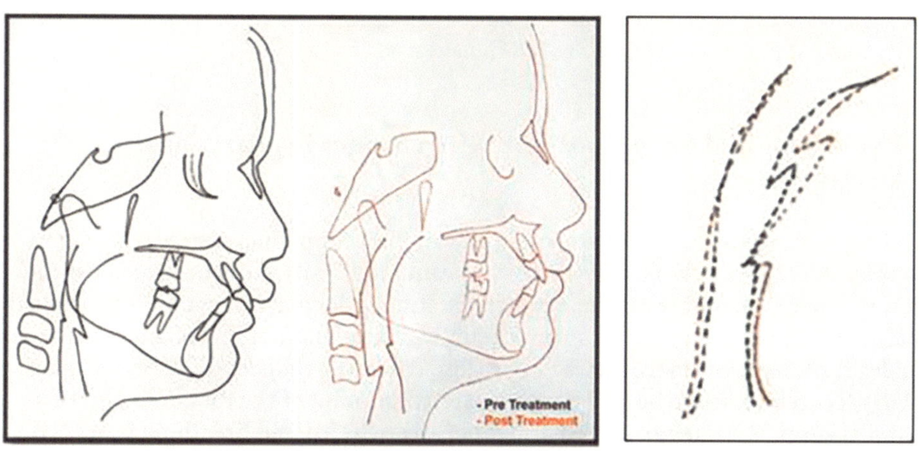

Figure 4.
Changes in the dimension of pharyngeal aiway width using functional appliance therpy [9].

8. Effect of various functional appliances on pharyngeal airway

Twin block is considered to be one of the most patient compliant myofunctional appliance. Therefore prominent results can be drawn with this appliance [21]. According to Jena et al. [21] when twin block was compared with Mandibular protraction appliance MPA, the improvement of oropharynx dimension by twin-block appliance was significantly more. Another study showed significant increase in the dimensions of nasopharynx, oropharynx and hypopharynx following twin-block treatment [22]. Although the growth itself had very minor contribution in the improvement of oropharyngeal dimension, but the advancement of mandible through myofunctional orthopedic correction was evidentally beneficial. The anterior relocation of mandible by the functional appliances places the tongue more forward and thus increases the overall dimension of oropharynx [23]. The improvement in the dimension of oropharynx was more with removable functional appliance (twin block) compared to fixed functional appliance [21, 24]. An increase in oropharyngeal volume was found after functional appliance treatment in Class II patients, leading to an increase in final volume of the upper airway.

Forsus Fatigue Resistence Device (FFRD) brought about improvement in the oropharyngeal airway significantly when compared the untreated subjects. Post treatment, the mean values of Superior Pharyngeal Space and Middle Pharyngeal Space increased by 1.06 mm and 1.28 mm respectively in the FFRD group. Aksu et al. [25] measured the airway space equivalent to the depth of hypopharynx andconcluded that there was no significant improvement in the width of hypopharynx. Bavbek et al. [26] measured CV3 projection in FFRD group and control group and found that FFRD did not increase the hypopharyngeal width. Whereas the other three studies had not measured the hypopharyngeal airway dimension.

The following were the conclusions drawn from the systematic review [27]:

> *Functional appliances help in improving the pharyngeal airway dimensions in Class II malocclusion subjects with retrognathic mandibles. But it is also evident that minimum effect on nasopharyngeal airway passage and the minor improvement is mainly due to growth. Improvement of oropharyngeal airway passage dimensions is a very prominent effects of functional appliance treatment. Removable functional appliance prove to be more efficient than fixed functional appliance in the improvement of positive airway pressure (PAP) dimension.*

9. Hyoid bone and tongue position with changes in pharyngeal airway space

The results obtained by treatment with functionalappliances are mainly dentoalveolar in nature, there ishowever a significant modification of the oropharyngeal airway dimension is observed in most of the studies. Hypothesiscould be presumed that, the dentoalveolar modifications occurringafter functional appliance treatment, guides the tongue to amore forward position, enlarging theposterior airway space (PAS). Therefore, it can be said that forward positioningof the tongue is part of a planned surgical strategywhen treatment of sleep disordered breathing is needed. Changes observed in the hyoid bone distance are moreprominent horizontally than that in the vertical direction [27].

The conclusions drawn with respect to hyoid bone position are as follows:

Hyoid bone is found to be posteriorly and superiorly placed in patients with Class II skeletal malocclusion when compared to Class III and Class I skeletal cases. The hyoid bone position in males is foundto be more inferiorly and anteriorly when compared to females. Also the anterior cranial base is very strongly related to the nasal fossa length and a moderately related to positive correlation with the hyoid bone vertical position and lower airway width. The hyoid bone vertical position had a strong positive correlation with the length of the nasal fossa [4].

10. Changes in pharyngeal airway space with various surgical procedures

Orthognathic surgery is a common method to treat dentofacial deformities. It changes the position of facial skeletal structures and also affects the morphology of the pharynx drastically. Structures such as soft palate, tongue, hyoid bone and some surrounding tissues are attached directly or indirectly to the maxilla and mandible, therefore any desired movement of the jaws by orthognathic surgery affects these tissues, causing changes in the dimensions of the pharyngeal area [28].

11. Mandibular set back surgery

In a thesis by Jain et al. [29], statistically significant increase in the nasopoharyngeal airway dimension was observed. This finding has also been reported by Kitagawara et al. [30] and has been explained as a biological adaptation against postoperative swelling and edema, and for airway maintenance. It is a compensatory mechanism after the hypopharyngeal airway collapses. According to Susarla et al. [31], the upper airway length (UAL) contributes to resistance to airflow. Longer airways have more resistance to airflow than shorter airways [31].

12. Bimaxillary surgeries

Chen et al. [32] found that patients undergoing bimaxillary surgery had changes at the three levels, with increase at the nasopharynx and decreases at the oropharynx and hypopharynx. Bimaxillary operations mostly decrease the narrowing effect of the mandibular setback operations [33]. This indicates that Upper Airway Length increases along with narrowing of the airway, in patients who undergo bimaxillary surgery.

13. Mandibular advancement

Statistically significant increase in the oropharyngeal and hypopharyngel airway dimension was observed according to Jain et al. [29] and Turnbull et al. [34].

14. Pharyngeal airway in cleft lip and palate patients

Cleft patient presents more frequently with large adenoids than do the non-cleft population. This has been regarded as a compensatory phenomenon to decrease the pharyngeal depth and make velopharyngeal competence possible. After palatal operation, soft tissue is sometime short and scarred and frequently the uvula is missing, tissue deficit results in incompetence to velopharyngeal sphincter mechanism.

Gohilot et al. [35] in a study noted that adenoidal tissue size was larger in the juvenile and adolescent cleft group as compared to the adolescent cleft group and airway passage was decreased in juvenile subjects. The thickness of adenoidal tissues decreases with age in both subjects with and without CLP. Conversely, the upper airway dimensions increase in those with and without CLP.

15. Effect of expansion on pharyngeal airway

Iwasaki et al. [36] evaluated the effect of rapid maxillary expansion (RME) on nasal airway ventilation condition, tongue posture, and pharyngeal airway volume. They found that RME enlarges the pharyngeal airway bothways with and without improvement in nasal obstruction. Another study by Malkoç et al. [37] derived that expansion does not cause any significant change in the dimension of pharyngeal airway.

16. Cervical spine posture

Various researchers have been taking prime interest in finding the correlation between the cervical spine posture, head position and pharyngeal airway space, but significant evidence still needs to be procured through proper research.

17. Effect of different growth patterns on pharyngeal airway

A study by Kocakara et al. [38] showed that, the pharyngeal airway dimensions and hyoid bone position are similar in individuals in the sagittal direction. The vertical airway length is significantly shorter in Class III patients with hypodivergent patterns. Another study by Ucar et al. [39] concluded that the nasopharyngeal airway space and upper pharyngeal airway space in Class I subjects is larger in low angle cases than in high angle cases.

18. Conclusions

Impactful evaluation of orthodontic treatment on the pharyngeal airway dimensions is considered one of the prime aspects of orthodontic diagnosis and treatment planning. The protocol helps in emboldening the impersonation of what the nature had planned i.e. by fitting all the teeth early enough through various habit breaking appliances, expansion appliances, and functional jaw orthopedics. Although maxillomandibular advancement surgeries are very well known to improve the airway dimensions along with improvement in dento-facial esthetics. But the hypothetical percentage of cases undergoing this beneficial modality is far less due to its invasive nature. Although Orthodontia at the present juncture, recognizes the importance of evaluating and treating airway, sleep disorders, there are yet tremendous scope untouched.

Author details

Tejashri Pradhan[1] and Aarti Sethia[2]*

1 Department of Orthodontics and Dentofacial Orthopedics, KLE VK Institute of Dental Sciences, KLE Academy of Higher Education and Research, Belagavi, Karnataka, India

2 Department of Orthodontics and Dentofacial Orthopedics, Dr. D.Y. Patil University School of Dentistry, Nerul, Navi Mumbai, Maharashtra, India

*Address all correspondence to: aarti2701@gmail.com

References

[1] Jayan B, Kadu A, Kumar RR. Airway centric orthodontics: A view point. Indian Journal of Sleep Medicine (IJSM). 2016;**11**(3):89-94

[2] Page DC. Your jaws—Your life. The Functional Orthodontist. 2002; **19**(3):36-38

[3] Kalha AS, Jayan B. Dental sleep medicine: An overview. In: Nangia V, Shivani S, editors. Sleep Related Breathing Disorders. 1st ed. 2015. pp. 151-168

[4] Acharya A, Mishra P, Shrestha RM. Pharyngeal airway space dimensions and hyoid bone position in various craniofacial morphologies. Journal of Indian Orthodontic Society. 2021;**13**:03015742211007621

[5] Redner H, Dondale D. Assessment of the nasopharyngeal airway: A rhinomanometric and radiographic study in children with adenoids. Acta Oto-Laryngologica. 1980;**89**:227-332

[6] Harvold EP, Tomer BS, Chierici G. Primate experiments on oral respiration. American Journal of Orthodontics. 1981;**79**(4):359-372

[7] Yamada T, Tanne K, Miyamoto K. Influences of nasal respiratory obstruction on craniofacial growth in young Macaca fuscata monkeys. American Journal of Orthodontics and Dentofacial Orthopedics. 1997;**111**(1): 38-43

[8] Ricketts RM. Respiratory obstruction syndrome. American Journal of Orthodontics. 1968;**54**:495-507

[9] Dedhiya N, Pradhan T, Sethia A. Assessment of airway dimensions and hyoid bone position in class II patients treated with fixed twin block and forsus fatigue resistant device—A retrospective cephalometric study. Journal of Orofacial Sciences. 2020;**12**:131-138

[10] Siddiqui H, Rizwan S, Faisal SS, Hussain SS. Correlation between pharyngeal airway space and sagittal skeletal malocclusions. Journal of Pakistan Dental Association. 2020;**29**(4):217

[11] Saeed G et al. Comparative study of airways in the saggital plane with mcnamara analysis on lateral cephalometric analysis. International Journal of Dental and Health Sciences. 2016;**3**:868-875

[12] Pirilä-Parkkinen K, Löppönen H, Nieminen P, Tolonen U, Pääkkö E, Pirttiniemi P. Validity of upper airway assessment in children: A clinical, cephalometric, and MRI study. The Angle Orthodontist. 2011;**813**:433-439

[13] Vizzotto MB, Liedke GS, Delamare EL, Silveira HD, Dutra V, Silveira HE. A comparative study of lateral cephalograms and cone-beam computed tomographic images in upper airway assessment. The European Journal of Orthodontics. 2012;**34**(3):390-393

[14] Robin P. Glossoptosis due to atresia and hypotrophy of the mandible. American Journal of Diseases of Children. 1934;**48**:541-547

[15] Clark GT, Arand D, Chung E, Tong D. Effect of anterior mandibular positioning on obstructive sleep apnea. The American Review of Respiratory Disease. 1993;**147**:624-629

[16] Antonarakis GS, Kiliaridis S. Short-term anteroposterior treatment effects of

functional appliances and extraoral traction on class II malocclusion. A Meta-Analysis. Angle Orthodontist. 2007;77:907-914

[17] Ozbek MM, Memikoglu TU, Gogen H, Lowe AA, Baspinar E. Oropharyngeal airway dimensions and functional-orthopedic treatment in skeletal Class II cases. The Angle Orthodontist. 1998;**68**:327-336

[18] Temani P, Jain P, Chaudhary S, Rathee P, Pachori Y, Temani R. Computed tomographic evaluation of three dimensional changes in pharyngeal airway in class II division 1 patients treated with Twin Block Appliance. Journal of Indian Orthodontic Society. 2014;**48**:439-445

[19] Kannan A, Sathyanarayana HP, Padmanabhan S. Effect of functional appliances on the airway dimensions in patients with skeletal class II malocclusion: A systematic review. Journal of Orthodontic Science. 2017;**6**:54-64

[20] Godt A, Koos B, Hagen H, Goz G. Changes in upper airway width associated with Class II treatments (headgear vs activator) and different growth patterns. The Angle Orthodontist. 2011;**81**:440-446

[21] Mohamed RN, Basha S, Al-Thomali Y. Changes in upper airway dimensions following orthodontic treatment of skeletal class II malocclusion with twin block appliance: A systematic review. Turkish Journal of Orthodontics. 2020;**33**(1):59-64

[22] Jena AK, Singh SP, Utreja AK. Effectiveness of twin-block and mandibular protraction appliance-4 in the improvement of pharyngeal airway passage dimensions in class 2 malocclusion subjects with a retrognathic mandible. The Angle Orthodontist. 2013;**83**:728-734

[23] Elfeky HY, Fayed MM. Three-dimensional effects of twin block therapy on pharyngeal airway parameters in class 2 malocclusion patients. Journal of World Federation of Orthodontists. 2015;**4**:114-119

[24] Isidor S, Di Carlo G, Cornelis MA, Isidor F, Cattaneo PM. Three-dimensional evaluation of changes in upper airway volume in growing skeletal Class II patients following mandibular advancement treatment with functional orthopedic appliances. The Angle Orthodontist. Sep 2018;**88**(5):552-559

[25] Aksu M, Gorucu-Coskuner H, Taner T. Assessment of upper airway size after orthopedic treatment for maxillary protrusion or mandibular retrusion. American Journal of Orthodontics and Dentofacial Orthopedics. 2017;**152**: 364-370

[26] Bavbek NC, Tuncer BB, Turkoz C, Ulusoy C, Tuncer C. Changes in airway dimensions and hyoid bone position following class 2 correction with forsus fatigue resistant device. Clinical Oral Investigations. 2016;**20**:1747-1755

[27] Anusuya V, Jena AK, Sharan J. Effects of functional appliance treatment on pharyngeal airway passage dimensions in Class II malocclusion subjects with retrognathic mandibles: A systematic review. APOS Trends in Orthodontics. 2019;**93**:138-148

[28] Nguyen M, Visuttiwattanakorn S, Truong D, Wongsirichat N. Effects of orthognathic surgery on pharyngeal airway space: A literature review. Mahidol Dental Journal. 2014;**34**(2):165-173

[29] Isha J, Tejashri P, Keluskar KM, Aarti S. Evaluation of the effect of

bimaxillary, mandibular setback and advancement surgeries on the pharyngeal airway space and positions of the hyoid bone, soft palate and tongue. Thesis. Belagavi, Karnataka, India: KAHER'S KLE VK Institute of dental sciences; 2021

[30] Kitagawara K, Kobayashi T, Goto H, Yokobayashi T, Kitamura N, Saito C. Effects of mandibular setback surgery on oropharyngeal airway and arterial oxygen saturation. International Journal of Oral and Maxillofacial Surgery. 2008;**37**(4):328-333

[31] Susarla S, Abramson Z, Dodson T, Kaban L. Upper airway length decreases after maxillomandibular advancement in patients with obstructive sleep apnea. Journal of Oral and Maxillofacial Surgery. 2011;**69**(11):2872-2878

[32] Chen F, Terada K, Hua Y, Saito I. Effects of bimaxillary surgery and mandibular set back surgery on pharyngeal airway measurements in patients with Class III skeletal deformities. American Journal of Orthodontics and Dentofacial Orthopedics. 2007;**131**:372-377

[33] Aydemir H, Memikouglu U, Karasu H. Pharyngeal airway space, hyoid bone position and head posture after orthognathic surgery in Class III patients. The Angle Orthodontist. 2012;**82**(6):993-1000

[34] Turnbull N, Battagel J. The effects of orthognathic surgery on pharyngeal airway dimensions and quality of sleep. Journal of Orthodontics. 2000;**27**(3): 235-247

[35] Gohilot A, Pradhan T, Keluskar KM. Cephalometric evaluation of adenoids, upper airway, maxilla, velum length, need ratio for determining velopharyngeal incompetency in subjects with unilateral cleft lip and palate. Journal of Indian Society of Pedodontics and Preventive Dentistry. 2014;**32**(4):297

[36] Iwasaki T, Saitoh I, Takemoto Y, Inada E, Kakuno E, Kanomi R, et al. Tongue posture improvement and pharyngeal airway enlargement as secondary effects of rapid maxillary expansion: A cone-beam computed tomography study. American Journal of orthodontics and Dentofacial Orthopedics. 2013;**143**(2):235-245

[37] Malkoç S, Üşümez S, İşeri H. Long-term effects of symphyseal distraction and rapid maxillary expansion on pharyngeal airway dimensions, tongue, and hyoid position. American Journal of Orthodontics and Dentofacial Orthopedics. 2007;**132**(6):769-775

[38] Kocakara G, Buyukcavus MH, Orhan H. Evaluation of pharyngeal airway dimensions and hyoid bone position according to craniofacial growth pattern. CRANIO®. 2020;**1**:1

[39] Ucar FI, Uysal T. Orofacial airway dimensions in subjects with Class I malocclusion and different growth patterns. The Angle Orthodontist. 2011;**81**(3):460-468

Chapter 14

Orthodontic Management of Adult Sleep Apnea: Clinical Case Reports

Lahcen Ousehal, Soukaina Sahim, Hajar Bouzid, Hakima Aghoutan, Asmaa El Mabrak, Mohamed Mahtar and Mohamed El Fatmi Kadri Hassani

Abstract

Obstructive sleep apnea (OSA) is a serious public health problem that has important impacts on the quality and life expectancy of affected individuals. It is characterized by repetitive upper airway collapse during sleep. OSA requires a multidisciplinary plan of treatment. There is increasing interest in the role of the orthodontist both in screening for adult obstructive sleep apnea and its management. Dental appliances and orthognathic surgery are two strategies that are currently used in the treatment of sleep apnea. This chapter focuses on the orthodontic management of sleep apnea in adults through three clinical cases with varying degrees of severity of sleep apnea. It provides a background on OSA treatment approaches and discusses the potential risks and benefits of each.

Keywords: adult sleep apnea, orthodontics, management, oral appliances, orthognathic surgery

1. Introduction

Obstructive sleep apnea (OSA) is a common sleep disorder resulting from repetitive narrowing and collapsing of the upper airway [1]. Its prevalence has increased worldwide and affects about one in four men and one in 10 women [2]. OSA is characterized by repeated episodes which lead to sleep fragmentation and oxygen desaturation. Clinically, OSA is defined by the occurrence of daytime sleepiness, loud snoring, witnessed breathing interruptions, or awakenings due to gasping or choking [3, 4]. Polysomnography (PSG) is the gold standard for OSA diagnosis and it allows to assess the apnea/hypopnea index (AHI) that is the expression of OSA severity [5]. The AHI is the mean number of sleep apneas and hypopneas per hour of sleep. The American Academy of Sleep Medicine (AASM) defines mild OSAH as an AHI of 5–15 events per hour; moderate OSAH as 15–30 events per hour; and severe OSAH as an AHI of greater than 30 events per hour [6].

The complexity of OSA is exemplified by its multifactorial etiology such as craniofacial structures and neuromuscular tone [7]. Many risk factors are associated with the occurrence of OSA: obesity (BMI > 35) with increased neck circumference, sleeping in the supine position, smoking, alcohol, type 2 diabetes, nasal obstruction (septal deviation and rhinitis), endocrine abnormalities (hypothyroidism and acromegaly), genetics (family history of OSA), and menopause [8].

Untreated OSA is associated with a range of adverse health outcomes such as cardiovascular diseases, cerebrovascular events, diabetes, and cognitive impairment in addition to impaired quality of life [9, 10].

The treatments of OSA can range from weight loss to maxillomandibular advancement. The treatment of choice is influenced by the etiology of the problem, but also by its severity and the personal yearnings [2].

The orthodontist may play an important role in both screening for OSA and the multidisciplinary management of OSA in adults. The contribution of orthodontists to the study and treatment of respiratory disorders associated with sleep focus on three aspects: the diagnosis of the structural changes often present in these diseases, the treatment of mild to moderate forms using intraoral appliances, and presurgical orthodontic treatment of patients programmed for orthognathic surgery [11]. This chapter aimed to discuss, through three clinical cases, the role of the orthodontist in the management of adult sleep apnea according to the severity of the disorder.

2. Case reports

2.1 Case 1

A 63-year-old female was referred to the Department of Dento-Facial Orthopedics of the Dental Consultation and Treatment Center (CCTD) of the Ibn Rochd University Hospital in Casablanca, Morocco. She was diagnosed with moderate OSA based on polysomnography analysis that showed an apnea-hypopnea index (AHI) of 24. Her body mass index (BMI) was 32 kg/m^2. She exhibited severe snoring and excessive daytime sleepiness. She had no history of temporomandibular disorder.

Facial examination revealed a convex profile with protrusive upper lip, retruded chin, and short throat length (**Figure 1A**). Intraoral examination revealed a full set of teeth with maxillary anterior diastema, Class I molar and canine relationships, shallow overbite, and an important overjet (**Figure 1B**). Lateral cephalometric analysis showed skeletal Class II relationship with mandibular retrusion (SNB = 74°), hyperdivergent vertical pattern (GoGn/Sn = 45°), proclined lower incisors as well as low hyoid bone position, and narrow oropharyngeal airway space, particularly at the retroglossal airway (**Figure 1C**).

The primary objective was to relieve the symptoms of OSA by using a mandibular advancement device (MAD). The dental appliance chosen was the "KASPERSKY" appliance which corrects the retroposition of the mandible and, consequently, repositions the tongue (**Figure 2**). Initially, the mandibular position of the MAD was preset at 60% of maximal protrusion. Afterward, its position was advanced by 0.5–1 mm every 1–2 weeks until the patient was satisfied with the symptoms. The anterior interocclusal space was kept at 7 mm so that the oropharyngeal airway was opened during sleep, as a result of the anterior displacement of the tongue and hyoid bone, and in turn, the mouth was inhibited from opening wide. The device was worn overnight for 4 months. Regular follow-up visits were conducted to check for any dental problems or side effects (tissue and joint pain), device wear, and to make appropriate adjustments to optimize the desired clinical effect. The patient was seen once every 6 months the first year and once annually afterward. The patient was very positive

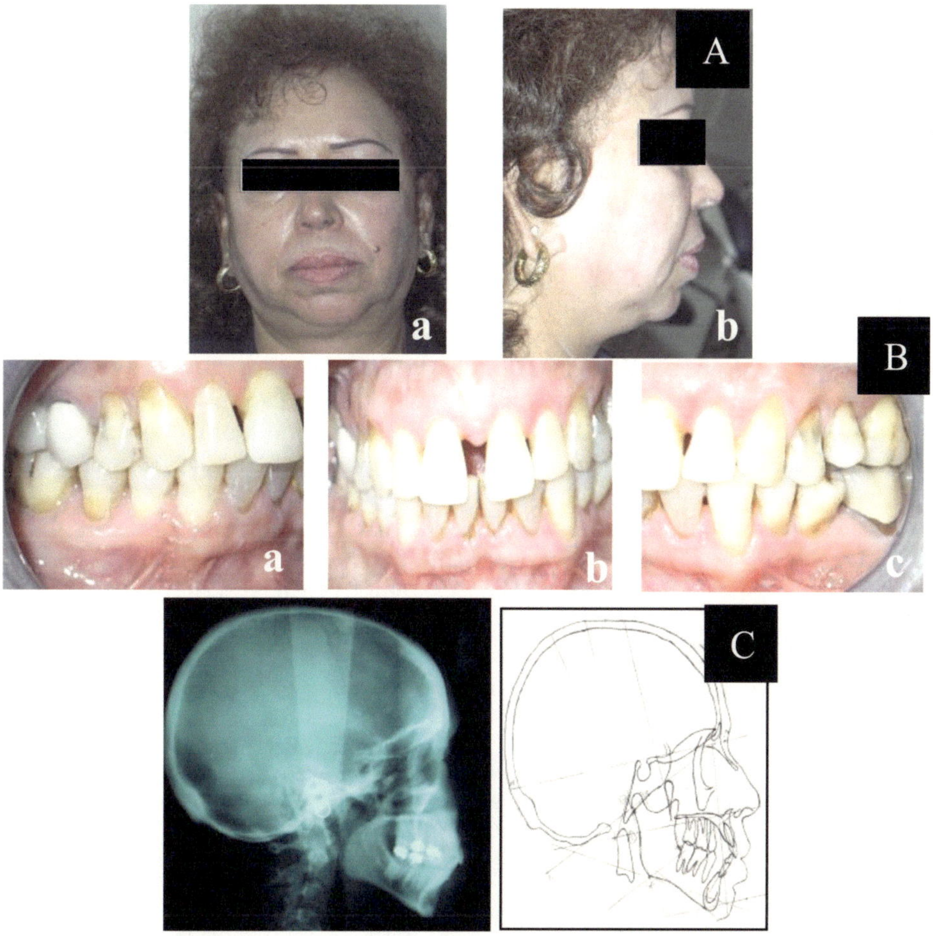

Figure 1.
(A) Pretreatment extraoral photographs: (a) frontal at rest and (b) profile. (B) Pretreatment intraoral photographs: (a) right lateral, (b) frontal, and (c) left lateral. (C) Pretreatment lateral cephalogram.

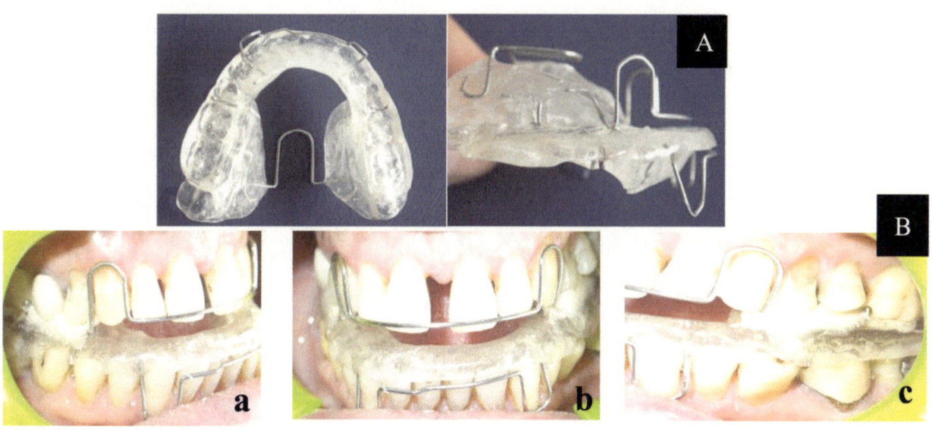

Figure 2.
(A) "KASPERSKY" appliance. (B) Intraoral photographs with the oral appliance: (a) right lateral, (b) frontal, and (c) left lateral.

about the treatment effects. Subjective improvement was noticed with the reported absence of snoring, reduction of daytime sleepiness, and reduction of tiredness. A subsequent sleep test revealed no evidence of OSA with an AHI = 2.5.

2.2 Case 2

A 35-year-old male presented to the Department of Dento-Facial Orthopedics of the Dental Consultation and Treatment Center (CCTD) of the Ibn Rochd University Hospital in Casablanca complaining of chronic loud snoring, restless sleep, and daytime somnolence. His body mass index (BMI) was 27 kg/m^2. The diagnostic polysomnography (**Figure 3D**) revealed a severe OSA with AHI of 30 events/hour. The patient was otherwise healthy and did not smoke nor drink.

Extraoral examination revealed a long symmetrical face, a convex profile with the protrusive lower lip and retruded chin (**Figure 3A**). Intraoral examination showed a full set of teeth except for the first lower left permanent molar, Class II canine relationship in both sides, and right Class I molar relationship. A slight dental crowding in the upper arch was also noted (**Figure 3B**). Lateral cephalometric analysis showed skeletal Class II relationship with mandibular retrognathia (decreased Sella-Nasion-B point (SNB) angle of 70°), hyperdivergent vertical pattern (GoGn/Sn angle of 55°), and proclined lower incisors as well as narrow oropharyngeal airway space (**Figure 3C**).

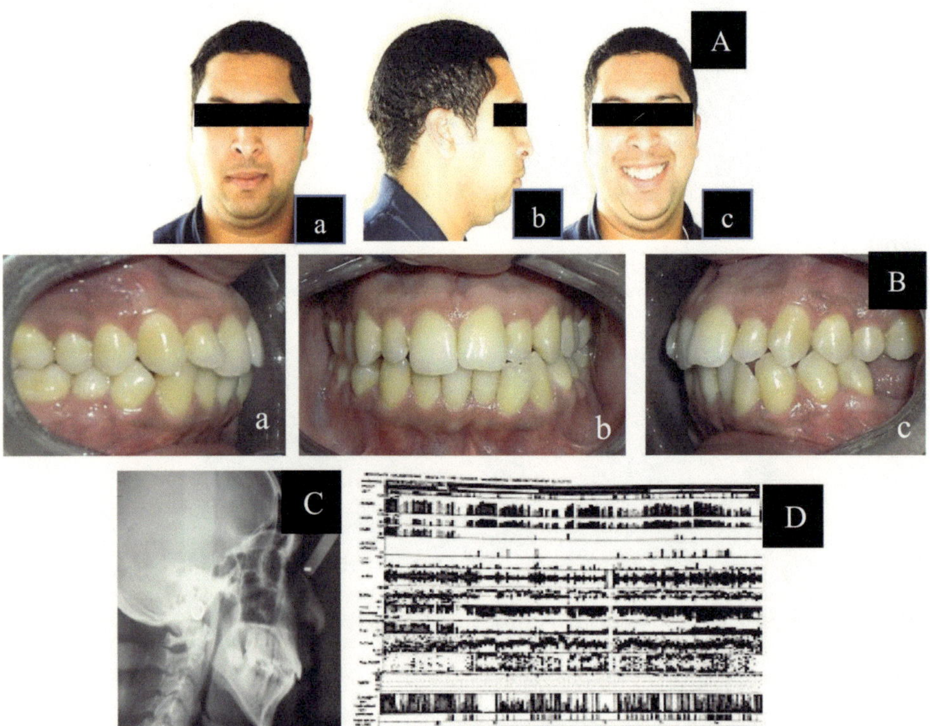

Figure 3.
(A) Pretreatment extraoral photographs: (a) frontal at rest, (b) profile, and (c) frontal smiling. (B) Pretreatment intraoral photographs: (a) right lateral, (b) frontal, and (c) left lateral. (C) Pretreatment lateral cephalogram. (D) Pretreatment polysomnography.

The primary objective was to relieve the symptoms of the severe OSA by mandibular and genioglossus advancement surgery. The presurgical orthodontic aimed to decompensate the teeth within arches and to correlate both arches. A treatment plan with the extraction of four premolars was set. After orthodontic preparation, a 9 mm mandibular advancement was performed by a bilateral sagittal split ramus osteotomy using rigid bone plate fixation associated with advancing genioplasty.

The main outcome measures were assessed by the functional, occlusal, radiographic, and esthetic changes achieved and also by a reduction in the AHI. A normal over-jet and over-bite were established, the inferior pharyngeal airway space was increased, and there was a profound esthetic profile enhancement (**Figure 4**). The patient snoring and overall AHI significantly improved; he was more rested with easy breathing.

2.3 Case 3

A 29-year-old male presented to the Department of Dento-Facial Orthopedics of the Dental Consultation and Treatment Center (CCTD) of the Ibn Rochd University Hospital in Casablanca for repetitive nocturnal apneas, gummy smile as well as unesthetic profile. His body mass index (BMI) was 22.3 kg/m^2. The diagnostic polysomnography (**Figure 5D**) revealed a severe OSA with AHI of 54.4 events/hour. The patient was otherwise healthy and neither smoke nor drink.

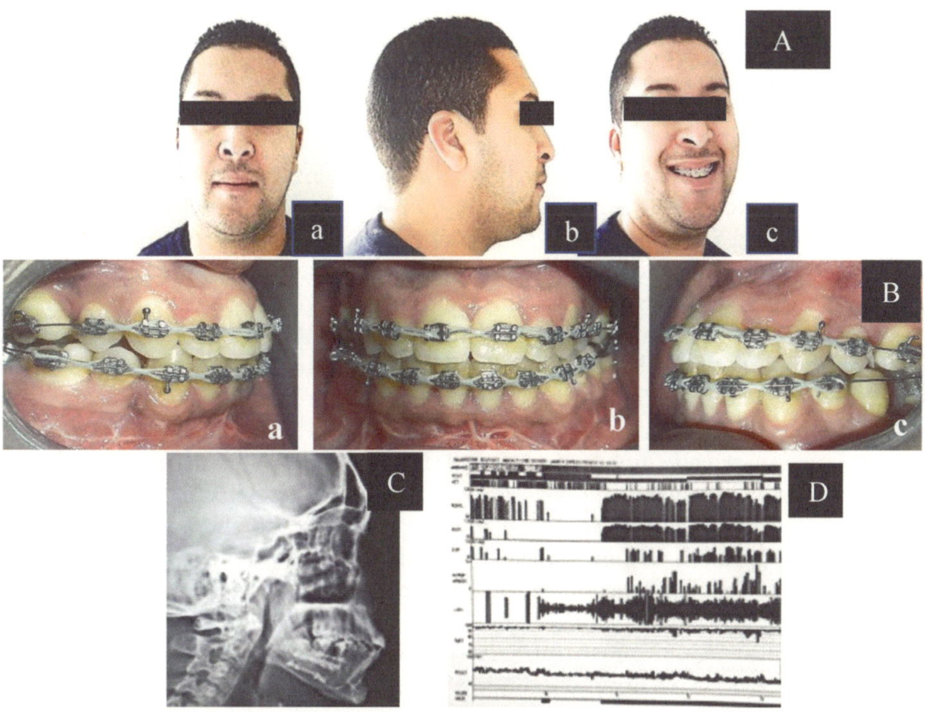

Figure 4.
(A) Posttreatment extraoral photographs: (a) frontal at rest, (b) profile, and (c) frontal smiling. (B) Posttreatment intraoral photographs: (a) right lateral, (b) frontal, and (c) left lateral. (C) Posttreatment lateral cephalogram. (D) Posttreatment polysomnography (Surgery performed by Professor Kadiri).

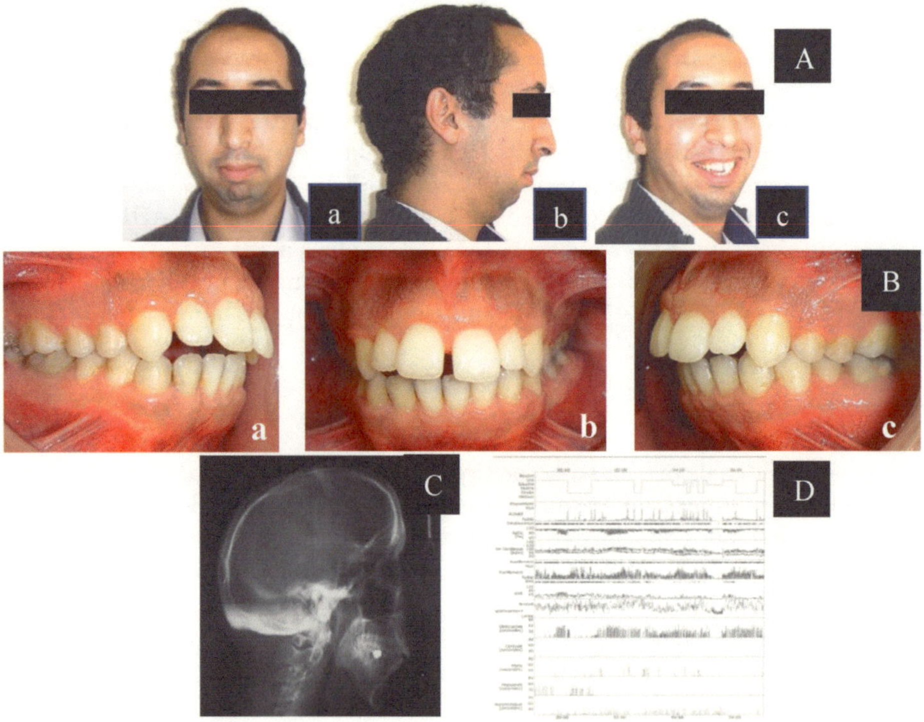

Figure 5.
(A) Pretreatment extraoral photographs: (a) frontal at rest, (b) profile, and (c) lateral smiling. (B) Pretreatment intraoral photographs: (a) right lateral, (b) frontal, and (c) left lateral. (C) Pretreatment lateral cephalogram. (D) Pretreatment polysomnography.

The patient reported a previous orthodontic treatment that relapsed. The clinical examination showed a long symmetrical face, a convex profile with lip incompetence, retruded chin, and a very poor chin-neck contour (**Figure 5A**). Intraoral examination revealed Class II canine and molar relationships in both sides, anterior open bite, important overjet, and maxillary interincisal diastema (**Figure 5B**).

Lateral cephalometric analysis showed skeletal Class II relationship with mandibular retrognathia (decreased Sella-Nasion-B point (SNB) angle of 68°), hyperdivergent vertical pattern (GoGn/Sn angle of 62°), proclined upper and lower incisors, as well as narrow oropharyngeal airway space (**Figure 5C**).

The patient received combined orthodontic and surgical treatment of his skeletal malocclusion to advance the mandible, manage the retroglossal obstruction and ensure an esthetically pleasing appearance. Presurgical orthodontic aimed to decompensate the teeth within arches and to correlate both arches, then maxillomandibular rotational advancement and advancing genioplasty were planned. The treatment led to good esthetics and well-settled occlusion (**Figure 6A** and **B**). The maxillomandibular advancement surgery (MMA) was very effective in nearly eliminating the obstructive events and in improving nocturnal breathing as evidenced by the postoperative polysomnography (**Figure 6D**). On lateral cephalometry, the posterior airway space was increased postoperatively (**Figure 6C**). The patient reported easier breathing, undisturbed sleep, and complete resolution of excessive daytime sleepiness.

DOI: http://dx.doi.org/10.5772/intechopen.101193

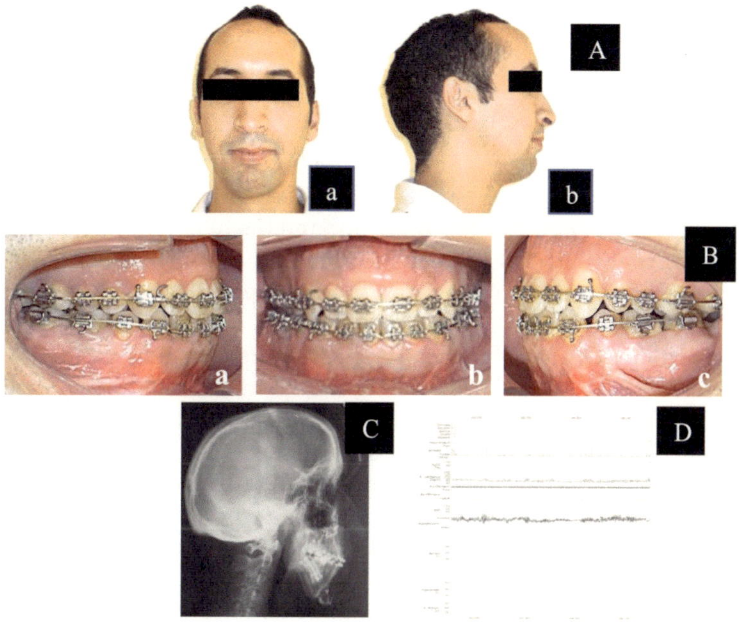

Figure 6.
(A) Posttreatment extraoral photographs: (a) frontal at rest and (b) profile. (B) Posttreatment intraoral photographs: (a) right lateral, (b) frontal, and (c) left lateral. (C) Posttreatment lateral cephalogram. (D) Posttreatment polysomnography (Surgery performed by Professor Kadiri).

3. Discussion

Obstructive sleep apnea (OSA) is a sleep disorder characterized by repeated interruption of breathing during sleep due to episodic collapse of the pharyngeal airway. The diagnostic strategy includes a sleep-oriented history, physical examination, and objective testing of the patient [12]. The gold standard for diagnosis of OSA is overnight polysomnography. The AHI, which is the mean number of sleep apneas and hypopneas per hour of sleep, is an objective and specific measure of the severity of OSA. The American Academy of Sleep Medicine (AASM) defines mild OSA as an AHI of 5–15 events per hour; moderate OSA as 15–30 events per hour; and severe OSA as an AHI of greater than 30 events per hour [6].

The orthodontist is well-positioned to perform an OSA screening assessment and refer at-risk patients for diagnostic evaluation [7]. Besides the clinical examination, some important anatomic features observed radiographically in patients with OSA include, narrow mandible arch; maxillary and mandibular retrognathism; increased lower facial height; the lower and more anterior position of the hyoid bone; reduced pharyngeal area; increased cranio-cervical angle; decreased distance between the base of the tongue and the posterior pharyngeal wall; hypertrophied tonsils and adenoids; over-erupted maxillary and mandibular dentition and enlarged tongue [4].

Besides lifestyle modification (weight loss, smoking cessation, reduction of alcohol intake, position management, and sleep hygiene), there are three major interventions for obstructive sleep apnea: positive airway pressure (CPAP) therapy, oral appliance therapy (OAT), or surgery [6, 13]. The treatment of choice is influenced by the etiology of the problem, its severity, and the patient's individual needs.

Although CPAP is widely used as a first-line treatment for OSA, OAT mainly mandibular advancement devices (MAD) are an alternative to CPAP in the treatment of mild to moderate OSA. Their lower cost, relative comfort, and ease of use lead to greater patient compliance [8]. Worn intraorally during sleep, the MAD can prevent upper airway collapse by holding the mandible and tongue forward [6].

The devices may vary in construction, material, coverage of the teeth, and the possibility of vertical and lateral movements of the mandible [14]. There are two main types of oral appliances namely: the monobloc and the bibloc appliance. A retrospective comparative study by Isacsson et al. [15] found that both the monobloc and bibloc appliances were equally effective and significantly reduced the AHI by a mean of about 12–14 events per hour.

Candidates for a MAD require adequate healthy teeth, no important TMJ disorder, adequate jaw range of motion, and adequate manual dexterity and motivation to insert and remove the OA [12]. A meta-analysis by Sharples et al. [6] found that the most important patient feature is the ability to protrude the mandible 6 mm or more. Oral appliances initially are delivered with the mandible advanced to a position approximating two-thirds of the maximum protrusion [7]. The amount of protrusion can be titrated or increased until optimum symptom relief is obtained as in the first clinical case.

Short-term side effects of MAD are common but most resolve within 2 months. They include dental and gingival tenderness, hypersalivation, dry mouth, TMJ discomfort or sounds, and myofascial pain, [16]. Skeletal changes occur soon after the onset of treatment (6 months). Small but statistically significant increases in face height are accompanied by a significant downward position of the mandible secondary to dental changes [17]. Occlusal changes start happening later on, and they will be significant at the 30-month follow-ups [4]. They include a decrease in overjet, proclination of mandibular incisors, retroclination of the maxillary incisors, decreased occlusal contacts, and mesial shift of the molar and cuspid occlusion [16]. Some effects can lead to beneficial orthodontic changes in Class II division one patients, as in the first clinical case, especially decreasing in overjet and the tendency toward a mesiocclusion [17]. The dental situation needs to be carefully checked during regular visits. In cases of unacceptable, progressive occlusal alterations, the indication for therapy with an OA has to be re-evaluated and might be changed to CPAP or even surgery [18].

If MADs are preferentially indicated for mild or moderate OSA, orthognathic surgery may be an effective and safe treatment in patients with severe sleep apnea as in cases 2 and 3 or in patients who do not desire or cannot tolerate long-term CPAP therapy. The principle of surgical treatment is to get a physical airway by a permanent skeletal change that leads to soft tissue adaptation [3]. Of the surgical procedures, mandibular advancement, maxillomandibular advancement (MMA), and genioplasty are the most frequently performed. In OSA patients with micrognathia or retrognathia the surgical mandibular advancement may be considered. In case two, mandibular and genioglossus advancement surgery illustrated objective improvement in the symptoms associated with severe OSA. With this type of surgical intervention, the entire body of the mandible is brought forward [19]. Presurgical orthodontics is mandatory, otherwise, the width of the maxilla is typically too narrow to accommodate the advanced mandible [20]. However, little evidence is present for isolated mandibular advancement. Currently, osteotomy of maxillo-mandibular advancement (MMA) is the first-choice treatment for severe OSA. Chang et al. [9] reported success rate of MMA ranges from 75 to 100%. Moving the jaw stretches the palatine tissue, which in turn exerts traction upon the palatoglossal muscle and increases lingual support, favoring pharyngeal patency [11]. MMA predictably leads to significant improvements in daytime sleepiness, QOL, sleep-disordered breathing, and neurocognitive performance, as well as a reduction in cardiovascular risk (blood pressure) [21]. The AHI score is improved over the long term and the results remain stable over time.

According to Calero et al. [11], two characteristics must be fulfilled to indicate MMA. First, there must be multiple sites of obstruction, or blockage must be diffuse and inaccessible. Second, the patient must present skeletal class II malocclusion, and MMA surgery must offer multiple benefits for the patient. Presurgical orthodontic therapy aims to obtain complementary maxillary and mandibular dental arches. Patients with a Class II malocclusion, as in the third clinical case, undergo surgical mandibular advancement to achieve a Class I dental and skeletal relationship. Advancement of the maxillomandibular complex by 8–12 mm is generally required to obtain the intended result [22]. According to Lee et al. [23], a non-extraction approach is preferred in patients with OSA to retain expanded pharyngeal volume after surgery. An additional procedure for completing MMA is genioglossal muscle advancement (GA). This technique expands the magnitude of genioglossal, geniohyoid, and digastric muscle replacement [11].

4. Conclusion

Adult sleep apnea is a complex sleep-related breathing disorder that decreases quality of life and increases morbidity and mortality in patients. It is a highly prevalent disease and requires long-term and multidisciplinary management.

Orthodontists should recognize the signs and symptoms of this disorder to identify patients at risk of developing the complications of sleep apnea and guide the selection of appropriate treatment. Various oral appliances can be applied with good results in mild to moderate cases. In severe OSA, a surgical orthodontic approach is indicated. Maxillomandibular advancement surgery is a safe, very effective, and highly skeletally stable procedure.

Long-term management of OSA and regular follow-up are required to monitor compliance to therapy, treatment efficacy, side effects, and development of medical complications related to OSA.

Author details

Lahcen Ousehal[1*], Soukaina Sahim[1], Hajar Bouzid[1], Hakima Aghoutan[1], Asmaa El Mabrak[2], Mohamed Mahtar[3] and Mohamed El Fatmi Kadri Hassani[4]

1 Faculty of Dentistry, Department of Dentofacial Orthopedics, University Hassan II, Casablanca, Morocco

2 Dental Consultation and Treatment Center, Ibn Rochd University Hospital, Casablanca, Morocco

3 Faculty of Medicine, Department of Otorhinolaryngology, University Hassan II, Casablanca, Morocco

4 Private Practice, Casablanca, Morocco

*Address all correspondence to: lahcen2228@yahoo.fr

References

[1] Ramar K, Dort LC, Katz SG, Lettieri CJ, Harrod CG, Thomas SM, et al. Clinical practice guideline for the treatment of obstructive sleep apnea and snoring with oral appliance therapy: An update for 2015. Journal of Clinical Sleep Medicine. 2015;**11**(7):773-827. DOI: 10.5664/jcsm.4858

[2] Faber J, Faber C, Faber AP. Obstructive sleep apnea in adults. Dental Press Journal of Orthodontics. 2019;**24**(3):99-109. DOI: 10.1590/2177-6709.24.3.099-109.sar

[3] Kim YK, Kim JW, Yoon IY, Rhee CS, Lee CH, Yun PY. Influencing factors on the effect of mandibular advancement device in obstructive sleep apnea patients: Analysis on cephalometric and polysomnographic parameters. Sleep & Breathing. 2014;**18**(2):305-311. DOI: 10.1007/s11325-013-0885-5

[4] de Oliveira Almeida MA, de Britto Teixeira AO, Vieira LS, Quintão CC. Treatment of obstructive sleep apnea and hipoapnea syndrome with oral appliances. Brazilian Journal of Otorhinolaryngology. 2006;**72**(5): 699-703. DOI: 10.1016/s1808-8694(15)31028-4

[5] Bartolucci ML, Bortolotti F, Corazza G, Incerti Parenti S, Paganelli C, Alessandri Bonetti G. Effectiveness of different mandibular advancement device designs in obstructive sleep apnoea therapy: A systematic review of randomised controlled trials with meta-analysis. Journal of Oral Rehabilitation. 2021;**48**(4):469-486. DOI: 10.1111/joor.13077

[6] Sharples LD, Clutterbuck-James AL, Glover MJ, Bennett MS, Chadwick R, Pittman MA, et al. Meta-analysis of randomised controlled trials of oral mandibular advancement devices and continuous positive airway pressure for obstructive sleep apnoea-hypopnoea. Sleep Medicine Reviews. 2016;**27**:108-124. DOI: 10.1016/j.smrv.2015.05.003

[7] Behrents RG, Shelgikar AV, Conley RS, Flores-Mir C, Hans M, Levine M, et al. Obstructive sleep apnea and orthodontics: An American association of orthodontists white paper. American Journal of Orthodontics and Dentofacial Orthopedics. 2019;**156**(1): 13-28.e1. DOI: 10.1016/j.ajodo.2019.04.009

[8] Şimon IM, Băciuţ M. Orthodontic appliances in the management of obstructive sleep apnea syndrome—Types and therapeutic indications. Pneumologia. 2018;**67**(2):62-66

[9] Chang HP, Chen YF, Du JK. Obstructive sleep apnea treatment in adults. The Kaohsiung Journal of Medical Sciences. 2020;**36**(1):7-12. DOI: 10.1002/kjm2.12130

[10] Geoghegan F, Ahrens A, McGrath C, Hägg U. An evaluation of two different mandibular advancement devices on craniofacial characteristics and upper airway dimensions of Chinese adult obstructive sleep apnea patients. The Angle Orthodontist. 2015;**85**(6):962-968. DOI: 10.2319/040314-245.1

[11] Azagra-Calero E, Espinar-Escalona E, Barrera-Mora JM, Llamas-Carreras JM, Solano-Reina E. Obstructive sleep apnea syndrome (OSAS). Review of the literature. Medicina Oral, Patología Oral y Cirugía Bucal. 2012;**17**(6):e925-e929. DOI: 10.4317/medoral.17706

[12] Epstein LJ, Kristo D, Strollo PJ Jr, Friedman N, Malhotra A, Patil SP, et al.

Adult obstructive sleep apnea task force of the american academy of sleep medicine. Clinical guideline for the evaluation, management and long-term care of obstructive sleep apnea in adults. Journal of Clinical Sleep Medicine. 2009;**5**(3):263-276

[13] Mintz SS, Kovacs R. The use of oral appliances in obstructive sleep apnea: A retrospective cohort study spanning 14 years of private practice experience. Sleep & Breathing. 2018;**22**(2):541-546. DOI: 10.1007/s11325-018-1643-5

[14] Wojda M, Jurkowski P, Lewandowska A, Mierzwińska-Nastalska E, Kostrzewa-Janicka J. Mandibular advancement devices in patients with symptoms of obstructive sleep apnea: A review. Medical Science and Research Advances in Experimental Medicine and Biology. 2019;**1153**:11-17. DOI: 10.1007/5584_2019_334

[15] Isacsson G, Fodor C, Sturebrand M. Obstructive sleep apnea treated with custom-made bibloc and monobloc oral appliances: A retrospective comparative study. Sleep & Breathing. 2017;**21**(1):93-100. DOI: 10.1007/s11325-016-1377-1

[16] Jacobowitz O. Advances in oral appliances for obstructive sleep apnea. Advances in Oto-Rhino-Laryngology. 2017;**80**:57-65. DOI: 10.1159/000470865

[17] Martins OFM, Chaves Junior CM, Rossi RRP, Cunali PA, Dal-Fabbro C, Bittencourt L. Side effects of mandibular advancement splints for the treatment of snoring and obstructive sleep apnea: A systematic review. Dental Press Journal of Orthodontics. 2018;**23**(4):45-54. DOI: 10.1590/2177-6709.23.4.045-054.oar

[18] Rose EC, Staats R, Virchow C Jr, Jonas IE. Occlusal and skeletal effects of an oral appliance in the treatment of obstructive sleep apnea. Chest. 2002;**122**(3):871-877. DOI: 10.1378/chest.122.3.871

[19] Alami S, Aghoutan H, Diouny S, El Quars F, Bourzgui F. In: Motamedi MHK, editor. Orthodontic Considerations in Obstructive Sleep Apnea—State of the Art, A Textbook of Advanced Oral and Maxillofacial Surgery. Vol. 2. Mohammad Hosein Kalantar Motamedi. IntechOpen; 2015. IntechOpen, DOI: 10.5772/59086. Available from: https://www.intechopen.com/chapters/47489

[20] Conley RS. Evidence for dental and dental specialty treatment of obstructive sleep apnoea. Part 1: The adult OSA patient and Part 2: The paediatric and adolescent patient. Journal of Oral Rehabilitation. 2011;**38**(2):136-156. DOI: 10.1111/j.1365-2842.2010.02136.x

[21] Boyd SB, Chigurupati R, Cillo JE Jr, Eskes G, Goodday R, Meisami T, et al. Maxillomandibular advancement improves multiple health-related and functional outcomes in patients with obstructive sleep apnea: A multicenter study. Journal of Oral and Maxillofacial Surgery. 2019;**77**(2):352-370. DOI: 10.1016/j.joms.2018.06.173

[22] Cillo JE Jr, Dattilo DJ. Maxillomandibular advancement for severe obstructive sleep apnea is a highly skeletally stable long-term procedure. Journal of Oral and Maxillofacial Surgery. 2019;**77**(6):1231-1236. DOI: 10.1016/j.joms.2019.01.009

[23] Lee KH, Kim KA, Kwon YD, Kim SW, Kim SJ. Maxillomandibular advancement surgery after long-term use of a mandibular advancement device in a post-adolescent patient with obstructive sleep apnea. Korean Journal of Orthodontics. 2019;**49**(4):265-276. DOI: 10.4041/kjod.2019.49.4.265

Chapter 15

Accidental Aspiration of Orthodontic Components or Appliances

Siddharth Sonwane

Abstract

Background: Contemporary orthodontic practice consists of innovative appliances for ease, safe, and quick results. However, the associated potential disadvantages are rarely published. **Objective** is to publish the literature on the accidental swallow of foreign objects such as orthodontic appliances or parts of fixed orthodontic appliances in patients. **Method:** An electronic search was performed on PubMed, Medline, Scopus, The Cochrane Library, and EMBASE until March 15th 2019. Methodological quality and synthesis of case series and case report tool (MQCC) was applied to determine the quality of these case reports and series. The outcome variable was to assess its effect on airway and gastrointestinal tract; methods of removal of these foreign bodies. Meta-analysis was not performed as the study included case reports and case series in which no control groups were present **Results:** Out of 113 case reports and series, twenty-nine articles were included in this systematic review. Only 31% of articles have satisfied the MQCC scale and maintained as high-quality case reports, 43% of articles were medium to high quality and 26% designated as low quality. **Conclusions:** An orthodontic appliance accidentally detaches from its position, and patient can engulf due to patient's negligence, lack of its maintenance education and awareness. Orthodontist should educate, instruct and provide a written format of management, precautions. Accidental ingested foreign body can be managed in two methods, first is noninvasive, check forth airway obstruction, encourage for fiber-rich diet and laxatives. Second method is the use of endoscopically and laparoscopy with use magill's forceps.

Keywords: accidental swallow, orthodontic appliances, arch wire, mini-screw

1. Introduction

Accidental ingestion of a foreign body is more often seen in children. Contemporary studies have reported that 1500 subjects die per year [1]. However, data published on a death rate depends upon the nature of the aspirated object, i.e. size, shape, and finishing [2]. Dhandapani et al. (2009) illustrate that 80% - 90% of the aspirated foreign bodies pass through the gastrointestinal tract routinely, approximately 10–20% need to be removed endoscopically, and 1% requires surgery [3].

IntechOpen

Most researchers have described that high intake of fibrous diet; water and laxatives are the regular methods in the management of ingested blunt objects. But, accidental swallow of sharp objects always associates with a high rate of airway obstruction and gastrointestinal (GI) perforation corresponding to treatment dilemmas [1–4].

To date, various innovative appliances are being used in dentistry and orthodontics but very rare among these material limitations have been published. Through this chapter, I would like to present the associated drawbacks of such appliances to "GI" and airway systems, their clinical presentations, recommendations, and management. For a better understanding of readers, this chapter is divided into introduction, incidences; Types of appliances ingested or aspirated, Pathophysiology and associated symptoms of ingested "FBs", Management, Retrieval of accidental swallowed "FBs", Recommendations to prevent accidental swallow, Basic measures to prevent accidental swallow and Conclusion.

2. Incidences of accidental ingestion of different orthodontic appliances reported in the literature

In general, incidence of accidental aspiration of foreign body occurs in children (80%), elderly, mentally impaired, or alcoholic individuals and sometimes it may occur deliberately in prisoners or psychiatric patients. Coins, meat boli, and button batteries; sewing needles, tooth picks, straightened paper clips and razor blades are the most often ingested foreign bodies [5].

In dentistry, accidental aspiration of foreign bodies is recognized as a hurdle in all clinical specialties of dentistry. A wide range of complications succeeding from foreign bodies ("FBs") has been recognized in clinical practice as a broken denture, single-tooth crowns, inlays, edndo files, and broken orthodontic appliance's reason for the majority of "FBs" ingested by adults in the dental setting [1–6].

Kurkciyan et al. (1996), Pavlidis et al., (2008) and Dhandapani et al.,(2009) have reported that the overall incidence of dental "FBs" aspiration is higher in adult than in children, among which 10–20% required endoscopic removal and 1% alarm for surgical removal [1–7].

In orthodontics, Wasundhara A. Bhad (2011), Uday Kumar Wizziyiane Ahmad, and Priya Balakrishnan (2012), Appasaheb Naragond et al. (2013), have reported that the most frequently aspirated FBs are brackets, wire fragment, activation key, and fractured twin block, removable retention appliances, and lingual retainers. However, Tamura et al., reported that the incidence of accidental swallowing of orthodontic appliances ranges from 3.6% to 27.7% among them 2% -3.7% require emergency treatment as these foreign bodies obstruct in "GI" or respiratory tract, and the rest of the material pass "GI" without complications [7–11].

3. Types of appliances or components of orthodontic appliance ingested or aspirated

While the existing incidence of this complication in orthodontics is hypothetical, there is significant variation as to the types of appliances involved [8]. The reported "FBs" includes a lower spring retainer; fractured twin block appliance, expansion keys, fragment of a maxillary removable appliance, retainer, trans-palatal arch, and

DOI: http://dx.doi.org/10.5772/intechopen.100397

		Object	Place	Immediate symptoms	Location	Complications	Basic treatment	Final outcome
Nazif, M.M.; 1983	9 yr./f	Activation of expansion key	Home	Vomiting	Stomach	No signs of bleedings	Fiber rich diet	child's excrement
Hinkle, F.G. 1987	18/f	Retention plate	Home	Vomiting	Esophagus	Nill	Not seen	Laproscopy
Parkh house 1991	15/m	Removable plate	Home	Breathing	Esophagus	Medical emergency	Life support	Surgical removed
Lee BW 1992	15/m	Retention wire	Fast	Stomach pain	Pylorus	Bleeding in excreta	Soft diet	Gastroscope
Absi et al. 1995	25/m	Wire of Trenspalatel bar	Home	Pain and vomiting	Upper part of iliac fosse	Pain	methylcellulose, stomach filler	Proctoscopy.
Debis et al. 2000	9 /f	Digit sucking appliance(habit braking appliance)	Home	Pain, palatel laceration,	Esophagus	Due to laceration during removal	Soft diet, antibiotics and analgesics	Without surgical intervention
Milton et al. 2001	14/f	Fixed bracket	Home	Pain, bleeding excreta	Abdominal region	Antibiotics and analgesics	Fiber rich diet	came out in large bowels
Queck et al. 2002	26/m	Coil spring	Dental office	Vomiting	Stomach	pain and blood spot in excreta	Fiber rich diet antibiotics	Gastroscope
Klein et al. 2002	15/m	Retainer	Home	Plural chest pain	Chest left side	Decreased count of WBC, cough	Broad-spectrum antibiotics	rigid bronchoscopy and removed

Table 1.
Summary of all case reports.

Author	Age/ sex	Object	Place	Immediate symptoms	Location	Complications	Basic treatment	Final outcome
Sfondrini, M.F.; 2003	23/f	Broken transpalatel bar	Fast food	Bleed during speech	Upper part of GI tract	Pain,		
Abdel-Kader 2003	26/m	Fixed bracket	Home	Nill	Stomach	Pain initiated after 13 day	Soft diet, antibiotics and analgesics	Gastroscope
Al-Wahadni et al. 2006	15/f	10 mm NITI 17X25 wire	Dental office	NILL	piriform recess	Pain during food intake	Post operative pyrexia	endoscopic retrieval
Allwork et al. 2007	13/m	Quad helix	Dental office	Bleeding, vomiting	lower esophagus.	visceral perforation	Post operative pyrexia	mini-laparotomy
Fiho et al. 2008	17/f	During orthognathic surgery	Operation theater	Nill	piriform recess	Soft diet, antibiotics and analgesics	removed with Magill forceps	MacIntosh laryngoscope
Sheridan 2009	16/f	Bracketa	DENTAL OFFICE	Nill	lower esophagus.	Nill	Soft diet, antibiotics and analgesics	Gastroscope
Nicolas et al. 2009	17/m	17x25 santilone	Dental office	Nasal bleeding	Floor at junction	Nasal spray otravin	antibiotics and analgesics	Nasal endoscopy
Rohida et al. 2011	12/M	Broken twin block	Home at sleep	Pain TMJ	Upper part esophagus.	NIll	Soft diet, antibiotics and analgesics	Endoscopy
Tripathi T et al. 2011	17/m	Hyrax activation key	Home	otorhinolaryngology emergency	hypopharynx	otorhinolaryngology emergency	Magill's forcep	fiber-optic nasopharyngoscope

Table 2.
Summary of all case reports.

		Object	Place	Immediate symptoms	Location	Complications	Basic treatment	Final outcome
Monini Ada et al. 2011	9/M	Expansion key	Home	Nill	Abdominal	Nill	Fiber food and drinks	Excrited after 4 days
Umesan et al. 2012	12/F	Arch wire 17x25NITI	Dental office	Sharp pain in throat region	Laryngeal region	Nill	Fiber food and drinks	Endoscope
Naragon et al. 2013	16/M	Molar band	Home	NILL	Left lower chest	Nill	Laxative, fiber food	Endoscop with grasper
Park et al. 2013	19/m	Arch wire 19x25NITI	Dental office	Momentary pain	piriform recess	Nill	Routine food	MacIntosh laryngoscope
Hoseini 2013	29/m	Premolar bracket	Home	Gastric irritations	lower stomach.	Pancreatitis,	Metronidazole, ceftriaxone, Pantoprazol	under sedation with Midazolam
Tiller et al. 2014	37/f	Khubyoshki wire	Home	Calcification in pancreatic	Head of papillae of pancraes	PANCREATITIS	Metronidazole, ceftriaxone, Pantoprazol	Endoscope
Wilmott et al. 2016	19/F	Bracket	Home	a scratch at side of throat	Lower left posterior teeth	Pain unable to chew food	five day course of Amoxicillin	Oral and maxillofacial surgeon removed
Nikhilesh vaidya et al. 2016	11/M	Mini-screw	Dental office	Nill	Not located	Nill	Observation	Observation
Ravi Kumar Mahto, 2019	15/M	Molar band	Home	Nill	Neck Region of esophagus	Nill	Observation	Endoscopy

Table 3.
Summary of all case reports.

pieces of the arch wire [9]. In orthodontics, Hinkle published the first case of accidental aspiration of removable retainer and its retrieval report in 1987 [8–12]. The detail of cases published on accidental ingestion of various components, and their management is illustrated in **Tables 1–3**.

4. Pathophysiology and associated symptoms of ingested "FBs"

The accidental ingestion of "FBs" and appearance of any symptoms or signs is highly inconstant and depends on the age of the subject (child or an adult), movement, or impaction of "FBs". According to Susini (2007), Yadav Yadav RK (2015), Thakral A,(2015) in 75% of children accidental aspirated "FBs" have impacted at the level of the upper esophageal sphincter, and in adults 70% of the ingested FBs lodge at the level of the lower esophageal sphincter. Thus, it's crystal clear that accidental ingested"FBs"travel across a long pathway from an oropharynx to a gastrointestinal system with providing the clinical features of each stage [5, 8, 10].

4.1 "FBs" impacted at the oropharyngeal level

60% of the foreign bodies become lodged at this level. Subject presents with clear sensation of impacted "FBs", discomfort, drooling of saliva, inability to swallow, airway compromise and also infection and perforation can also occur [5–13].

4.2 "FBs" impacted at the esophageal level

If the impacted "FBs" as expansion key, twin block, removable retainer, subject (child) represents with gagging, vomiting, recurrent aspiration pneumonia and due to tracheal impingement may develop stridor or respiratory embarrassment while in adults presents with, dysphagia, and salivary drooling/pooling [5, 7, 8, 11, 14]. Wasundhara bhad and Rohida reported that the use of a broken Twin-block appliance was accidentally ingested in sleep [11, 13, 15, 16]. The patient developed immediate symptoms as breathless with a severe cough. The patient's father tried Heimlich's Maneuver method to retrieve it but failed, immediately subject shifted to emergency medical service. Endoscopically removed and confirmed that broken part of twin block located in the esophageal region [15–20].

4.3 "FBs" impacted at a sub-esophageal level

At this level delayed, symptoms develop as recurrent vomiting, passing rectal blood, and melena. Ghori et al. published case report in which removable retainer was accidentally aspirated, passed uneventfully from the elementary canal and caused perforation of the sigmoid colon proving lethal to the patient [16, 18, 20–23].

4.4 "FBs" impacted at gastrointestinal perforation

Delayed symptoms presents as with acute mediastinitis with chest pain with signs of pleural effusion and acute/subacute peritonitis. Uday Kumar Umesan et al. 2012 reported a case of accidental aspiration of arch wire segment during adjustment and were located at the laryngeal region that necessitated endoscopic retrieval in the hospital [24–29].

4.5 "FBs" impacted at body in airway

Patient present with classic triad of wheezing, coughing, and dyspnea immediate after accidental swallow; It later may develop with signs of the respiratory arrest and stridor [5–39].

5. Management

The existing incidence of accidental ingestion of "FBs" complication in orthodontics is hypothetical; there is substantial dissimilarity as to the types of appliances involved [14, 17, 30]. The literature published on accidental swallowing of "FBs" includes a lower spring retainer; broken twin block appliance, expansion keys, quad helix, transpalatel arch, and pieces of arch wire (**Tables 1–3**). Although, there is scanty evidence to pinpoint appliance or procedure has been related with an augmented risk of aspiration; the minute size of orthodontic components and saliva, limited working access, apprehensive subject, chair position, operator knowledge are the contributing factors [2, 4, 5, 7–9, 13, 16–18].

5.1 Case history

If the incident occurs in resident (outside of the clinic), a positive history of accidental swallow could be elicited. Clinician should note that a high degree of disbelief should be maintained especially in children and impaired adult while recording case report with missing orthodontic appliance fragments or components. A wise clinician must have check for clinical signs and symptoms that could appears in subject, which helps for a clinician to advice further radiographic investigation or call medical emergency service [17–21, 31].

5.2 Diagnosis

Based on case history and appearance of clinical symptoms suspicious inspection of the complete oral cavity, pharynx, larynx, and esophagus should be the first step taken. As per the pathophysiology of "FBs", and clinical signs further investigations as abdominal and chest X-rays, endoscopy, and computed tomography scans of thorax should be advised to confirm the lodgment of "FBs" [2, 3, 6, 11, 13, 14, 16–18, 22, 23, 33].

5.3 Radiographic assessment

Generally, radiographic assessment designated for subject with a positive history of accidental swallow of "FBs" within a period of less than 24 hours and without appearance of any respiratory symptoms. A chest radiograph is mandatory, but the "FB" is acrylic (radiolucent object), becomes difficult in localization of its exact position. In such situation subjects are made to swallow to identify the precise site of impaction, and ask the patient for area of uneasiness [2–26, 30–36].

If both the attempt fail to locate "FBs", a small amount of barium sulfate suspension is mixed with cotton wool pallets given to subjects to form a radio-opaque bolus around the object; this method significantly allow to track "FBs" radiographically. Also, gastrografin (a contrast agent), "CT" and "CBCT" scans have proved to be highly useful in locating the radioluscent foreign bodies [26, 38, 39].

6. Retrieval of accidental swallowed "FBs"

If accidental swallowing of FB occurred in a dental office, there are two methods to retrieve FB, the first line of action is the use for the Heimlich maneuver technique, abdominal or chest thrusts; secondly, turn the patient head one side and ask to spite; if an object does not spill out check in the oral cavity and oropharynx, supra-tonsillar recess, epiglottic vallecula and the piriform recess under good illumination and if the object is visible, it should be retrieved with forceps or high-volume suction [1, 5, 9, 12].

If the incidence occurs outside the clinic or in resident, based on case history, symptoms, diagnosis, and location of aspirated FBs subjects can be managed as Non-invasive emergency measures, Invasive emergency measures, and Surgical intervention [1, 2, 4, 9, 12, 16, 20, 24].

6.1 Non-invasive emergency measures

Size of the ingested "FBs" (larger than 6 cm in children and longer than 10 cm in adults) cause cyanosis, loss of consciousness, and permanent brain damage occurs within 4 to 6 minutes alarming a medical emergency if the obstruction is not relieved [1, 3, 6, 8, 16, 20, 34]. Therefore, speed and updated cardiopulmonary resuscitation (CPR) skills are vital for the clinician. If the "FBs" is obstructive and the patient is in respiratory distress, dislodgement should initially be attempted with back blows and abdominal thrusts (Heimlich maneuver). If this cannot dislodge the object, positive airway pressure needs to be maintained by artificial respiration until emergency services arrive [4, 5, 7, 11, 14, 21, 32, 35].

6.2 Invasive emergency measures

In this stage, "FBs" has passed the vocal cords uneventfully, but the subject requires medical attention. Few authors have reported that in 1–2% of subjects ingested "FBs" spontaneously expel, still do not wait for this to happen. Consider the entire subject as in an extreme emergency and to be escorted to the hospital for radiographic investigation to locate the position of "FBs", because 6% mortality has been reported with such subjects [4, 11, 16, 25, 32]. In this phase of emergency if the "FB" lodged in esophageal and tracheal region endoscopy is the best method to retrieve "FBs". Flexible pan endoscopy under local anesthesia is preferred for "FBs" lodged in intrathoracic areas and is accessible in tertiary medical centers. However, in this situation rigid endoscopy is recommended to reduce complication rates. Most commonly available armamentarium is Foley's catheter, passed distal to ingested "FB" under fluoroscopic guidance, inflating the balloon object can be retrieved [14, 16, 17, 21, 31, 34, 36].

6.3 Surgical intervention

This method to be opted last measure to retrieve accidental ingested "FBs". Subject gives all the clinical signs and symptoms of vital organ damage. Few authors have reported that the mortality and morbidity rates are very high in this stage. However, surgery is relatively successful opted during gastrointestinal perforation or lodgment in the airway [23, 26, 33, 36, 38].

7. Recommendations to prevent accidental swallow

During orthodontic treatment, there is always a high risk of accidental swallow or aspiration of appliance components. So the aim of the orthodontist must be to prevent and secure loose orthodontic components during treatment procedures.

Measures to be taken to minimize accidental swallow of orthodontic components include the following recommendations.

7.1 Case selection

The clinician needs to be more alert during the first consult appointment with young children, at this age group subject cannot understand and follow the instructions given by the clinician. The principal responsibility of an orthodontist is to assess the amount of cooperation that can be achieved from the patients and their parents during treatment. So an orthodontist must check complete cooperation and persistent controlling of their children to confirm that professional instructions are respected [10, 16, 23, 24, 26, 27].

The medico-legal point of that an orthodontist must opt to delay treatment until a patient's parent should give consent about their awareness of risks involved during a course of orthodontic treatment to avoid fallouts later [1, 23, 24, 27, 38].

8. Basic measures to prevent accidental swallow

8.1 Removable appliances

Operate with textured latex gloves to have a firm grip on orthodontic components. Routine visits for appliance adjustment should ensure adequate retention and its integrity. The clinician must give patient instruction in both verbal and written forms, also warn or alert them not to self-adjust or repair broken fragments instead should visit the orthodontist to ensure the appliance uprightness [11, 13, 16, 30, 33].

Use of contrast color to gastrointestinal mucosal color, in case of accidental swallows, can be identified easily during its retrieval through endoscopy [16].

During the night, wares of appliance tie a silk thread knot to either clasp assembly or active components [1–27, 30–39].

In-office, on chairside adjustment of an appliance, 7'o'clock should be the operator's position and make the patient comfortable before doing any adjustment [37].

Tie a silk thread knot to the activation key, quad helix at the time of activation, if any accidental aspiration occurs, the appliance can be securely retrieved through tied silk thread [29].

8.2 Fixed appliances

During bonding brackets, the operator should be at 7'o'clock position; use of a high-intensity light cure unit is always recommended and a high-vacuum section should be used.

Molar bands should be preferred over bondable tubes; especially in the second molar figure of ligature (. 009) should be tied to the first molar and second pre-molar [21, 26, 31, 39].

During the cutting of excessive distal end of archwire segment, use the gauze pad as protection distal tissue, adjust the length of wire outside the mouth on study models, or cinch the excess wire.

During debonding should be carried along with its base wire attachments.

9. Conclusion

Accidental swallowing of orthodontic appliances or components of it can occur often. The orthodontist must be skillful, knowledgeable, and cautious during treatment procedures. To counteract such an emergency, someone must well equip the orthodontic office, well-trained nurse staff; the medical emergency number should be maintained.

At the first consultation, an orthodontist must well educate and must make aware of demerits and accidental situations, management protocol in such as condition. The clinician must follow a protocol of prevention is better than cure.

Abbreviations used

"FB"/"FBs"	foreign bodies
"GI"	gastrointestinal Track
"CT"	cone been technique
"CBCT"	computed cone been technique
"CPR"	cardiopulmonary resuscitation

Author details

Siddharth Sonwane
Department of Orthodontics, People's College of Dental Sciences and Hospital
Bhopal, Madhya Pradesh, India

*Address all correspondence to: siddharth5678@gmail.com

References

[1] W. W. Barkmeier, R. L. Cooley, and H. Abrams, "Prevention of swallowing or aspiration of foreign objects," The Journal of the American Dental Association, vol. 97, no. 3, pp. 473-476, 1978.

[2] Amagasa, T" Iwaki, H., Watanabe, A. & Siiimizu, M.: Accidental swallowing and aspiration during dental practice. Nippon Dent, Rei', 1979: 438: 121-129.

[3] Awataguciu, S., Miyano, K., Maruyama, H. & Hakamada, M.: A clinical study of 63 cases with foreign bodies of the tracheobronchial tree. I. Jpn. Bronchoesophagol. Soc. 1980: 31: 315-321.

[4] Nazif, M.M.; Ready, M.A. Accidental swallowing of orthodontic expansion appliance keys: Report of two cases. ASDC J. Dent. Child. 1983, 50, 126-127.

[5] N. Tamura, T. Nakajima, and S.Matsumoto, "Foreign bodies of dental origin in the air and food passages," International Journal of Oral and Maxillofacial Surgery, vol. 15, no. 6, pp. 739-751,1986.

[6] Hinkle, F.G. Ingested retainer: A case report. Am. J. Orthod. Dentofac. Orthop. 1987, 92, 46-49.

[7] Parkhouse, R.C. Medical complication in orthodontics. Br. J. Orthod. 1991, 18, 51-57.

[8] Lee, B.W. Case report. Swallowed piece of archwire. Aust. Orthod. 1992, 12, 169-170.

[9] Kharbanda OP, Varshney P, Dutta U. Accidental swallowing of a gold cast crown during orthodontic tooth separation. J Clin Pediatr Dent 1995; 19: 289-92.

[10] E. G. Absi and J. G. Buckley, "The location and tracking of swallowed dental appliances: the role of radiology," Dentomaxillofacial Radiology, vol. 24, no. 2, pp. 139-142, 1995.

[11] Kürkciyan I, Frossard M, Kettenbach J et al. Conservative management of foreign bodies in the gastrointestinal tract. Z Gastroenterol 1996; 34(3): 173-77

[12] Aytac¸, Y. Yurdakul, C. Ikizler, R. Olga, and A. Saylam, "Inhalation of foreign bodies in children. Report of 500 cases," Journal ofThoracic and Cardiovascular Surgery, vol. 74,no. 1, pp. 145-151, 1977.

[13] T. Henderson, J. Engel, and P. Schlesinger, "Foreign body ingestion: review and suggested guidelines for management," Endoscopy, vol. 19, no. 2, pp. 68-71, 1987.

[14] T.M.Milton, S. D. Hearing, andA. J. Ireland, "Ingested foreign bodies associated with orthodontic treatment: report of three cases and review of ingestion/aspiration incident management," British Dental Journal, vol. 190, no. 11, pp. 592-596, 2001.

[15] Quick, A.N.; Harris, A.M. Accidental ingestion of a component of a fixed orthodontic appliance—A case report. SADJ 2002, 57, 101-104.

[16] Klein AM, Schoem SR. Unrecognized aspiration of a dental retainer: a case report. Otolaryngol Head Neck Surg 2002; 126(4): 438-39.

[17] Sfondrini MF, Cacciafesta V, Lena A. Accidental ingestion of a rapid palatal expander. J Clin Orthod 2003; 37(4): 201-202.

[18] Tiwana KK, Morton T, Tiwana PS. Aspiration and ingestion in dental practice: a 10-year institutional review. J Am Dent Assoc 2004; 135(9): 1287-91.

[19] Coulier B, Tancredi MH, Ramboux A. Spiral CT and multidetector-row CT diagnosis of perforation of the small intestine caused by ingested foreign bodies. Eur Radiol 2004; 14: 1918 25.

[20] Al-Wahadni, A.; Al-Hamad, K.Q.; Al-Tarawneh, A. Foreign body ingestion and aspiration in dentistry: A review of the literature and reports of three cases. Dent. Update 2006, 33, 561-570.

[21] Uyemura MC. Foreign body ingestion in children. Am Fam Physician 2006; 73(8): 1332

[22] Allwork JJ, Edwards IR, Welch IM. Ingestion of a quadhelix appliance requiring surgical removal: A case report. J Orthod Sep 2007; 34(3): 154-57.

[23] Laureano Filho JR, Godoy F, O'Ryan F. Orthodontic bracket lost in the airway during orthognathic surgery. Am J Orthod Dentofacial Orthop 2008; 134(2): 288-90.

[24] Obinata K, Satoh T, Towfik AM et al. An investigation of accidental ingestion during dental procedures. J Oral Sci 2011; 53: 495-500.

[25] Umesan UK, Chua KL, Balakrishnan P. Prevention and management of accidental foreign body ingestion and aspiration in orthodontic practice. Therapeutics and Clinical Risk Management 2012; 8: 245-52.

[26] Naragond, A.; Kengenal, S.; Rajasigamani, K.; Kumar, N.S. Accidental ingestion of molar band and its management: Maintenance is better than management. Case Rep. Dent. 2013.

[27] Tiller, M.; Schepp,W.; Gundling, F.; Tuerck, J. Chronic pancreatitis caused by a swallowed orthodontic device. Endoscopy 2014, 46, E667–E668.

[28] Murad MH,Sultan S, Haffar S, et al. Methodological quality and synthesis of case series and case reports BMJEvidence-Based Medicine 2018;23:60-63.

[29] Nikhilesh V, Pratik S, Meghna V. Oops! There goes my miniscrew!. APOS Trends Orthod 2016;6:277-80.

[30] Dibiase, A.T.; Samuels, R.H.A.; Ozdiler, E.; Akcam, M.O.; Turkkahraman, H. Hazards of orthodontic appliances and the oropharynx. J. Orthod. 2000, 27, 295-302.

[31] Nicolas R, Eggers G, Komposch G. Orthodontic archwire in the nasal cavity: A case report (in English, German). J Orofac Orthop 2009; 70(1): 92- 97.

[32] Sheridan, A. Orthodontic Bracket lost in airway. Am. J. Orthod. Dentofac. Orthop. 2009, 135.

[33] Rohida,N.S.; Bhad,W.A.Accidental ingestion of a fractured Twin-block appliance. Am. J.Orthod. Dentofac. Orthop.2011, 139, 123-125.

[34] Tipathi, T.; Rai, P.; Singh, H. Foreign body ingestion of orthodontic origin. Am. J. Orthod. Dentofac. Orthop.2011, 139, 279-283.

[35] Monini Ada, C.; Maia, L.G.; Gandini, L.G. Accidental swallowing of an orthodontic expansion appliance key. Am. J. Orthod. Dentofac. Orthop. 2011, 140, 266-268.

[36] Hoseini M, Mostafavi SMS, Rezaei N et al. Orthodontic wire ingestion during treatment: Reporting a case and review

the management of foreign body ingestion or aspiration (emergencies). Case Reports in Dentistry 2013; Article ID 426591

[37] Park, J.H.; Owtad, P.; Milde, B. Incident Management guidelines for an Ingested Orthodontic Object. IJO 2013, 24, 43-47.

[38] Ozturk K, Turhal G, Gode S et al. Migration of a swallowed blunt foreign body to the neck. Case Rep Otolaryngol 2014: 646785.

[39] Wilmott, S.E.; Ikeaqwuani, O.; McLeod, N.M. An orthodontic bracket embedded in the medial pterygoid surface: A case report. J. Orthod. 2016, 43, 65-67.

Section 4

Early Treatment

Chapter 16

A Removable Class III Traction Appliance for Early Class III Treatment

Kristin N. Moore, David R. Musich, Donald Taylor, Budi Kusnoto and Carla A. Evans

Abstract

Maxillary, mandibular, and dental effects resulting from the use of a removable intraoral Class III traction appliance as well as the protraction facemask in treatment of Class III malocclusion were assessed. This is a retrospective study comparing measurements from pre-treatment and post-treatment lateral cephalometric radiographs of two groups. Group 1 consisted of 25 patients treated with rapid palatal expansion followed by a removable intraoral Class III traction appliance. Group 2 consisted of 25 patients treated with rapid palatal expansion followed by a protraction facemask. The subjects were Caucasian, both male and female, with an age range of 3 to 12 years. The only significant differences were in length of treatment time and the skeletal change of angle SNA. The mean treatment times were 6.96 months and 10.96 months in the removable Class III traction appliance and protraction facemask groups, respectively. The mean increase in SNA was 0.46 degrees in the removable Class III traction appliance group and 1.81 degrees in the protraction facemask group. A removable Class III traction appliance provides orthodontists with another useful Class III treatment modality.

Keywords: Class III malocclusion, Class III treatment, protraction facemask, traction, orthodontics

1. Introduction

Class III malocclusion can result from mandibular prognathism, maxillary skeletal retrusion or a combination of both [1]. Many treatment philosophies and appliances have been used to treat this problem, such as protraction facemask, chin cup, and Frankel's FR-III appliance and orthognathic surgery. Miniplates and temporary anchorage devices are also being used in order to minimize the negative side effects that can occur with treatment. In Class III malocclusion, an accurate diagnosis and timing of treatment are considerations in order to achieve optimal results.

The orthopedic facemask was developed in the 1960's by Delaire [2] and has been shown to be effective in treatment of Class III malocclusion in early mixed or late mixed dentition. It can assist in correction of maxillary skeletal retrusion, maxillary

 IntechOpen

dentoalveolar retrusion, mandibular prognathism, and decreased lower facial height. It can produce the following effects: correction of a centric occlusion to centric relation (CO-CR) discrepancy, forward movement of the maxilla, forward movement of the maxillary dentition, lingual tipping of the lower incisors, and the downward and backward movement of the mandible [3]. The protraction facemask applies an anterior force on the circummaxillary sutures and stimulates bone apposition in suture areas [4]. Generally the facemask is prescribed to be worn by the patient for 12 to 16 hours per day with forces ranging between 180 g and 500 g [4, 5]. It has been suggested that the facemask be worn until the patient achieves approximately 4-5 mm of positive overjet [3]. It is often used in combination with a rapid palatal expander.

Macdonald et al. [6] found that facemask treatment increased the convexity of the facial profile due to the forward displacement and downward and backward rotation of the maxilla as well an opening rotation of the mandible. The maxillary incisors moved forward as the mandibular incisors retruded. Ngan et al. [7] found that the maxilla moved forward an average of 2.1 mm and the molar relationship corrected to Class I or even Class II relationship. In addition, the lower face height increased and the overbite decreased by an average of 1.5 mm. Nartallo-Turley and Turley [8] found an increase in SNA, maxillary depth, and ANB as well as forward movement of A-point and ANS. The maxilla moved forward and rotated counter-clockwise and the mandible rotated clockwise as the SNB and facial depth decreased.

Intraoral devices for treatment of Class III malocclusions [9, 10] have been described. A removable Class III traction appliance using elastics to produce the desired vector of force (**Figures 1a** and **1b**) was developed in the 1980's to overcome issues of patient compliance with the protraction facemask. It can be used in conjunction with rapid palatal expansion or fixed appliances in Class III treatment. This removable appliance can be used at any age and aids in disclusion of the dentition as well as directional traction as it addresses maxillary skeletal retrusion, maxillary dentoalveolar retrusion, and functional shifts associated with mandibular prognathism [11]. Similar to protraction facemask, it is said to have the following effects: correction of a CO-CR discrepancy, forward and downward displacement of the maxilla, forward movement of the maxillary dentition, lingual tipping of the lower incisors, and the downward and backward movement of the mandible. The appliance is worn by the patient full time (20–22 hours per day) sometimes in conjunction with a rapid palatal expander and/or partial or full braces treatment until 3-4 mm of positive overjet is achieved [10].

The main advantages for the removable Class III traction device are the capacity to have light, continuous, full-time forces acting to disarticulate the occlusion and allow correction of the posterior and anterior crossbites with minimal occlusal interference. 4–8 ounce elastics are recommended for younger patients and heavier forces are recommended for older patients. 10–12 ounce elastics are sometimes recommended at night based on individual patient needs. If needed, a removable appliance could be used in conjunction with a facemask at night. Another advantage of the removable appliance is that it is easy to gain optimal compliance in patients and is tolerated well by the patient.

Some disadvantages have been reported with the removable orthodontic traction device. In the mixed dentition, strong retention from the composite ridges can accelerate exfoliation of the primary canines, compromising the anchor teeth and causing some discomfort to the patient. For this reason, it is recommended that the retentive ridges be used on teeth with the best root structure. The appliance can also experience significant wear if patients have a nocturnal bruxism habit. However, replacement of the appliance is simple and inexpensive.

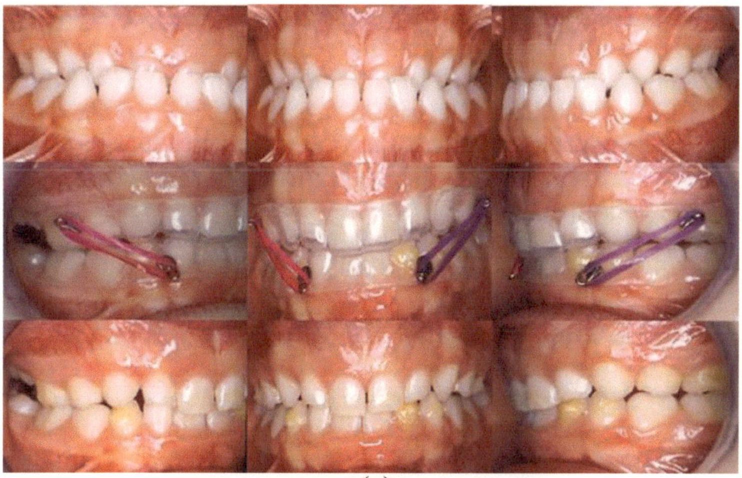

(a)

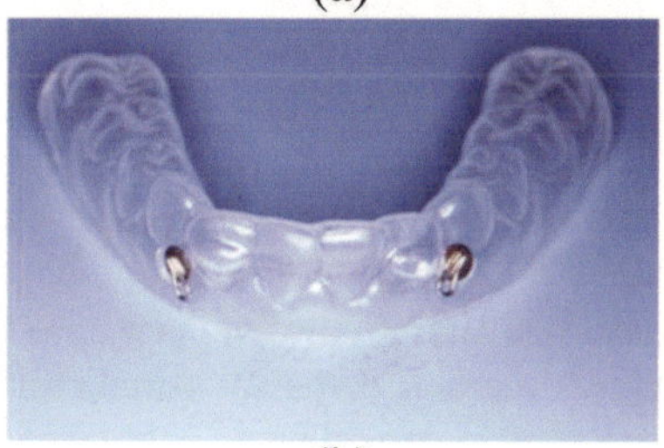

(b)

Figure 1.
(a) Anterior crossbite correction using the removable traction appliance followed by a retention phase using the same appliance. Retention ridges can be seen in the bottom row. (b) Location of hooks on the lower removable traction appliance.

This study was designed to determine whether treatment of Class III malocclusion with a removable Class III traction appliance has outcomes similar to a protraction facemask. Specifically, the objectives were to compare maxillary, mandibular, and dental effects resulting from use of both appliances.

2. Comparison of removable traction appliance and protraction facemask

2.1 Methods

The removable orthodontic traction device described in this chapter (**Figures 1a** and **1b**) is relatively inexpensive and easy to fabricate. The first step in making this appliance is the application of retentive ridges to several of the patient's mandibular teeth especially in the anterior region. This is done by etching the tooth and then applying a composite resin to the surface of the tooth in a ridge shape, about 75% of the mesial-distal tooth width and 2-3 mm in height. Next, an impression is taken of the arch and a stone model is fabricated. Separating medium is applied to the cast and allowed to dry. A vacuum formed type retainer using C+ plastic from DENTSPLY Raintree Essix (DENTSPLY Raintree Essix, Sarasota, Florida, USA) is fabricated on the model. Durasoft® or Biocryl® from Great Lakes Orthodontics

(Great Lakes Orthodontics, Ltd., Tonawanda, New York, USA) can also be used. If a hygienic fixed expander is in place, a similar removable appliance can be made for attachment of elastics to the maxillary arch. After trimming, Caplin hooks (DENTSPLY GAC International, Bohemia, NY, USA) are added to the retainers in the upper molar and lower canine regions by heating each hook with a torch and pressing it into the appropriate area on the appliance, ensuring it does not melt completely through the plastic (**Figure 1b**). After ensuring the hooks are secure, the appliance is inserted into the patient's mouth and traction is initiated using Class III elastics. The patient is instructed to wear the appliance full time. Monthly visits are recommended to monitor for progress [10].

In this retrospective study, Group 1 consisted of 25 Caucasian patients from a private orthodontic practice who had been treated with rapid palatal expansion (hygienic Hyrax™ expander) followed by the removable intraoral Class III traction appliance and 180 g force from Class III elastics. Group 2 consisted of 25 Caucasian patients treated with a rapid palatal expansion (hygienic Hyrax™ expander) followed by a protraction facemask (AD Protraction Facemask; Ormco, Orange, CA, USA) with 350-400 g traction, taken from a different private orthodontic practice. Patient data from both offices were collected, de-identified, and assigned case numbers by the private practice orthodontists. Patients from both groups were treated until positive overjet was achieved. The inclusion criteria for both groups were an initial diagnosis of a dental and skeletal Class III malocclusion based on an ANB angle less than 0 degrees, Wits appraisal less than 0, and at least 25% Class III molar relationship in permanent or primary molars. If any functional shifts were present, they were not recorded and thus not taken into consideration. Patients were excluded if any of the following were present: dentofacial deformities (i.e. cleft lip and palate), missing teeth, periodontal disease, or prior treatment elsewhere.

The patients' pre-treatment (T1) and post-treatment (T2) lateral cephalometric radiographs were collected, scanned and digitized. The radiographs were uploaded and traced using Dolphin software (Dolphin, Chatsworth, CA, USA). Skeletal and dental measurements were collected. The landmarks seen in **Figure 2** were used in the cephalometric analysis. The following cephalometric measurements were used: SNA, SNB, ANB, Wits appraisal, Y axis, angle of convexity, mandibular plane angle, facial angle, cant of occlusal plane, upper incisor to SN, lower incisor to mandibular plane, interincisal angle, upper incisor to NA, lower incisor to NB, overbite, overjet, millimeter measurement from sella perpendicular to palatal plane to maxillary molar, millimeter measurement from sella perpendicular to palatal plane to maxillary incisor, millimeter measurement from sella perpendicular to palatal plane to mandibular molar, millimeter measurement from sella perpendicular to palatal plane to mandibular incisor, millimeter measurement from sella to A point, millimeter measurement from PTM to ANS.

A statistical power analysis determined that a sample of 20–25 subjects would yield a power of 0.8 which would provide statistically significant results. Intra-reliability and inter-reliability tests all had a correlation of 0.8 or above and those values were considered to be reliable. An independent *t*-test was used to compare sample descriptives, and to compare T1 values. An independent *t*-test for parametric data and a Mann–Whitney test for non-parametric data was utilized to evaluate mean differences between groups. Also, as another indicator of similarity of samples, cervical vertebral maturation (CVM) stage for T1 and T2 for both groups, means and standard deviations were calculated according to the method of Baccetti et al. [12].

DOI: http://dx.doi.org/10.5772/intechopen.99885

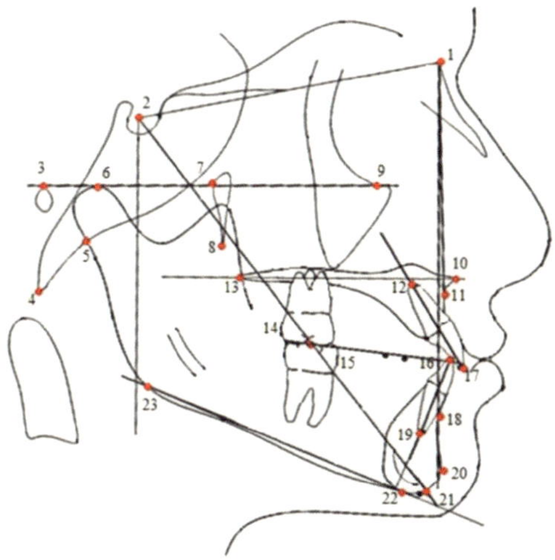

Figure 2.
Landmarks: 1-Nasion (N); 2-Sella (S); 3-Porion (Po); 4-Basion (Ba); 5-Articulare (Ar); 6-Condylion (Co); 7-PT point; 8-Pterygomaxillare (PTM); 9-Orbitale (or); 10-anterior nasal spine (ANS); 11-Subspinale (a); 12-upper central incisor root tip; 13-posterior nasal spine (PNS); 14-upper first molar occlusal; 15-lower first molar occlusal; 16-lower central incisor crown; 17-upper central incisor crown; 18-Supramentale (B); 19-lower central incisor root; 20-Pogonion (Pog); 21-Gnathion (Gn); 22-Menton (me); 23-Gonion (go).

2.2 Results

2.2.1 Sample descriptives

Means and standard deviations were calculated for both T1 and T2 chronological ages for both groups (**Table 1**). The mean age for Group 1 at T1 was 8 years, 8 months and at T2 was 10 years, 6 months. The mean age for Group 2 at T1 was 8 years, 9 months and at T2 was 11 years, 1 month. An independent *t*-test showed that no significant differences existed among the T1 and T2 chronological ages between groups ($p>0.05$). To examine cervical vertebral maturation (CVM) stages for T1 and T2 for both groups, means and standard deviations were calculated. The mean CVM

Group	Traction	Protaction facemask
Total number of patients	25	25
Number of males	13	13
Number of females	12	12
Average age (years)	8.74	8.87
Age range (years)	3.11–12.1 (SD 2.08)	6.9–12.1 (SD 1.47)
Average CVM	2	2
CVM range	2–3	2–5
Average treatment time (months)	6.96*	10.96*
Range of treatment time (months)	2–20	4–18
*Indicates $p < 0.001$.		

Table 1.
Sample characteristics.

for group 1 at T1 was 2.1 and at T2, 2.8. The mean CVM for group 2 at T1 was 2.4 and at T2, 3.1. An independent *t*-test showed that no significant differences occurred at T1 and T2 between groups. For length of treatment of both groups, an independent *t*-test was used and showed that significant differences existed between groups ($p<0.05$).

2.2.2 Comparison of T1 values and T2 values between groups

Independent *t*-tests were used to evaluate if any differences existed among the T1 values and the T2 values between groups. It was found that no significant differences existed among the T1 values between groups ($p>0.05$).

2.2.3 Comparison of T2-T1 differences between groups

Differences between T2 and T1 were calculated for each variable within each group (**Tables 2** and **3**). An independent *t*-test was used to evaluate if any significant differences existed among the changes from T1 to T2 between groups for parametric data. A Mann–Whitney test was used for non-parametric data (group 2 for sella to A point and millimeter measurement of Ptm to ANS). SNA showed that significant differences existed between groups ($p<0.05$). All other values showed no significant differences between group 1 and group 2 ($p>0.05$).

2.3 Discussion

Both groups started and ended treatment at similar chronologic ages. Since chronologic age is only a rough indicator of maturity, cervical vertebral maturation stage was examined for both groups. Peak mandibular growth or the pubertal growth spurt has been found to occur between stages 3 and 4 with active growth having been completed at stage 6 [12]. Baccetti et al. [12] suggested that Class III treatment with rapid maxillary expansion and protraction facemask therapy should be started during stages 1 and 2 in order to produce the most effective results on the maxilla. Both groups had a mean initial CVM of stage 2 which correlates to pre-pubertal growth peak. No significant differences in CVM stage existed at T1 and T2 between groups suggesting that both groups were similar with regards to skeletal maturation before and after treatment.

The significant difference in treatment times may have affected the outcomes between groups. The protraction facemask was used for a greater period of time on average than the removable Class III traction appliance and has a direct effect on the maxilla. Thus, with a greater treatment time one could expect more change at SNA, which may have contributed to the significantly increased SNA in the protraction facemask treated group when compared with the removable Class III traction appliance treated group. The outcomes of the protraction facemask treated group were consistent with studies conducted by Nartallo-Turley and Turley [8], Ngan et al. [7], and Macdonald et al. [6].

No significant differences were found between groups comparing Wits appraisal, ANB, FMA, Y-axis, cant of the occlusal plane, Sella to A point, PTM to ANS, and angle of convexity. This may suggest that both appliances produced similar results in the maxilla and rotation of the mandible. It was also found that both groups exhibited proclination of the upper incisors, mesial movement of the upper and lower dentition, uprighting of the lower incisors, increase in interincisal angle, increase in overjet and increase in overbite similar to the studies by Nartallo-Turley and Turley [8], Ngan et al. [7], and Macdonald et al. [6].

Angular measurements (degrees)	Group	Mean	Standard deviation	t	df	Significance (2-tailed)
Facial angle	1	0.41	2.49	0.23	48	0.82
	2	0.24	2.62			
Angle of convexity	1	−0.28	2.41	−1.66	32.74	0.11
	2	1.73	5.55			
SNA	1	0.46	1.71	−2.61	48	0.01*
	2	1.81	1.96			
SNB	1	0.15	1.48	−1.71	48	0.09
	2	0.92	1.71			
ANB	1	0.30	1.35	−1.04	36.71	0.31
	2	0.90	2.53			
FMA	1	0.02	3.23	−0.03	48	0.97
	2	0.05	2.92			
Y axis	1	0.36	2.50	−0.11	48	0.91
	2	0.44	2.42			
Cant of occlusal plane	1	−1.24	4.00	1.16	48	0.25
	2	−2.47	3.52			
Interincisal angle	1	−2.70	7.08	0.15	42.80	0.88
	2	−3.07	10.19			
U1-SN	1	4.25	6.04	−0.67	48	0.51
	2	5.58	7.82			
U1-NA	1	3.81	5.97	0.02	43.51	0.98
	2	3.76	8.33			
L1-MP	1	−1.40	5.28	0.28	48	0.78
	2	−1.82	5.55			
L1-NB	1	−1.41	4.88	0.13	48	0.90
	2	−1.59	5.13			

**Indicates $p < 0.05$.*

Table 2.
Comparison of T2-T1 angular differences between groups ($N = 25$).

The strength of this study is that it evaluated the effects of using a removable Class III traction appliance. Since the results showed that no statistical differences existed for dental and all but one of the skeletal variables between groups, the removable Class III traction appliance could be used as another minimally invasive Class III treatment modality for patients. Further studies of removable Class III traction appliances should implement a randomized patient assignment prospectively as well as obtain long-term results in order to evaluate their overall effectiveness.

Conventional protraction facemask therapy has been found in multiple studies to be effective; however, compliance is a major limitation. Patients often view the protraction facemask as awkward at best and complain about it being difficult to wear and interfering with sleep. Cole [13] evaluated patient compliance using headgear to treat Class II malocclusion; patients were fitted with a commercially available timing

Linear measurements (mm)	Group	Mean	Standard deviation	t	df	Significance (2-tailed)
Wits appraisal	1	1.28	4.38	−0.25	48	0.80
	2	1.56	3.41			
U1-NA	1	1.09	2.03	−0.45	48	0.66
	2	1.37	2.38			
L1-NB	1	−0.32	1.30	0.08	48	0.93
	2	−0.35	1.44			
Overbite	1	1.19	2.47	0.71	48	0.48
	2	0.78	1.49			
Overjet	1	1.88	2.80	−1.19	48	0.24
	2	2.73	2.19			
Distance from sella ⊥ to maxillary molar occlusal	1	2.32	3.26	−1.70	48	0.10
	2	3.90	3.32			
Distance from sella ⊥ to maxillary incisor	1	3.52	4.26	−0.39	48	0.70
	2	3.95	3.52			
Distance from sella ⊥ to mandibular molar occlusal	1	2.41	2.45	−1.89	48	0.06
	2	3.72	2.45			
Distance from sella ⊥ to mandibular incisor	1	1.19	2.64	−1.08	40.67	0.29
	2	1.87	1.68			

$p < 0.05$.

Table 3.
Comparison of T2-T1 linear differences between groups (N = 25).

headgear that measured the amount of headgear wear. Compliance levels varied from 5.6% to 107.7% with a mean of 74.4%. It was found that most patients reported more headgear wear than what actually took place. Poor patient compliance with headgear or facemask can contribute to poor outcomes in treatment.

Since the removable orthodontic traction device is an intraoral appliance, it is possible for patients to adapt to wearing the appliance full time. Patients may not view this removable intraoral appliance with the same annoyance as they do the protraction facemask. If any minimally invasive treatment modalities can be used with predictability, it has great benefit as significant risk and cost is reduced in the care of the patient.

Based on the outcomes of this study comparing a removable Class III traction appliance and protraction facemask for the treatment of Class III malocclusion, it seems that both appliances are effective treatment modalities. Each appliance has its advantages and disadvantages and each treatment modality should be selected on a patient-by-patient basis.

3. Conclusion

A removable intraoral Class III traction appliance provides orthodontists with a useful noninvasive treatment alternative to protraction facemask in young patients presenting with Class III malocclusions. Both treatments resolved the Class III dental relationships; only slight differences in outcomes were found between the protraction facemask and removable Class III traction appliance, namely, time in treatment and change in angle SNA were both slightly larger in the protraction facemask patients. It is common for orthodontists to treat using a protraction facemask, but if similar results can be achieved by using a removable Class III removable traction appliance, then it may be advantageous to consider this appliance as an option for some Class III patients.

Conflict of interest

The authors declare no conflict of interest.

Abbreviations

CO	centric occlusion
CR	centric relation
CVM	cervical vertebral maturation
mm	millimeter
T1	pre-treatment
T2	post-treatment

Author details

Kristin N. Moore[1], David R. Musich[2], Donald Taylor[3], Budi Kusnoto[4] and Carla A. Evans[5]*

1 Lake Zurich, IL, USA

2 Schaumburg, IL, USA

3 Montreal, QC, Canada

4 University of Illinois at Chicago, Chicago, IL, USA

5 Boston University, Boston, MA, USA

*Address all correspondence to: caevans@bu.edu

References

[1] Guyer EC, Ellis EE, McNamara JA, Behrents RG. Components of class III malocclusion in juveniles and adolescents. Angle Orthod 1986;56:7-30.

[2] Delaire J. L'emploi physiologique des tractions extra-orales postero-anterieures sur masque orthopedique dans Ie traitement des classes III. Orthod Fr 1988;59:577-589.

[3] McNamara JA. Treatment of patients in the mixed dentition. In: Orthodontics: Current Principles and Techniques, ed. TM Graber, RL Vanarsdall, KWL Vig, Elsevier Mosby, St. Louis, 2005, pp. 543-577.

[4] Şar Ç, Arman-Özçipici A, Uçkan S, Yazici AC. Comparative evaluation of maxillary protraction with or without skeletal anchorage. Am J Orthod Dentofacial Orthop 2011;139:636-649.

[5] Yepes E, Quintero P, Rueda ZV, Pedvoza A. Optimal force for maxillary protraction facemask therapy in the early treatment of class III malocclusion. Eur J Orthod 2014;36:586-594.

[6] Macdonald KE, Kapust AJ, Turley PK. Cephalometric changes after the correction of class III malocclusion with maxillary/facemask therapy. Am J Orthod Dentofacial Orthop 1999;116:13-24.

[7] Ngan, P., Yiu, C., Hu, A., Hägg, U., Wei, S.H., and Gunel, E. Cephalometric and occlusal changes following maxillary expansion and protraction. Eur. J. Orthod. 20:237-254, 1998.

[8] Nartallo-Turley PE, Turley PK. Cephalometric effects of combined palatal expansion and facemask therapy on class III malocclusion. Angle Orthod 1998;68:217-224.

[9] Vanlaecken R, Williams MO, Razmus T, Gunels E, Martin C, Ngan P. Class III correction using an inter-arch spring-loaded module. Prog Orthod 2014;15:32.

[10] Musich DR, Busch MJ. Clinical management of the class III growing patient. Int Orthod Kieferorthop 2008;40:13-26.

[11] White LW. Orthodontic Pearls: A Clinician's Guide. Self-Published, 2011, p. 115.

[12] Baccetti T, Franchi L, McNamara JA. The cervical vertebral maturation (CVM) method for the assessment of optimal treatment timing in dentofacial orthopedics. Semin Orthod 2005;11:119-129.

[13] Cole W. Accuracy of patient reporting as an indication of headgear compliance. Am J Orthod Dentofacial Orthop 2002;121:419-423.

Chapter 17

Bridging the Gap: Nasoalveolar Moulding in Early Cleft Palate Rehabilitation

Amanda Nadia Ferreira

Abstract

Orofacial clefts (OFC) are among the commonest birth defect in developed and developing countries alike. In underdeveloped and developing countries, babies born with oral clefts are generally anaemic with low birth weight and may be unfit for surgery. The surgical reconstruction is also challenging and the aesthetic outcome cannot be guaranteed by the surgeon. Presurgical nasoalveolar moulding (PNAM) has been suggested to bridge the gap between the clefted segments before surgical repair. It is a simple yet effective technique that needs to be initiated at the right time and age to achieve ideal functional and aesthetic outcomes. This chapter highlights the effectiveness of the nasoalveolar moulding technique and details the manner in which the appliance is fabricated and activated.

Keywords: presurgical nasoalveolar moulding, feeder plate, clept lip and palate

1. Introduction

Each year, around 250,000 babies are born with some form of orofacial clefts [1]. Worldwide, the incidence of cleft is reported in one of every 600–800 newborns [2]. A vast majority of these babies are born in underdeveloped or developing countries. This already deplorable situation is aggravated by the fact that most of these cases are concentrated in rural areas where access to health care is severely inadequate or unavailable as compared to urban cities [3, 4].

In developed countries, cleft lip/palate (CL/P) is identified before birth by ultrasonography, which gives the parents much needed time for education and counselling regarding the additional care needed after birth. Consequently, due to the widespread access to medical care and scientific data, aetiology is scientifically understood to be due to a combination of genetic and environmental factors. In contrast, in developing countries prenatal care is less advanced or limited, a CL/P is usually unexpected and families rely less on medical explanations for the cleft and rely more on religion and folklore to explain the deformity [5].

Veau [6] classified clefts into (**Figure 1**).

Group I: Cleft involving the soft palate alone.

Group II: Cleft involving the hard and soft palate up to the incisive foramen.

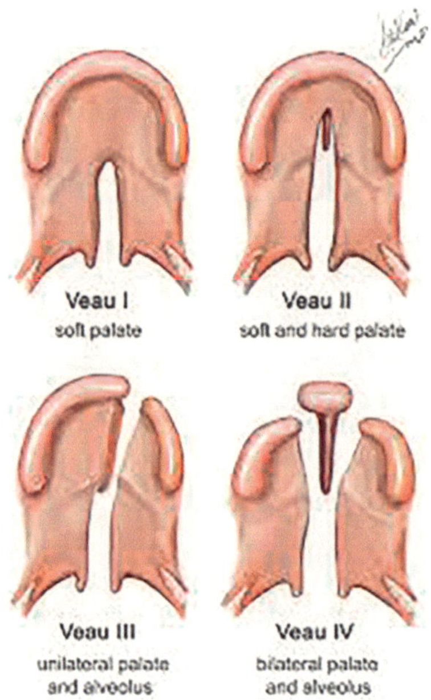

Figure 1.
Veau's classification.

Group III: Complete unilateral cleft involving the soft and hard palate, the lip and alveolar ridge on one side.

Group IV: Complete bilateral cleft involving the soft and hard palate, the lip and alveolar ridge on both sides.

Successful rehabilitation of all these cases requires a multidisciplinary approach. Patients with orofacial clefts need to be treated at the right time and age to achieve functional and aesthetic well-being. The management of the child born with a cleft lip and palate requires coordinated care provided by a cleft care team [7], comprising of different individuals belonging to several specialities in:

1. Dental specialities (orthodontics, oral surgery, paediatric dentistry and prosthodontics),

2. Medical specialities (genetics, otolaryngology, paediatrics, plastic surgery and psychiatry),

3. Allied health care fields (audiology, nursing, psychology, social work and speech pathology)

In many developing countries, there are several unrepaired cleft patients due to the mismatch between the volume of patients and resources. Furthermore, babies who are born underweight or anaemic are not suitable for surgery. There is also an acute shortage of qualified surgeons available to treat them [8]. This results in patients who cannot reach their full social and economic potential [9]. Surgical repair alone cannot address the multiple issues encountered in patients with cleft lip and palate. One specific task is the aesthetic recreation of the deficient columella. The earliest mention of presurgical infant orthopaedics was in the 1950s. This adjunctive therapy reduced the severity of the initial cleft deformity before surgery. This enabled the surgeon to enjoy the benefits associated with surgical repair in an infant with a minimal cleft deformity and reduced the need for a secondary surgery [10].

This chapter describes the technique of presurgical nasoalveolar moulding (PNAM), which was first described by Grayson et al. [11] in 1993 and had several modifications made over the years by Brecht et al. [12] in 1995, Grayson and Santiago [13] in 1997 and Cutting et al. [14] in 1998. This approach involves the active moulding and repositioning of the deformed nasal cartilages and alveolar process and lengthening the deficient columella, using the NAM appliance which consists of nasal stents attached to an intraoral moulding plate to aid in the moulding of the clefted alveolar ridge and nasal cartilage. The primary goal of PNAM is to achieve good arch form and eventually stabilisation.

The concept of NAM works on Matsuo's principle that a high degree of plasticity is seen in the cartilages of infants in the first few months after birth. A high amount of circulating maternal oestrogen causes an increase in the amount of hyaluronic acid in the fetal cartilage, rendering it plastic. Hence, active soft tissue and cartilage moulding are most successful if initiated within the first 6 weeks of life [15].

2. Unilateral orofacial cleft lip and palate

Clinical examinations of babies born with unilateral cleft lip and palate often show significant nasal deformities. The lower lateral alar cartilage is concave and

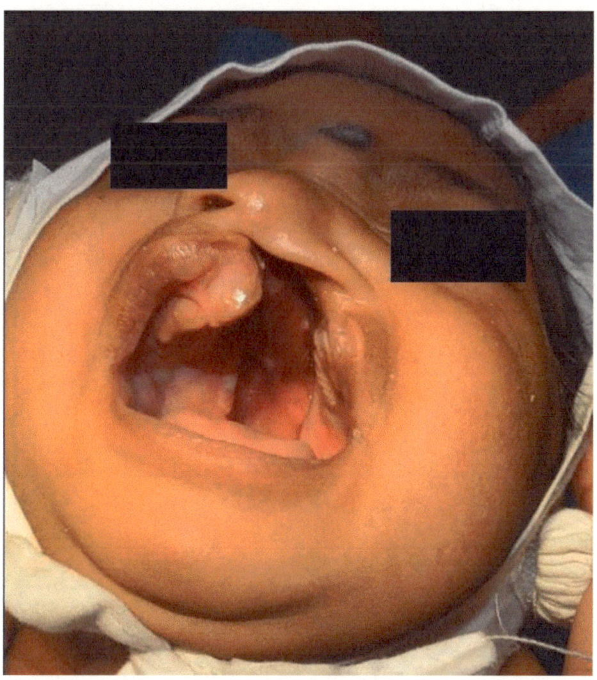

Figure 2.
Unilateral orofacial cleft lip and palate.

depressed in the alar rim and separated from the contralateral cartilage. This results in a depressed nasal tip and possibly an overhang of the apex of the nostril. The columella and nasal septum are deviated towards the cleft, and the base towards the non-cleft side. Furthermore, the orbicularis oris muscle in the lateral lip segments contracts into a bulge with some fibres running superiorly along the margins of the cleft towards the nasal tip (**Figure 2**) [16, 17].

3. Bilateral orofacial cleft lip and palate

Babies born with bilateral cleft lip and palate often present a challenge to the cleft care team. In these cases, the alar cartilages have failed to migrate up into the nasal tip and stretch the columella. So, the cartilages are positioned along the alar margins and are stretched over the cleft as flaring alae. The prolabium also lacks muscle tissue and is positioned directly on the end of the shortened columella. In the complete bilateral cleft, the premaxilla is suspended from the tip of the nasal septum, while the clefted alveolar segments stay behind (**Figure 3**) [18, 19]. The primary issue in these cases is that the premaxilla is unattached laterally and is positioned far too anteriorly by the time lip surgery is scheduled. Secondly, in some cases, the lateral width of the premaxilla exceeds the anterior space between the two lateral maxillary segments. A combination of these two challenges may also exist.

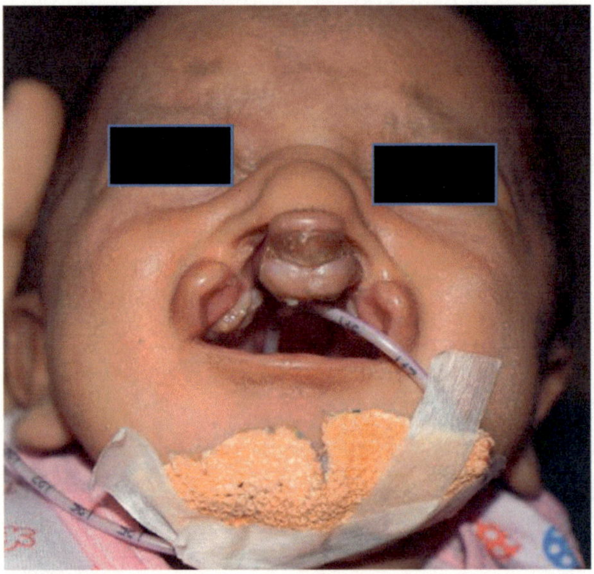

Figure 3.
Bilateral orofacial cleft lip and palate.

4. Procedure

Before commencing any treatment procedures, the parents/caregivers are counselled about PNAM therapy. The procedure, goals, possible complications and their role is explained to them.

5. Impressions

Several impression materials and techniques have been advocated for making the impression of the clefted alveolar segments. Grayson and Shetye [20] advised keeping the child nil orally for about 4 hours and making the impression while holding the baby upside down to prevent aspiration in the event of vomiting and asphyxia due to airway obstruction. A thick mix of tissue conditioning material was loaded onto the tray and inserted intraorally. The impression is allowed to set while the baby is making suckling actions in order to create the desired border seal and ensure the baby's ability to perform nasal breathing. The baby's oxygen level was monitored during the entire duration of impression making.

Retnakumari et al. [21] used heavy body silicone impression material with the baby in a supine position during the procedure. Dubey et al. [22] kept the baby in the mother's lap with the head facing downward and her hands supporting the baby's chest and lap region while making the impression. Yang et al. [23] advised alginate impressions using a beaded pretrimmed paediatric tray. Splengler et al. [24] made intraoral and extraoral alginate impressions with the baby under general anaesthesia. This method is generally not recommended as the patient is subjected to hospitalisation for an impression procedure.

Irrespective of the material and technique used, the sole objective of including all the available undercuts in the dental cast should be met. An ideal impression material must be rigid and set fairly quickly in the baby's mouth. The baby is positioned in an upright position, fully awake on the caregiver's lap. It is preferable if the baby is crying, as it allows better visuals of the extent of the cleft. The entire clefted palate should be recorded (**Figure 4**) and the size of the cleft should be determined on the resultant cast using a Vernier calliper.

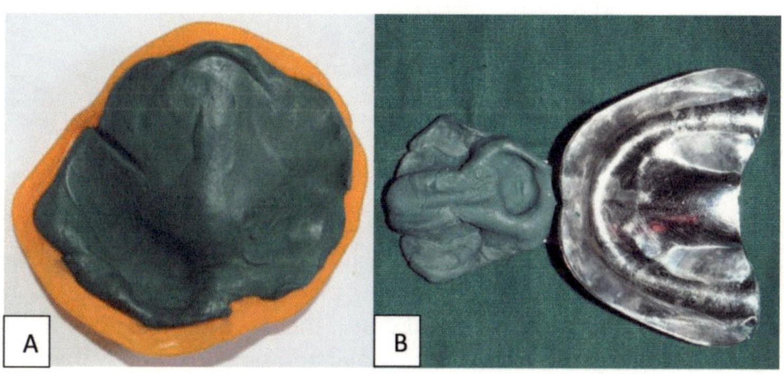

Figure 4.
Impression of the clefted segments in a unilateral cleft (A) and a bilateral cleft (B).

6. Appliance fabrication and design

The moulding plate is fabricated on the dental stone cast obtained from the impression. All the undercuts and the cleft space are blocked with wax. The moulding plate is made up of clear acrylic. A 5 mm hole is incorporated to facilitate breathing in case of accidental dislodgement (**Figure 5**). The plate must be 2–3 mm in thickness to provide structural integrity and permit adjustments during the process of moulding.

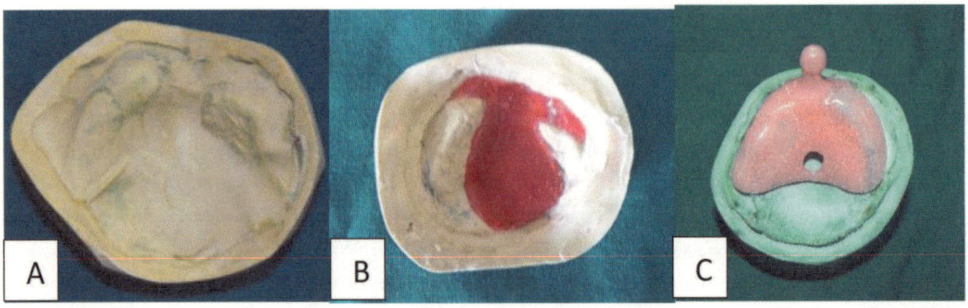

Figure 5.
On the obtained cast (A), cleft space is blocked out with wax (B) and the moulding plate is fabricated with a breathing hole (C).

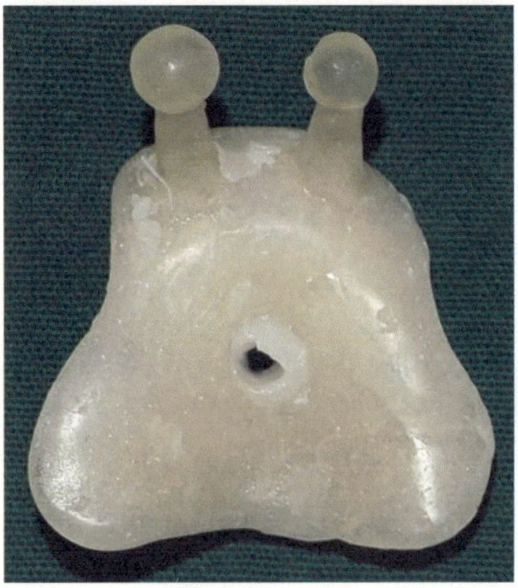

Figure 6.
Two retentive arms are incorporated in bilateral cases.

A retentive acrylic arm is fabricated and positioned labially at an angle of 40 degrees to the plate. It should be placed at the junction of the upper and lower lip. The retentive arm adequately secures the moulding plate in the mouth with the help of orthodontic elastics and tapes. In bilateral cases, there is a need for two retentive arms (**Figure 6**) [13]. The appliance has to be finished and polished ensuring that no sharp borders are present.

7. Appliance insertion and moulding

The NAM appliance was tried on the baby. The intaglio surface of the plate was then modified to allow for selective pressure on the two segments of the arch using tissue conditioner. There is selective removal of acrylic in the region into which the movement of alveolar bone is desired; and tissue conditioner was added to regions from which, the alveolar bone needed to be reduced. Selective pressure was applied on the greater and lesser alveolar segments to permit moulding. 1 mm thickness of tissue conditioner was applied onto the outer surface in the region of the greater segment and the inner surface was relieved by 1 mm. Tissue conditioner was also applied on the inner surface in the region of the lesser segment and the outer region was relieved by 1 mm (**Figure 7**). This caused a force that was directed inward on the greater segment and outward on the lesser segment that would cause approximation of alveolar tissue [25].

The NAM appliance is secured extra orally to the cheeks and bilaterally by surgical tapes with orthodontic elastic bands at one end. A muslin head cap with Velcro strips at the side is tailor-made for the baby (**Figure 8**). The Velcro strips provided attachment of the elastic bands, as well as facilitated their placement and removal. The elastic band is looped on the retentive arm of the moulding plate and secured with tape to the cheeks. The elastics with an inner diameter of 0.25 inch, and heavy wall thickness, should be stretched to about twice their resting diameter in order to achieve an ideal activation force of about 100 g. The amount of force could vary depending on the clinical objective and the mucosal tolerance to ulceration. Additional tapes may be necessary to secure the horizontal tape to the cheeks.

The infant may require time to adjust to feeding with the NAM appliance in the first few days. The baby is seen weekly to make adjustments to the moulding plate. These adjustments are made by selectively removing the hard acrylic and adding the

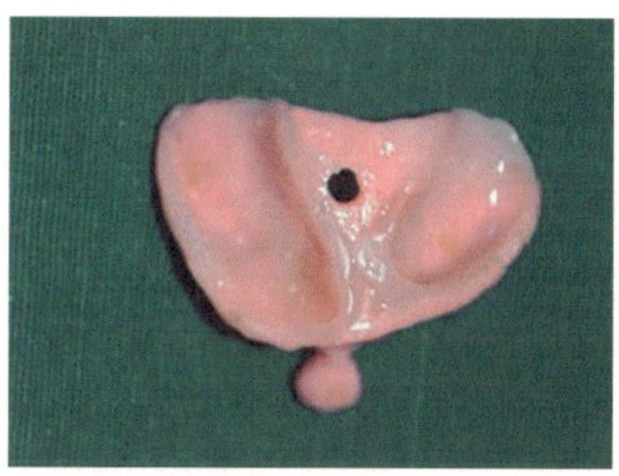

Figure 7.
Selective pressure applied on the clefted alveolar segments.

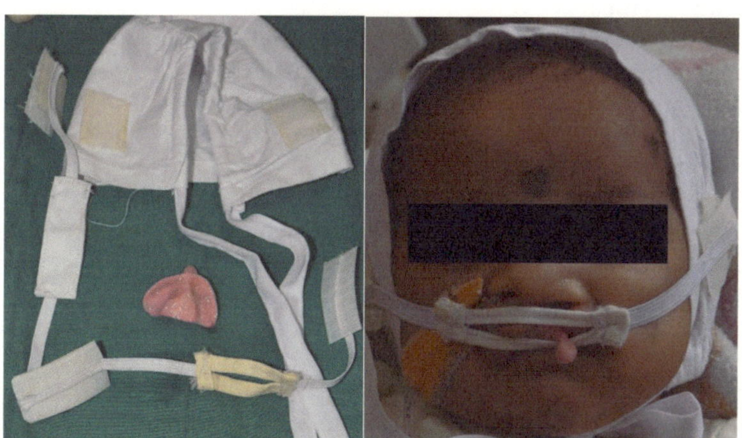

Figure 8.
A custom made muslin head cap used to secure the NAM appliance.

soft tissue conditioner to the moulding plate. No more than 1 mm of modification of the moulding plate should be made per visit. The desired movement can usually be accomplished within 6 to 8 weeks.

The NAM appliance needs to be worn 24 hours a day and removed only for daily cleaning, and needs to be inserted back soon afterwards. Even after 3 weeks, most cases did not show any clinical evidence of tissue irritation or accumulation of debris.

The effectiveness of the selective moulding is enhanced by adequately supporting the appliance against the palatal tissues and taping the lip segments across the cheek. This tight apposition of the lip segments provides the same benefit of traditional lip adhesion, but without the consequent scarring. It also serves to improve the alignment of the nasal base by bringing the columella towards the midsagittal plane, thereby improving the symmetry of the nostrils. Lip adhesion in isolation produces an uncontrolled orthopaedic movement. However, if carried out along with the moulding plate, the movements can be more precise and controlled.

8. Nasal stent

The nasal stent is added to the NAM appliance when the width of the cleft is reduced to a size of ≥6 mm. The reasoning behind delaying the addition of the nasal stent is that when the cleft size reduces, the alignment of the base of the nose and the lip segment also improves. The alar rim, which was initially stretched over the clefted segments at birth, will show some laxity, now that the cleft size has reduced and thus can be elevated into a symmetrical and convex form with the nasal stent. Any attempt to correct this deformity before reducing the cleft size may result in an undesirable increase in the lateral alar wall [26].

Matsuo and Hirose [27] suggested a silicone nasal conformer, which can be used for presurgical nasal moulding. The height of the conformer is adjusted by gradually adding some soft resin or flat silicone sheets on the domes. It can be used for presurgical elongation of the columella in incomplete clefts or postoperative maintenance of the nostril configuration. Blanching occurs at the nasal tip as infant suckles and activates the appliance. It also exerts a reciprocal intraoral moulding force against the clefted alveolar segments.

Grayson and Shetye [20] adapted nasal stent to extend from the anterior flange of an intraoral moulding plate. The greatest advantage of NAM is that it enables the practitioner to apply force skilfully to shape the nasal cartilage. Figueroa's technique [28] involves the simultaneous moulding of the alveolar cleft and nasal cartilage using a rigid acrylic nasal extension attached to an acrylic plate. Elastics are attached to the acrylic plate to allow gentle retraction of the premaxilla. A soft resin ball may also be attached to the acrylic plate across the prolabium in order to maintain the nasolabial angle. In bilateral cases, there is a need for two retentive arms as well as two nasal stents which are similar in shape to the unilateral stent.

The nasal stent is made from 19 gauge (0.36 inch), round stainless-steel wire, in the shape of a 'Swan Neck' (**Figure 9**). The base of the stent should be located midway between the clefted lip segments. The superior loop is adjusted to fit passively in the nostril on the cleft side. The nasal portion of the wire is then covered with self-cure clear acrylic and then by a layer of the tissue conditioner until mild blanching is evident. This superior lobe gently lifts the nasal dome forward, while the lower lobe lifts the tip of the nose and defines the top of the columella.

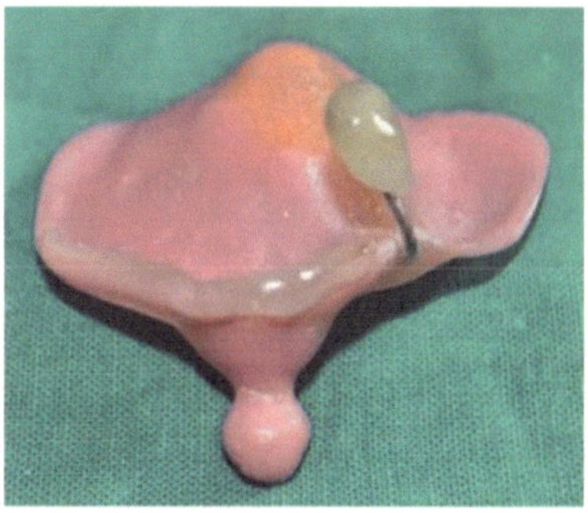

Figure 9.
Nasal stent.

Through gradual increments of tissue conditioner, the nostril on the cleft side is lifted to achieve acceptable elevation, and symmetry moulding continued until the desired nasal cartilage and alveolar shape is achieved.

Shetty et al [29] used the following protocol for presurgical NAM therapy:

1. **First visit:**

- Parent education and counselling: Use of audiovisual aids and live demonstrations
- Interaction with parents of older NAM patients
- Diet counselling
- Detailed documentation: Photographs and Dentofacial impressions
- Medical evaluation of patients
- Demonstration of daily appliance care
- Awareness and management of possible complications

2. **Second visit (1 week after the first visit):**

- Evaluation of patient and parent compliance
- Detailed documentation
- Evaluation of fit of the appliance and required modifications
- About 8–10 mm gap between the clefted segments—aggressive alveolar moulding

3. **Periodic 3 weeks recall visits:**

- Evaluation of patient and parent compliance
- Detailed documentation

- Comparison of dentofacial impressions recorded before treatment outcome and assessment.
- Fit of the appliance and required modifications
- Nasal moulding
- Active alveolar moulding continued till completion
- Passive alveolar moulding started once complete approximation of alveolar segment achieved
- Fabrication of new appliance every 2 months
- Parents participation in periodic NAM workshops

4. **Care and instructions**

- Washing of plate should be with warm water
- Never use a brush to clean the plate that will damage the resin
- Never drop the plate
- Clean after every feeding to avoid fungal infection
- Feed the baby at an upright position not sleeping

5. **Troubleshooting for parents**

- In case of rash – discontinue plate – apply cream – continue plate wearing
- In case of gag inform doctor
- In case of incessant crying—discontinue plate
- In case of bleeding areas discontinue plate – inform the doctor

6. **Troubleshooting for cleft care team:**

- Gag—trim posterior ends
- Bleeding—trim sharp ends
- Bleeding from skin—stop wearing the plate—use soothing lotions
- Plate gets dislodged—reduce force or change direction of tapes, change angulations of the handle
- Baby dislodges the plate by tongue—flatten the palatal surface so that the tongue does not get a grip

9. Lip and nose surgery

The success of PNAM depends upon the surgical procedure and the treating surgeon's skill. The surgical procedure, most commonly recommended is the modified gingivoperiosteoplasty (GPP), described by Millard and Lantham [30] carried out usually within 12–16 weeks of age. The surgery may be delayed in cases where additional weeks of PNAM therapy is needed. The surgical procedure involves a first stage primary lip nose repair to close the alveolar defect followed by one-stage palatal repair at 11–13 months of age when speech begins to develope (**Figure 10**) [31].

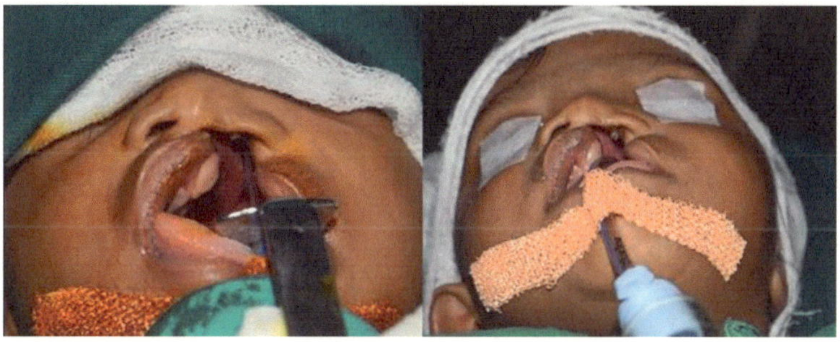

Figure 10.
Lip and nose surgery.

10. Extraoral nasal stent

Postsurgery, an additional external nasal stent can be given for 1 year to improve the nasal morphology if it did not resemble the unaffected side and also maintain the nasal correction if needed. The postsurgical external nasal stent is fabricated by making an impression of the unaffected nostril using tissue conditioner, and using it to mould the nasal contour on the cleft side [32].

11. Complications

The most common complication with the NAM therapy is irritation of the oral mucosa, gingival tissue and nasal mucosa. These issues arise due to the forces applied by the appliance [20]. They can be avoided by careful examination and modification of the extent and fit of the appliance. Fungal infection is another complication that can occur due to poor oral hygiene and continuous wear of the appliance. This can be avoided by following a meticulous oral hygiene routine and following the wash care instructions for the NAM plate. In severe cases, local nystatin or systemic amphotericin can be used [33].

12. Conclusion

Presurgical infant orthopaedics by means of nasoalveolar moulding enables the surgeon to carry out gingivoperiosteoplasty, which decreases the need for a second surgery. Bilateral cases, especially benefit as columella lengthening is carried out nonsurgically. It also minimises scar tissue formation and provides for more consistent outcomes. PNAM is most successful when initiated early and through meticulous planning and collaboration between the various disciplines.

Author details

Amanda Nadia Ferreira
Department of Prosthodontics, Crown and Bridge, Goa Dental College and Hospital, Goa, India

*Address all correspondence to: dr.amandaferreira@gmail.com

References

[1] Mars M, Sell D, Habel A, editors. Management of Cleft Lip and Palate in the Developing World. West Susex, England: John Wiley & Sons, Ltd; 2008

[2] Gaurishankar S. Textbook of Orthodontics. 1st ed. Hyderabad, India: Paras Medical Publication; 2011

[3] Cubitt JJ, Hodges AM, Van Lierde KM, Swan MC. Global variation in cleft palate repairs: An analysis of 352,191 primary cleft repairs in low- to higher-middle-income countries. The Cleft Palate-Craniofacial Journal. 2014;**51**(5):553-556. DOI: 10.1597/12-270

[4] Mossey P, Little J. Addressing the challenges of cleft lip and palate research in India. Indian Journal of Plastic Surgery. 2009;**42**(Suppl):S9-S18

[5] Medwick L, Synder J, Schook C, Blood E, Brown S, White W. Casual attributes of cleft lip and palate across cultures. The Cleft Palate-Craniofacial Journal. 2013;**50**:655-667

[6] Veau V. Division Palatine. Paris: Masson; 1931. Cited in Whitaker et al. A proposed new classification of craniofacial anomalies. Cleft Palate Journal. 1981;**18**(3):161-76

[7] Dean JA, Mcdonald RE, Avery DR. Dentistry for the Child and Adolescent. 9th ed. Missouri, United States: Elsevier Mosby; 2012

[8] Sommerlad BC. A technique for palate repair. Plastic and Reconstructive Surgery. 2003;**112**:1542-1548

[9] Roberts-Thomson K. Epidemiology of cleft lip and palate. In: Peres MA, Antunes JLF, Watt RG, editors. Oral Epidemiology. Textbooks in Contemporary Dentistry. Cham: Springer; 2021

[10] Dinh TTN, Van Nguyen D, Dien VHA, Dong TK. Effectiveness of presurgical nasoalveolar molding appliance in infants with complete unilateral cleft lip and palate. The Cleft Palate-Craniofacial Journal. 2021. DOI: 10.1177/10556656211026493

[11] Grayson BH, Cutting CB, Wood R. Preoperative columella lengthening in bilateral cleft lip and palate. Plastic and Reconstructive Surgery. 1993;**92**: 1422-1423

[12] Brecht LE, Grayson BH, Cutting CB. Columellar elongation in the bilateral cleft lip and nose patient. Journal of Dental Research. 1995;**74**:257

[13] Grayson BH, Santiago PE. Presurgical orthopedics for cleft lip and palate. In: Aston SJ, Beasley RW, CHM T, editors. Grabb and Smith's Plastic Surgery. 5th ed. Philadelphia: Lippincott-Raven; 1997. pp. 237-244

[14] Cutting CB, Grayson BH, Brecht LE, Santiago PE, Wood R, Kwon S. Presurgical columellar elongation and primary retrograde nasal reconstruction in one-stage bilateral cleft lip and nose repair. Plastic and Reconstructive Surgery. 1998;**101**:630-639

[15] Matsuo K, Hirose T, Tomono T, Iwasawa M, Katohda S, Takahashi N, et al. Nonsurgical correction of congenital auricular deformities in the early neonate: A preliminary report. Plastic and Reconstructive Surgery. 1984;**73**:38-51

[16] Huffman WC, Lierle DM. Studies on the pathologic anatomy of the unilateral harelip nose. Plastic and Reconstructive Surgery. 1949;**4**:225-234

[17] Hogan VM, Converse JM. Secondary deformity of unilateral cleft lip and nose. In: Grabb WC, Rosentein SE, Bzoch KR, editors. Cleft Lip and Palate-Surgical, Dental and Speech Aspects. Boston: Little Brown; 1971. pp. 245-264

[18] Broadbent TR, Woolf RM. Cleft lip and nasal deformity. Annals of Plastic Surgery. 1984;**12**:216-234

[19] Millard DR. Embryonic rationale for the primary correction of the classical congenital clefts of the lip and palate. Annals of the Royal College of Surgeons of England. 1994;**76**:150-160

[20] Grayson BH, Shetye PR. Presurgical nasoalveolar moulding treatment in cleft lip and palate patients. Indian Journal of Plastic Surgery. 2009;**42**:S56-S61

[21] Retnakumari et al. Nasolveolar molding in presurgical infant orthopedics. Archives of Medicine and Health Sciences. 2014;**2**(1)

[22] Dubey RK, Gupta DK, Chandraker NK. Presurgical nasoalveolar moulding: A technical note with case report. Indian Journal of Dental Research. 2012:67-68

[23] Yang S, Stelnicki EJ, Lee MN. Use of nasoalveolar moulding appliance to direct growth in newborn patient with complete unilateral cleft lip and palate. Pediatric Dentistry. 2003;**25**:253-256

[24] Splengler LA, Chavarria C, Teichgraber FJ, Gatenes J, Xia JJ. Presurgical nasoalveolar moulding therapy for the treatment of bilateral cleft lip and palate: A preliminary study. The Cleft Palate-Craniofacial Journal. 2006;**43**:321-328

[25] Sarin SP, Parkhedkar RD, Deshpande SS, Patil PG, Kothe S. Journal of Indian Prosthodontic Society. 2010;**10**:67-70

[26] Grayson BH, Cutting CB, Santiago PE, Brecht LE. Presurgical nasoalveolar moulding in infants with cleft lip and palate. The Cleft Palate-Craniofacial Journal. 1999;**36**:486-498

[27] Matsuo K, Hirose T. Preoperative non surgical overcorrection of cleft lip nasal deformity. British Journal of Plastic Surgery. 1991;**44**:5-11

[28] Figueroa A. Orthodontics in cleft lip and palate management. In: Mathes SJ, Hentz UR, editors. Plastic Surgery. 2nd ed. Philadelphia, PA: Saunders; 2006. pp. 271-310

[29] Shetty V, Vyas HJ. A comparison of results using nasoalveolar moulding in cleft infants treated within 1 month of life versus those treated after this period: Development of a new protocol. International Journal of Oral and Maxillofacial Surgery. 2012;**41**:28-36

[30] Millard DR, Lanthum RA. Improved primary surgical and dental treatment of clefts. Plastic and Reconstructive Surgery. 1990;**86**:856-871

[31] Grayson BH, Wood RJ, Cutting CB. Gingivoperostoplasy and midfacial growth. The Cleft Palate-Craniofacial Journal. 1997;**34**:17-20

[32] Bhutiani N, Tripathi T, Verma M, Bhandari PS, Rai P. Assessment of treatment outcome of presurgical nasoalveolar molding in patients with cleft lip and palate and its postsurgical stability. The Cleft Palate-Craniofacial Journal. 2020;**57**(6):700-706. DOI: 10.1177/1055665620906293

[33] Murthy PS, Deshmukh S, Bhagyalakshmi A, Srilantha KT. Presurgical nasoalveolar molding: Changing paradigms in early cleft lip and palate rehabilitation. Journal of International Oral Health. 2013; **5**(2):70-80

Chapter 18

Deleterious Facial Effects Caused by Noninvasive Ventilation Mask Early Treatment, in Congenital Muscular Dystrophy

David Andrade, Maria-João Palha, Ana Norton, Viviana Macho, Rui Andrade, Miguel Palha, Sandra Bussadori, Lurdes Morais and Manuela Santos

Abstract

Neuromuscular disorders is a general term that encompasses a large number of diseases with different presentations. Progressive muscle weakness is the predominant condition of these disorders. Respiratory failure can occur in a significant number of diseases. The use of devices to assist ventilation is quite frequent in these types of patients. Noninvasive ventilation can be applied by various means, including nasal, oronasal, or facial masks. Masks, type bilevel positive airway pressure, continuous positive airway pressure, and similar are generally supported on the maxilla. Oral health in pediatric neuromuscular diseases has some peculiar aspects that we must consider in these patients' follow-up. Based on a clinical case, this chapter provides a better understanding of these patients. It will focus on the oral and maxillofacial morphological alterations and preventive measures and strategies for oral pathologies management in this population. Despite always aiming at esthetics, treating these patients should always prioritize the possibilities of improving the oral and general functions of the body.

Keywords: neuromuscular diseases, congenital muscular dystrophy, noninvasive ventilation, clinical case, adverse effects, palatal expansion technique, extraoral traction appliances, pediatric dentistry, maxillary retrusion, airway obstruction

1. Introduction

Neuromuscular disorders (NMD) is a general term that encompasses a large number of diseases with different presentations.

Progressive muscle weakness is the predominant condition of these disorders. Respiratory failure can occur in a significant number of diseases. The use of devices to assist ventilation is quite frequent in these types of patients. Noninvasive ventilation (NIV) can be applied by various means, including nasal, oronasal, or facial masks.

Masks, type bilevel positive airway pressure (BiPAP), continuous positive airway pressure (CPAP), and similar are generally supported on the maxilla.

Long-term noninvasive ventilation (LTNIV) has been increasingly used in children to manage chronic respiratory failure and airway obstruction. Interfaces are of paramount importance for NIV effectiveness and patient compliance. Factors such as the child's age, disease, craniofacial conformation, type of ventilator and ventilation mode, and children's and family's preferences should be considered when selecting the appropriate mask. Adverse events such as skin lesions, facial growth impairment, and leaks must be prevented and promptly corrected. Humidification is a controversial issue on NIV, but it may be helpful in certain circumstances. Regular cleaning and disinfection of interfaces and equipment must be addressed. During follow-up, educational programs, close supervision, and continuous support to children and families are crucial to the success of LTNIV therapy [1].

Oral health in pediatric neuromuscular diseases has some peculiar aspects that we must consider in these patients' follow-up. Based on a clinical case, this chapter provides a better understanding of these patients. It will focus on the oral and maxillofacial morphological alterations and preventive measures and strategies for oral pathologies management in this population. Despite always aiming at esthetics, treating these patients should always prioritize the possibilities of improving the oral and general functions of the body.

Also, future research on the oral health of patients will be discussed.

2. Neuromuscular disorders

Neuromuscular disorders (NMDs) include conditions affecting the anterior horn cell (e.g., Spinal muscular atrophy = SMA), the peripheral nerve (e.g., Charcot–Marie–Tooth disease = CMT), the neuromuscular junction (e.g., Congenital myasthenia), or the muscle itself (e.g., Duchenne muscular dystrophy = DMD). NMDs are progressive, impair motor function, and often reduce life expectancy and quality of life [2]. Progressive muscle weakness is the predominant condition of these disorders. All muscles may be involved, such as facial muscles (including orbicularis oris) and bulbar muscles. In some of the patients, congenital high arched palate and even temporomandibular arthrogryposis can be present. Feeding problems are common, with the need for a feeding tube or gastrostomy. Speech problems with anarthria or dysphonia with nasal speech can be present.

The terms "muscle disease," "myopathy," "neuromuscular conditions," and "neuromuscular disorders" all describe a group of conditions that affect either the muscles, those in the arms and legs or the heart and lungs, or the nerves which control the muscles [3].

3. Noninvasive ventilation

Positive airway pressure (PAP) may be invasive or not, depending on the techniques we use. Furthermore, it can be used in acute or chronic situations.

Noninvasive ventilation can be applied by various means, including nasal, oronasal, or facial mask, among others [4]. Masks, type BIPAP, CPAP, VPAP, and similar, are generally supported over the jaw. A nasal interface (or nasal cannula) is the preferred interface, and a nasobuccal interface can be used with caution in case of mouth breathing.

Positive Long-term NIV is a highly efficacious type of noninvasive respiratory support that has transformed the scope of chronic respiratory failure and severe sleep-disordered breathing in children with NMD by avoiding tracheotomies and allowing the child to live at home with a good quality of life for a child and his family. The tremendous heterogeneity of the disorders, ages, prognosis, and outcomes of the patients underlines the necessity of management by experienced, multidisciplinary pediatric centers, having technical competencies in pediatric NIV, and expertise in sleep studies and therapeutic education [5].

4. Major groups of risk

If we look to the population that uses NIV, we identify the significant groups of risk, where respiratory muscles are weakened, or the airway is obstructed:

1. Neuromuscular disorders,

2. Obstructive sleep apnea,

3. Cystic fibrosis,

4. Children with obesity and Down syndrome.

5. Facial side effects during noninvasive positive pressure ventilation in children

Retrognathia is a physical misalignment of the upper (maxilla) and lower (mandibular) jawbones in which either or both recede relative to the frontal plane of the forehead. In the maxilla, we use the term maxillary retrusion as synonymous [6].

Facial side effects during noninvasive positive pressure ventilation (NPPV) in children are not a new effect. Brigitte Faroux [7], in 2005, concluded about the use of nasal masks that global facial flattening was present in 68% of the patients, and a maxillary retrusion was present in 37% of patients. In that time, she suggested systematic maxillofacial follow-up so that these effects may be identified. Remedial measures could include the change of the interface or reducing the daily use of NPPV.

Continuous positive airway pressure (CPAP) is a type of positive airway pressure used to deliver a set pressure to the airways maintained throughout the respiratory cycle during inspiration and expiration [8].

Bariani, in 2020, reports that most of the studies demonstrated that long-term use of nasal positive airway pressure in childhood/adolescence is associated with midface hypoplasia [9].

Ma, in 2021, tries the fit and comfort evaluation of custom mask designs using a randomized fit test with a series of three-dimensional (3D) printed versus commercial standard masks. Results indicate that custom masks are more comfortable than conventional continuous positive airway pressure (CPAP) masks, particularly on fit, contact pressure, and comfort [10].

Martelly, in 2021, also makes 3D masks (BiPAP and CPAP) and reports that while the custom-fit mask did not reduce the average measured leakage for subjects, subjects reported experiencing less leakage. Overall, results suggest that the custom-fit masks are more comfortable and tolerable than the provided off-the-shelf (OTS) mask option [11].

6. Case report—deleterious facial effects caused by noninvasive ventilation mask early treatment in congenital muscular dystrophy

With this clinical case, we want to familiarize professionals who work with these patients about the consequences that LTNIV may have in these children's face and oral functions and the importance of a pediatric dentist or an orthodontist in the team that treats these patients.

A 5-year-old child born with congenital muscular dystrophy type 1A (MDC1A) and total absence of merosin due to laminin α2 gene (*LAMA2*) mutation was referred by the pediatrician for the first time to the dentist. The child had a motor deficit, absence of gait, muscle hypotonia, feeding difficulty, breathing difficulties, sleep apnea, and normal intellectual development.

MDC1A is a rare autosomal recessive hereditary disease [12, 13] with severe consequences for its patients. It is characterized by motor deficits, muscle hypotonia, retractions, and progressive respiratory system impairment [14]. Affected individuals may show muscle hypertrophy [15]. The use of noninvasive ventilation devices is one of the strategies to manage the disease [16]. BiPAP and other similar units function as air compressor units and are used to treat respiratory insufficiencies [17], aiding ventilation with positive results in the pediatric population [18]. In this population, these devices are often used with a mask resting on the upper jaw.

Severe maxillary retrusion was diagnosed. Looking for the cause of such a severe facial deformity, it was hypothesized that force exerted by the noninvasive ventilation mask in this particular patient (with facial and bulbar weakness since birth) is one of the reasons for the deformity. The use of devices to assist ventilation is quite frequent in these patients. The use of these auxiliary ventilation devices, which are very important for the patient's well-being, must be carefully considered as they cause maxillary hypoplasia.

The retrusion of the middle floor of the face is maxillary hypoplasia or maxillary deficiency, which is an underdevelopment of the jawbones, with the greater concavity of the face and reduced nasolabial angle. This term represents underdevelopment of the maxilla (upper jaw) in length (decrease in the average height of the face) or depth (retrusion of the jaw) [19]. The maxillary retrusion resulting in non-development creates a pseudo-class III malocclusion resulting in esthetic disharmony, greater resistance of the nasal pathways [20, 21], narrowing of the pharyngeal airway, discomfort, and problems of eruption in mixed dentition [22, 23], with maxillary compression and crowding, in addition to pseudomacroglossia [24]. That is, the benefit obtained by the best oxygenation should always be equated with the relative anatomo-functional misfit that may result from prolonged use of the mask. Surveillance of the evolution of the maxilla development by pediatric dentists is necessary, and this professional should be part of the treatment and follow-up team.

The management of this disease and its comorbidity is predominant for the patient's quality of life, considering that there is no cure for it.

In this case, the use of the noninvasive ventilation device (BiPAP) occurred from the age of 15 months in the context of rest, nocturnal use (**Figure 1**). The device is used due to the child's ventilation difficulties, trying to compensate for the fragility of the respiratory muscles.

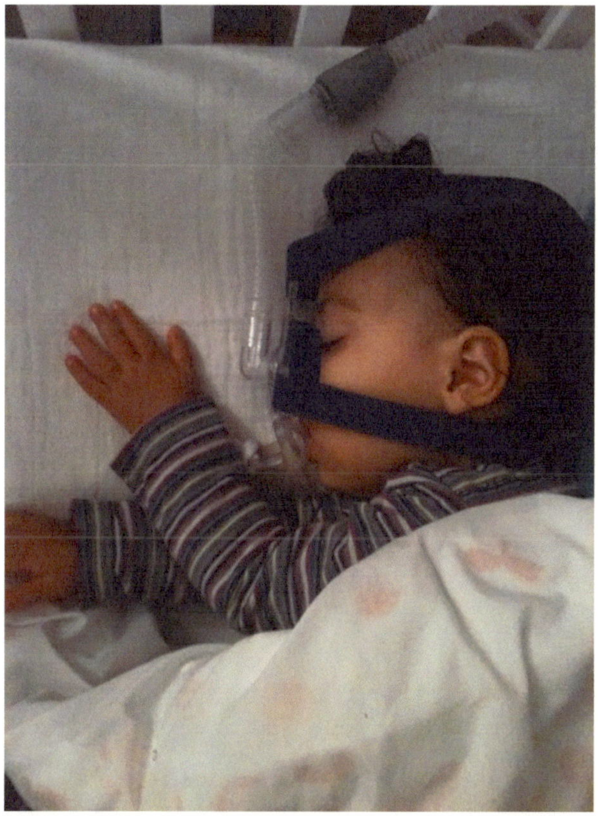

Figure 1.
At 15 months, the child started using noninvasive night ventilation with a nasal mask. So that there is a good adaptation of the nasal mask, without air escaping, a strap adapts the silicone to the face, anchored in the neck or nape, easily creating a retrusive force to the jaw.

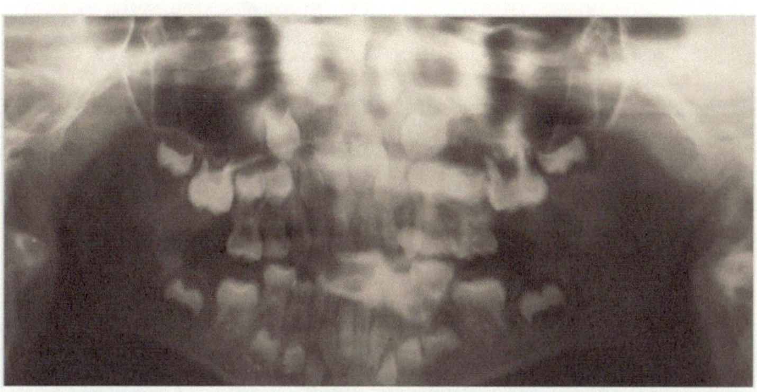

Figure 2.
The panoramic X-ray is the best exam to test the child and parent collaboration. For a child who does not walk and needs constant help from the mother to position himself, the radiograph is of sufficient quality and should not be repeated.

In our consultation, and despite the difficulties arising from age and the absence of gait that makes the child always dependent on the mother, good collaboration was achieved to perform a study [25], after obtaining additional diagnostic

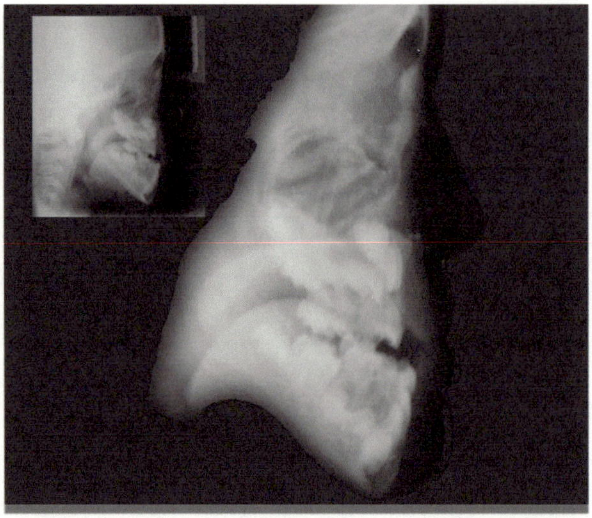

Figure 3.
Teleradiography - lateral radiography of the cranium from a 5-year-old female patient with Congenital Muscle Dystrophy. Severe maxillary retrusion, crossbite, open bite, and vertical growth of the mandible.

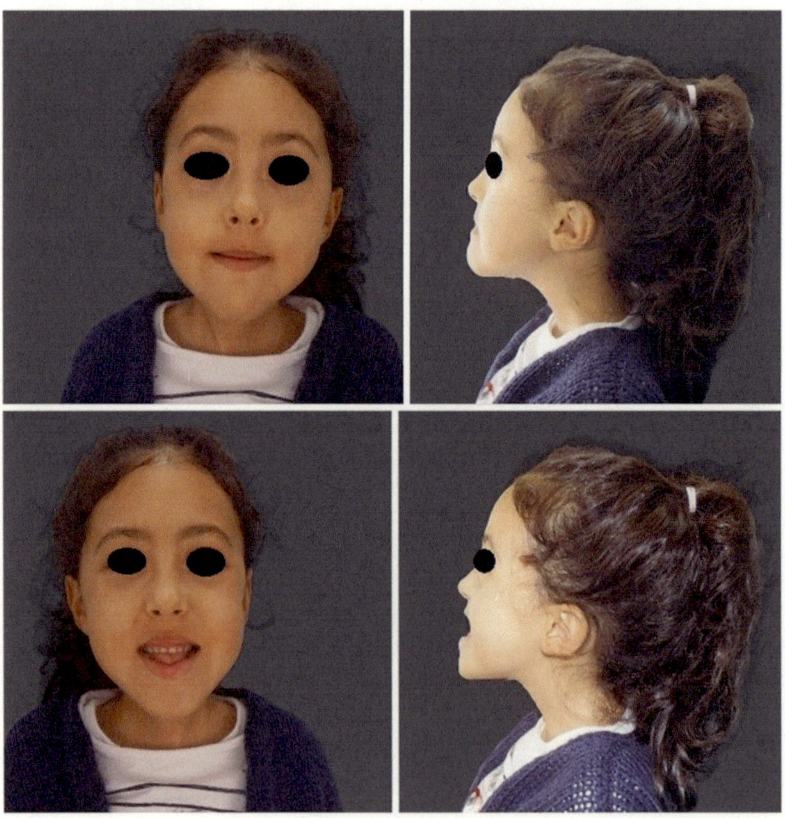

Figure 4.
Extra-oral photographs—as the child cannot hold herself standing, the photos were taken in the dental chair. The mother and child were very collaborative.

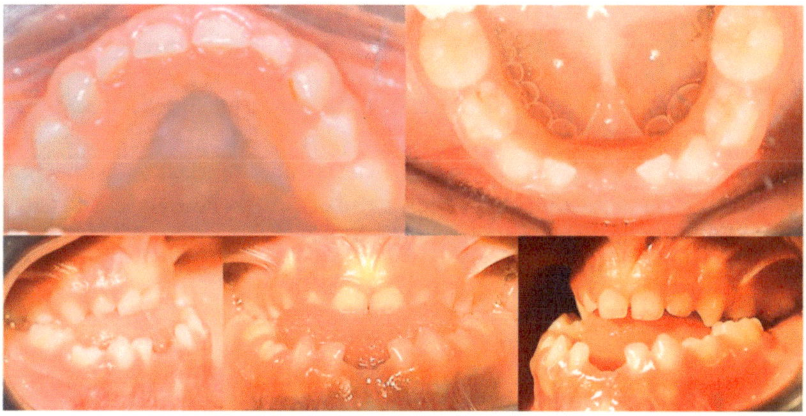

Figure 5.
Intra-oral photographs—the lips were previously moistened with a lip care balm to avoid the child's sensitivity and facilitate the placement of the lips and cheeks retractors.

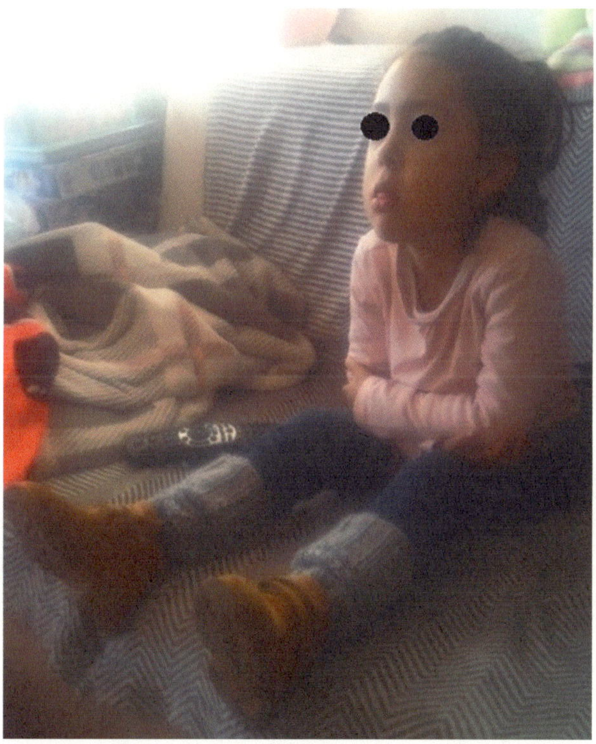

Figure 6.
On 22/01/2017—the educator's photo shows retrognathic profile and lingual protrusion (Pseudomacroglossia).

elements: orthopantomography (**Figure 2**), teleradiography (**Figure 3**), extra-oral (**Figure 4**), and intra-oral photographs (**Figure 5**), and upper and lower molds of the child's mouth.

The child does not present dental problems, all teeth being healthy.

The study allowed to suggest starting the first phase of the correction of this problem, using an orthopedic maxillary therapy, with the placement of a rapid maxillary expansion appliance to widen the maxilla, followed by the simultaneous use of a facial mask for maxillary traction. At all times, the use of noninvasive ventilation was maintained.

The child must be regularly followed, and other therapeutical measures may have to be considered with the evolution of the treatment. At this moment, the focus is to recover as soon as possible the oral physiological functions.

Severe maxillary hypoplasia with progeny disharmony greater than 1 cm with a retracted appearance of the middle face is notorious. Retrusion, anterior and posterior crossbite, open bite, vertical growth of the mandible, and pseudomacroglossia (**Figures 2–6**).

Concavo profile and pseudomacroglossia (**Figure 6**) are visible in the resting position of the photo taken by the educators.

Further investigation of the facial features pre-use of NIV allowed us to conclude that the face was harmonic, without any hypoplasia or retrusion, as seen from the observation of several photographs and videos pre NIV (**Figures 7** and **8**). The profile was convex, with slight dystocclusion.

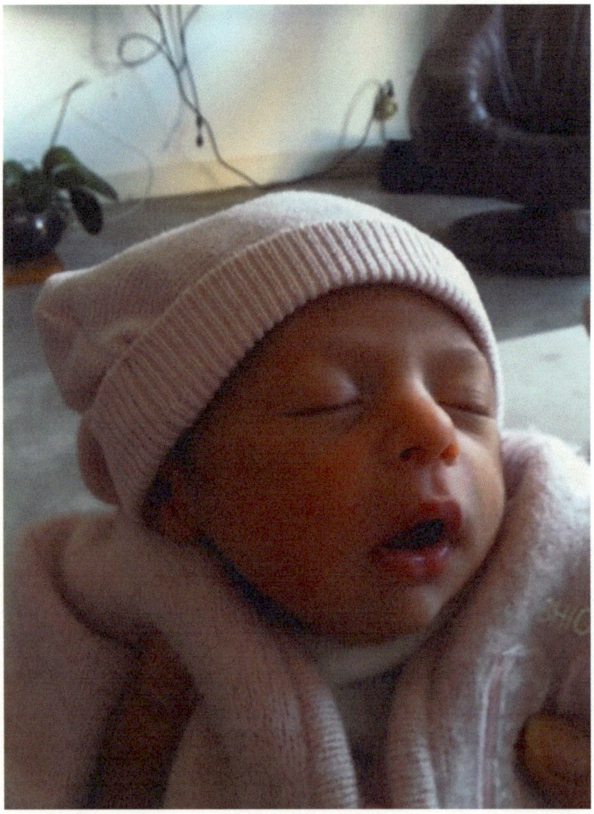

Figure 7.
Photo of the child on 17/11/2011, taken before using the noninvasive ventilation appliance; note the convex facial profile, without maxillary retrognathia problems.

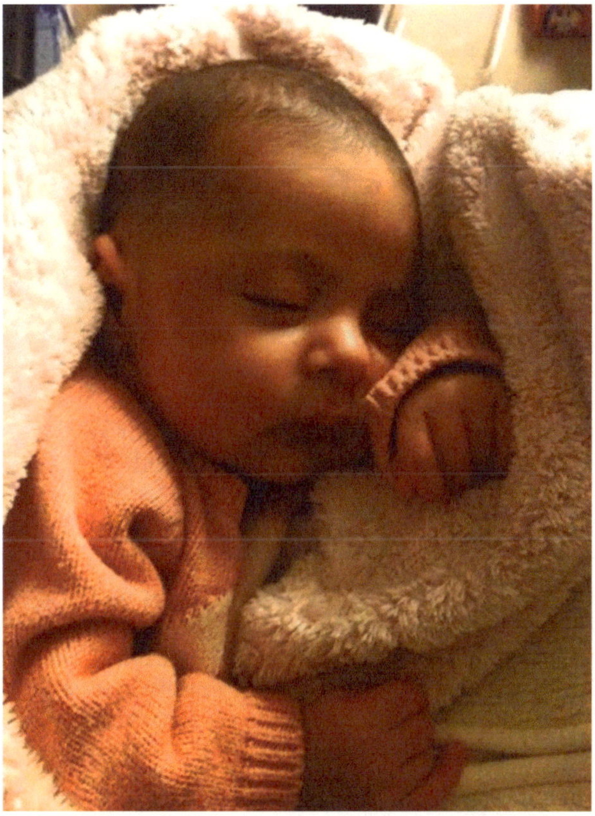

Figure 8.
Child's photograph on 10/01/2012, also taken before using the noninvasive ventilation device; note the convex face profile, with a noticeable distal occlusion of the mandible and the middle third of the face well developed and proportional.

7. Discussion

Noninvasive mechanical ventilation (NIV) is defined as a ventilatory support that does not require an orotracheal tube or tracheostomy, used through an interface, with the objective of promoting adequate ventilation, reducing respiratory work, preventing respiratory muscle fatigue, increasing alveolar ventilation, and improving gas exchange, thus avoiding intubation and promoting, in some cases, early extubation [26, 27]. The use of NIV may also reduce complications associated with invasive mechanical ventilation and, consequently, morbidity and mortality rates related to this ventilatory support [28].

Currently, NIV is considered an alternative ventilatory support in the Pediatric Neuromuscular Outpatient Clinic. It has good acceptability and high success rates. It is indicated in the presence of acute or chronic respiratory disorders, neuromuscular diseases, central nervous system disorders, obstructive sleep apnea, neuromuscular diseases, central nervous system disorders, obstructive sleep apnea, postoperative, post-extubation period, and early extubation [29, 30].

A certain type of patient needs to use a ventilation aid for different reasons and at different ages, sometimes in the first years of life. The use of these noninvasive ventilation masks (BiPAP, CPAP, and the like) is sometimes maintained for years and a considerable period of daily use (more than eight or even 12 hours). The masks allow patients better oxygenation, but closure must be obtained around the place where the mask touches so that there is no air leakage. This peripheral closure of the mask on the face is obtained by the traction pressure of the mask against the tissues, and the mask can be nasal, nasal and oral, or facial.

The harmful effects caused using the mask will depend on the type of mask applied, the places where the forces are applied, the intensity of the forces, their direction, and the time of action of the forces in question. If this mask does not rely on solid structures of the face causes severe deformations in patients, especially if they are young and with the skeleton to form and easily moldable. Also, the substrate on which the forces act is important because a hard bone of an adult male does not deform in the same way as the soft bone of a baby or child.

Looking for the possible causes for maxillary retrusion and hypoplasia found, the feasible one that can be related is the use of noninvasive nasal mask ventilation in a child with facial and bulbar weakness. In this clinical case, everything indicates that the deformation found was iatrogenic, caused by the masks used in noninvasive ventilation. That is one of the main reasons for the deformity due to the mask.

Using this device from an early age (15 months) exerts an anchoring force in the skull (more difficult to deform) that causes an inhibition reaction of the growth of the maxilla and its retrusion since the predominant force was exerted in the cranial calotte. In this sense, the absence of well-distributed facial supports caused the applied forces to retort the entire anterior sector.

Given what was observed, it seemed that the alternative would be to counteract all this movement. So, we associate with the retrusive force of BiPAP a protrusive force, through a facial mask, complemented by the transverse expansion of the maxillary disjunction.

Maxillary reverse traction therapy is indicated for the solution of orthodontic cases as a non-surgical alternative for correcting malocclusion, allowing movement of the maxilla forward and down through the remodeling of the maxillary sutures. At the same time, the mandible shows a clockwise rotation, which corrects the concavity of the soft tissue profile. The technique may be associated with surgical procedures and rapid maxillary expansion orthopedical movements. Better results are obtained when therapy is used in young patients when compared to older patients [31].

The technique used allowed the child to continue to use BiPAP, necessary for his health and metabolism of development, but at the same time counteract the forces exerted by the NIV.

In this case, maxillary hypoplasia was reported in a child with congenital muscular dystrophy and a total absence of merosin. These children have severe breathing problems and ventilation difficulties.

The obstruction of the nasal airways is related to their volume [32, 33]. Some authors believe that rapid maxillary expansion may result in greater ventilatory capacity [34, 35] resulting from increased permeability and nasal volume [36, 37] as well as different tongue positioning [38, 39] and changes in voice [40].

The correct anatomy, good airways permeability, and positioning of the teeth and tongue permit better oral functions, such as chewing, drinking, speaking, breathing, and even earing [41].

This procedure allowed an increase of the entire nasal pyramid, resulting from the rapid expansion of the maxillary, which in the future will allow better ventilation, tongue positioning, and drainage of secretions in addition to closer anatomy of normal. It allows better development and a smaller number of hours lost by parents in medical consultations.

Despite the importance of this intervention for the child's current development, the treatment must have a second phase, pluridisciplinary, that may involve pediatric dentistry, orthodontics, physiotherapy, speech therapy, and maxillofacial surgery.

The fact that we later found other cases in which the same etiological hypothesis is possible made us write this text as a starting point for investigation and as a warning to colleagues who put on auxiliary ventilation masks such as BiPAP device, CPAP, and similar, for the treatment of apnea, sleep apnea, or situations that require prolonged use of NIV. It is intended that this text is a warning so that the placement of these masks is supported whenever possible in an extensive area and with the involvement of multiple less deformable bones, besides making it necessary to control the forces used so that these masks do not act like an orthodontic device of maxillary retrusion. Whenever possible, use only nose tubes, or helmet-like devices, to avoid jaw pressure at early ages.

In NIV a mask supported by the maxilla is used. Suppose we hypothesized that its use since the age of 15 months might have retracted the jaw or prevented its growth, functioning as an orthodontic appliance and with an unequal distribution of forces. In that case, we are faced with a method of disease management that may end up being harmful in the long term, preventing the natural formation of the sinus and the consequent ventilatory improvement. The use of this method of disease management is a "two-beak stick" because it allows an improvement in ventilatory capacity when using the device but seems to decrease the typical anatomical characteristics necessary for adequate ventilation. In this sense, noninvasive ventilation devices with an average force distribution and forces supported in more extensive areas and independent bones should be preferred to prevent retrusion. The most extensive support surface can prevent retrusion by what would be ideal the realization of masks tailored to each face.

8. Patient perspective

The mother left a testimony, translated to English, after removing names:

Sharing: I, mother and primary caregiver, hereby share this testimony, with the greatest satisfaction of what this device gave to my child's mouth, as she has severe congenital muscular dystrophy, a total absence of merosin (strength protein).

As soon as the appliance was placed in her mouth, within days, there was massive notoriety in her teeth spacing, mouth opening, and "ogival" palate alteration (widening and less depth), to the point where the teeth fit (aligned) correctly, "teeth with teeth."

Something that had not happened before and that made chewing less effective, such as lack of muscle strength, which was another situation that made the situation worse.

After this situation was successful, we moved on to the next stage with the traction device. It rectifies the bite, which was misaligned, due to the BiPAP respiratory device for sleep apnea at a very early age. Bipap had a beneficial effect on oxygenation while sleeping, but at the jaw level, projected it backward.

The process was slower but managed to exceed expectations to the extent of the severity noted. Through this long but very advantageous process, the changes were notorious at all levels:

- respiratory (with better breath)
- speech (diction)
- eat (chews more firmly and quickly) (crack some foods)
- drinking (faster)

However, this could not happen if I had not chosen as an Orthodontist Prof. Doctor Casimiro de Andrade and his team in this very complex process. In this, there was a development of delivery, trust, and humanity par excellence, to which I fully thank.

He was gradually doing the treatment according to the child's condition, in the different phases, so that this process would not be invasive under any circumstances.

Moreover, the entire multidisciplinary team was delighted to see my daughter evolve and progress throughout her treatment (Dr. Lurdes Morais (pulmonologist), Dr. Julia Eça de Guimarães (pediatrician), and Physiotherapist Ana Moreira and her team.

Mother of the child. Grateful for everything.!!! Thank you all.

9. Informed consent

The patient responsible agreed to use and publish the disease-related article with personal information to be excluded.

10. Conclusions

Whenever VNI use is prolonged and at an early age, exclusively maxillary support should be avoided, if possible discarded, preferring the use of a mask with multi-site facial support, or in some instances, total and better-distributed loads, if necessary tailored to measure.

Pediatric dentistry and orthodontics play a vital role in promoting health and development in children with neuromuscular disorders.

A pediatric dentist is a vital element in the medical team that follows these patients and should always identify, prevent, and intercept these problems to achieve proper development.

Acknowledgements

We thank the fantastic collaboration of all the therapeutic teams that followed the child.

We thank the mother's child as an example of care and attention to her child.

Conflict of interest

The authors supported this investigation.

The authors declare no conflict of interest.

David Casimiro de Andrade, Maria João Palha e José Rui Andrade: responsible for the conception and design.

David Casimiro de Andrade, Maria João Palha, Viviana Macho and Ana Norton were responsible for the data collection and manuscript redaction.

Ana Norton, Viviana Macho were responsible for the critical revision of its contents.

Sandra Kalil Bussadori, Miguel Palha, Lurdes Morais and Manuela Santos were responsible for the critical revision of its intellectual contents.

David Casimiro de Andrade was responsible for graphics and photos, the critical revision of its intellectual contents, and the final approval of the version to be published.

All authors declare that written informed consent was obtained from the patient (or other approved parties) to publish this research paper.

Author details

David Andrade[1*], Maria-João Palha[2], Ana Norton[1], Viviana Macho[3], Rui Andrade[5], Miguel Palha[4], Sandra Bussadori[6], Lurdes Morais[7] and Manuela Santos[8]

1 Pediatric Dentistry, Faculty of Dental Medicine, University of Porto, Porto, Portugal

2 Pediatrics, Santa Maria Hospital, Centro Hospitalar Universitário Lisboa Norte, Lisboa, Portugal

3 Pediatric Dentistry, Faculty of Health Sciences, University Fernando Pessoa, Porto, Portugal

4 Developmental Pediatrician, Child Development Centre Diferenças, Lisbon, Portugal

5 Nutritionism, Clínica Dentária de Espinho, Espinho, Portugal

6 Pediatric Dentistry, Uninove, Campus Vila Prudente, São Paulo, Brazil

7 Pediatric Pneumology, North Maternal and Child Centre from Centro Hospitalar do Porto, Porto, Portugal

8 Neuropediatrics, North Maternal and Child Centre from Centro Hospitalar do Porto, Porto, Portugal

*Address all correspondence to: dandrade@fmd.up.pt

References

[1] Ferreira R. Interfaces, Circuits and Humidifiers. Front Pediatr. 2020 Dec 7;8:557301. doi:10.3389/fped.2020.557301. PMID:33365289; PMCID: PMC7750325.

[2] Flotats-Bastardas M, Hahn A. New Therapeutics Options for Pediatric Neuromuscular Disorders. Vol. 8, Frontiers in Pediatrics. Frontiers Media S.A.; 2020.

[3] Potikanond S, Nimlamool W, Noordermeer J, Fradkin LG. Muscular dystrophy model. In: Advances in Experimental Medicine and Biology [Internet]. Springer New York LLC; 2018 [cited 2021 Jul 3]. p. 147-72. Available from: https://pubmed.ncbi.nlm.nih.gov/29951819/

[4] Long-term non-invasive ventilation therapies in children: A scoping review | Elsevier Enhanced Reader [Internet]. [cited 2021 Jul 8]. Available from: https://reader.elsevier.com/reader/sd/pii/S1087079217300461?token=84E22C08CBF74E237DBCDC07D19C37F8BB65BE820300BE021454B02493F85DE3095AF1D652CD7AD2E4D4D52B26C6E8C1&originRegion=eu-west-1&originCreation=20210708061359

[5] Fauroux B, Khirani S, Griffon L, Teng T, Lanzeray A, Amaddeo A. Non-invasive Ventilation in Children With Neuromuscular Disease. Front Pediatr. 2020 Nov 16;8:482. doi:10.3389/fped.2020.00482. PMID: 33330262; PMCID: PMC7717941.

[6] MeSH | Cochrane Library [Internet]. [cited 2021 Jul 3]. Available from: https://www.cochranelibrary.com/advanced-search/mesh

[7] Fauroux, B, Lavis, JF., Nicot, F et al. Facial side effects during noninvasive positive pressure ventilation in children. Intensive Care Med 31, 965-969 (2005). https://doi.org/10.1007/s00134-005-2669-2.

[8] Pinto VL, Sharma S. Continuous Positive Airway Pressure. 2021 May 7. In: StatPearls [Internet]. Treasure Island (FL): StatPearls Publishing; 2021 Jan–. PMID: 29489216.

[9] Bariani RC, Guimarães TM, Cappellette Junior M, Moreira G, Fujita RR. The impact of positive airway pressure on midface growth: a literature review. Braz J Otorhinolaryngol. 2020;86:647---53. Available from: https://doi.org/10.1016/j.bjorl.2020.05.010 1808-8694.

[10] Ma, Z., Hyde, P., Drinnan, M., and Munguia, J. (March 12, 2021). "Custom Three-Dimensional-Printed CPAP Mask Development, Preliminary Comfort and Fit Evaluation." ASME. J. Med. Devices. June 2021; 15(2): 024501. https://doi.org/10.1115/1.4050201.

[11] Martelly, E., Rana, S., and Shimada, K. (March 12, 2021). "Design and Fabrication of Custom-Fit BiPAP and CPAP Masks Using Three-Dimensional Imaging and Three-Dimensional Printing Techniques." ASME. J. Med. Devices. June 2021; 15(2): 024502. https://doi.org/10.1115/1.4049981.

[12] Lista de doenças raras e de sinónimos, por ordem alfabética», Série de Relatórios da Orphanet, coleção de Doenças Raras, Janeiro 2021, Available from: http://www.orpha.net/orphacom/cahiers/docs/PT/lista_de_doen-as_raras_por_ordem_alfabetica.pdf

[13] Leitão TGM (2014). Distrofia Muscular Congénita com Deficiência de

Merosina - a propósito de um caso clínico (Dissertação de mestrado, Universidade Beira Interior, Covilhã, Portugal).

[14] Butterfield RJ. Congenital Muscular Dystrophy and Congenital Myopathy. Contin Lifelong Learn Neurol. 2019;25(6):1640-1661.

[15] Oliveira, J., Freixo, J. P., Santos, M., & Coelho, T. (2020). LAMA2 Muscular Dystrophy. GeneReviews®. https://www.ncbi.nlm.nih.gov/books/NBK97333/

[16] Nguyen Q, Lim KRQ, Yokota T. Current understanding and treatment of cardiac and skeletal muscle pathology in laminin-α2 chain-deficient congenital muscular dystrophy. Appl Clin Genet. 2019;12:113-130.

[17] David-João PG, Guedes MH, Réa-Neto Á, Chaiben VB d. O, Baena CP. Noninvasive ventilation in acute hypoxemic respiratory failure: A systematic review and meta-analysis. J Crit Care [Internet]. 2019;49:84-91. Available from: https://doi.org/10.1016/j.jcrc.2018.10.012

[18] Abramo T, Williams A, Mushtaq S, Meredith M, Sepaule R, Crossman K, et al. Paediatric ED BiPAP continuous quality improvement programme with patient analysis: 2005-2013. BMJ Open. 2017;7(1):1-14.

[19] Midface Retrusion, National Human Genome Research Institute; [Internet]. [cited 2021 Jul 3]. Available from: https://elementsofmorphology.nih.gov/index.cgi?tid=5b7ad34ab35682b5#:~:text=Definition%3A,and%2For reduced nasolabial angle.

[20] G Ottaviano, P Maculan, G Borghetto, V Favero, B Galletti, E Savietto, B Scarpa, A Martini, E Stellini, C De Filippis L Favero, Nasal function before and after rapid maxillary expansion in children: A randomized, prospective, controlled study, International Journal of Pediatric Otorhinolaryngology (2018), doi: https://doi.org/10.1016/j.ijporl.2018.09.029.

[21] de Moura CP, Vales F, Andrade D, Cunha LM, Barros H, Pueschel SM, et al. Rapid maxillary expansion and nasal patency in children with Down syndrome. Rhinology. 2005;43(2): 138-142.

[22] Ağlarcl C, Esenlik E, Flndlk Y. Comparison of short-term effects between face mask and skeletal anchorage therapy with intermaxillary elastics in patients with maxillary retrognathia. Eur J Orthod. 2016;38(3):313-323.

[23] Vidya VS, Sumathi FA. Rapid maxillary expansion as a standard treatment for obstructive sleep apnea syndrome: a systematic review. J Dental Med Sci. 2015;14:51-55.

[24] de Moura CP, Silveira H, Andrade D, Palha M, Clemente MP. Trissomia 21-Perspectiva Otorrinolaringológica. Arq Med. 2004;18(1/2):61-65.

[25] Macho V, Norton A, Areias C, Silva S, Silva CC, Macedo AP, Fraga C, Guedes-Pinto A, Andrade DC. A importância do Exame, Diagnóstico e Plano de Tratamento em Odontopediatria. In: Andrade DC, Guedes-Pinto AC. Textos Escolhidos de Odontopediatria. UP Editora, Porto, 2017. p.77- 102 p: il. color. e-ISBN: 978-989-746-138-5.

[26] Grande RAA, Fernandes GA, Andrade DP, Matsunaga NY, Oliveira T de, Almeida CCB, et al. Ventilação não invasiva em pacientes em uma Unidade de Terapia Intensiva Pediátrica: fatores associados à falha. J Bras Pneumol [Internet]. 2020 Aug 21 [cited 2021

Jul 8];46(6):1-8. Available from: http://www.scielo.br/j/jbpneu/a/ZsKwNhnPP6ddYtGyjhYTXrH/?lang=pt

[27] Viscusi CD, Pacheco GS. Pediatric Emergency Noninvasive Ventilation. Emerg Med Clin North Am. 2018 May 1;36(2):387-400.

[28] Ferreira S, Nogueira C, Conde S, Taveira N. Ventilação não invasiva. Rev Port Pneumol. 2009 Jul 1;15(4):655-667.

[29] Amaddeo A, Moreau J, Frapin A, Khirani S, Felix O, Fernandez-Bolanos M, et al. Long term continuous positive airway pressure (CPAP) and noninvasive ventilation (NIV) in children: initiation criteria in real life. Pediatr Pulmonol. 2016;51(9):968-974. http://dx.doi.org/10.1002/ppul.23416. PMid:27111113.

[30] Castro-Codesal ML, Dehaan K, Featherstone R, Bedi PK, Martinez Carrasco C, Katz SL, et al. Long-term non-invasive ventilation therapies in children: a scoping review. Sleep Med Rev. 2018;37:148-158. PMid:28410811.

[31] Primo, Bruno Tochetto et al. Terapia da tração reversa maxilar com máscara facial de Petit - relato de caso. RFO UPF [online]. 2010, vol.15, n.2, pp. 171-176. ISSN 1413-4012.

[32] G Ottaviano, P Maculan, G Borghetto, V Favero, B Galletti, E Savietto, B Scarpa, A Martini, E Stellini, C De Filippis L Favero, Nasal function before and after rapid maxillary expansion in children: A randomized, prospective, controlled study, International Journal of Pediatric Otorhinolaryngology (2018), doi: https://doi.org/10.1016/j.ijporl.2018.09.029.

[33] Andrade DC Macho V, Pinto M, Moura C., P. M., Andrade, C., Palha, M., Macho, V., Pinto, M., & Moura, C. (2009). Effects of Rapid Maxillary Expansion In Down Syndrome. O66 MH Abstracts and Proceedings Book of the 10th World Down Syndrome Congress. Dublin., O66 MH Abstracts and Proceedings book.

[34] Compadretti GC, Tasca I, Bonetti GA. Nasal airway measurements in children treated by rapid maxillary expansion. Am J Rhinol. 2006;20(4): 385-393.

[35] Moura, C., Vales, F., Andrade, D. J. C. de, Cunha, L., Barros, H., Pueschel, S., Pais-Clemente M. (2004). Rapid Maxillary Expansion and Nasal Permeability of a Down Syndrome Paediatric Population. Annual Meeting of American Academy of Otolaryngology, Head And Neck Surgery., 43(2), 138-142.

[36] De Felippe NLO, Da Silveira AC, Viana G, Kusnoto B, Smith B, Evans CA. Relationship between rapid maxillary expansion and nasal cavity size and airway resistance: short- and long-term effects. Am J Orthod Dentofacial Orthop 2008;134:370-382.

[37] Matsumoto MAN, Itikawa CE, Valera FCP, Faria G, Alnselmo-Lima WT. Long-term effects of rapid maxillary expansion on nasal area and nasal airway resistance. Am J Rhinol Allergy 2010;24:161-165.

[38] Areias C, Maia B, Macho V, Norton A, Macedo P, Andrade DC. Oral health in Down Syndrome, p. 45-68, 2015 in Health Problems in Down Syndrome. Intech open science|Open minds. Subrata Dey. 2015. ISBN 978-953-51-2154-1 DOI: 10.5772/60652 Available from: https://www.intechopen.com/books/health-problems-in-down-syndrome

[39] G Ottaviano, P Maculan, G Borghetto, V Favero, B Galletti, E Savietto, B Scarpa, A Martini, E

Stellini, C De Filippis L Favero, Nasal function before and after rapid maxillary expansion in children: A randomized, prospective, controlled study, International Journal of Pediatric Otorhinolaryngology (2018), doi: https://doi.org/10.1016/j.ijporl.2018.09.029.

[40] Moura C, Andrade DC, Cunha L, Cunha M, Vilarinho H, Barros H, Freitas D, Pais-Clemente M. Voice quality in Down syndrome children treated with rapid maxillary expansion. Interspeech. 6th 2005. (9th European conference on speech communication and technology) (5 vols); 1073-1076. Available from: www.isca-speech.org/archive/archive_papers/interspeech_2005/i05_1073.pdf

[41] de Moura, C. P., Andrade, D., Cunha, L. M., Tavares, M. J., Cunha, M. J., Vaz, P., Barros, H., Pueschel, S. M., & Pais Clemente, M. (2008). Down syndrome: Otolaryngological effects of rapid maxillary expansion. Journal of Laryngology and Otology, 122(12), 1318-1324. https://doi.org/10.1017/S002221510800279X.